SO-BLO-024

tear here

Twenty Questions to Help You Find Your Perfect Spa or Retreat

1. Does the facility have:
   - ➤ Spa-type beauty treatments; ask for list.
   - ➤ Fitness activities; ask for list.
   - ➤ Retreat-type programs/classes; ask for schedule.

2. What is the facility's primary approach, for example, is it yoga, fitness, pampering, solitude, or resort?

3. Does it target or are there special times for:
   - ➤ Singles?
   - ➤ Married people?
   - ➤ Couples?
   - ➤ Divorced, widowed people?
   - ➤ Families?
   - ➤ Men or women only?

4. How many guests are there each cycle?

5. What's the staff-to-guest ratio?

6. Are personal trainers available?

7. What's a sample day like?

8. What's the length of stay; is it flexible?

9. What lodging is available (private, semi-private, dormitory, camping, and so on)?

10. Are meals scheduled (set times only) or flexible? Are special diets accommodated?

11. Are sample menus available?

12. What is the atmosphere/setting of the facility?
    - ➤ Country/city
    - ➤ Grounds/gardens
    - ➤ Structured schedule of events
    - ➤ Free time
    - ➤ Relaxed/casual
    - ➤ Provide or are near to pools, golf courses, tennis courts, and so on

13. Does it have a religious or other affiliation? Does it provide:
    - ➤ Silent retreats?
    - ➤ Communal prayer?
    - ➤ Nondenominational chapel?

14. Is a spiritual advisor available?

15. Are there accommodations for special medical needs?

16. Ask about other personal considerations.
    - ➤ Is standard clothing provided?
    - ➤ Is it a clothing-optional program?
    - ➤ Are electronics permitted (specify)?
    - ➤ Is telephone/other contact permitted?
    - ➤ Are pets permitted?

17. Are there special weather needs?
    - ➤ Heating/air conditioning
    - ➤ Special gear requirements for rain or snow

18. What's the location?
    - ➤ Within/outside United States
    - ➤ Mountains, desert, water, or forest

19. Are there special timing considerations?
    - ➤ Time of year
    - ➤ Festivals
    - ➤ Religious observances

20. How about legalities?
    - ➤ Passport
    - ➤ Immunizations
    - ➤ Foreign currency

alpha
books

Ten Questions to Ask About Spa and Beauty Services and Fitness Classes

1. Which services and/or fitness classes are included in the base price?
2. Are descriptions of the treatments and classes available?
3. What's the cost of additional treatments and classes?
4. Do you need appointments to receive included services?
5. How are appointments made and how far in advance must they be made?
6. Are additional treatments and classes charged by the hour?
7. When are classes scheduled? If the times are inconvenient or unworkable, are substitutes available?
8. Is there a penalty for cancellation of a confirmed appointment?
9. Is a service charge or tax added to service's list price? Is a gratuity customary?
10. Must you provide any special clothing and equipment?

Basic Supply List for Turning Your Home into a Spa

With these few items, you are ready to give yourself facials and masks, massages, manicures, pedicures, soaks, steam baths, and wraps:

➤ Soft towels (splurge!)
➤ Candles (scented ones, too)
➤ Scrubbers: body brushes, loofahs, pumice, sea sponges, scrubbing mitts
➤ Cosmetic scrubs and jars of facial mud
➤ Moisturizers: foot and hand cream, body lotion, face lotion
➤ A few essential oils: perhaps lavender, peppermint, chamomile
➤ Herbs for tea and for bathing

To create a home retreat, you need:

➤ Quiet, hidden space defined by furniture, plants, or furnishings
➤ Candles, special pictures or objects, and a home altar
➤ A personal journal and meditative or spiritual readings

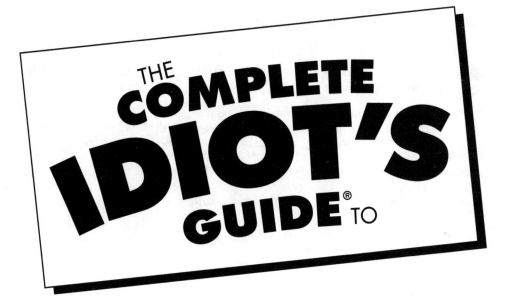

THE COMPLETE IDIOT'S GUIDE® TO

Self-Healing with Spas and Retreats

by Linda Short

**alpha
books**

Macmillan USA, Inc.
201 West 103rd Street
Indianapolis, IN 46290

A Pearson Education Company

To the spirit in each of us that guides us all to health and healing.

Copyright © 2000 by Linda Short

Appendix A, "The Spa Finder Directory of Spa Retreats and Spa Resorts," and Foreword by Frank van Putten © by Spa Finder

International Standard Book Number: 0-02-863662-7
Library of Congress Catalog Card Number: Available upon request.

02 01 00   8 7 6 5 4 3 2 1

Interpretation of the printing code: The rightmost number of the first series of numbers is the year of the book's printing; the rightmost number of the second series of numbers is the number of the book's printing. For example, a printing code of 00-1 shows that the first printing occurred in 2000.

Printed in the United States of America

Note: This publication contains the opinions and ideas of its author. It is intended to provide helpful and informative material on the subject matter covered. It is sold with the understanding that the author and publisher are not engaged in rendering professional services in the book. If the reader requires personal assistance or advice, a competent professional should be consulted.

The author and publisher specifically disclaim any responsibility for any liability, loss or risk, personal or otherwise, which is incurred as a consequence, directly or indirectly, of the use and application of any of the contents of this book.

Alpha Development Team

Publisher
Marie Butler-Knight

Editorial Director
Gary M. Krebs

Associate Managing Editor
Cari Shaw Fischer

Acquisitions Editors
Randy Ladenheim-Gil
Amy Gordon

Development Editors
Phil Kitchel
Amy Zavatto

Assistant Editor
Georgette Blau

Production Team

Development Editor
Carol Hupping

Production Editor
Christy Wagner

Copy Editor
Heather Stith

Cover Designer
Mike Freeland

Photo Editor
Richard H. Fox

Photo Researcher
J. Richard Seidel,
Artemis Picture Research Group

Illustrator
Jody P. Schaeffer

Book Designers
Scott Cook and Amy Adams of DesignLab

Indexer
Angie Bess

Layout/Proofreading
Angela Calvert
Mary Hunt

Contents at a Glance

Contents

xiii

Foreword

In my almost half century on this earth, I have been extremely fortunate. For the most part I have been healthy, successful, and blessed with a loving family. But still ... I've had my bad periods, times when I've felt bored with life, dissatisfied, and restless.

Yet, from my worst moments, I have often learned my best lessons. One of those lessons is that even though others may help me during difficult times, healing cannot take place without my active involvement.

Recently, I came across a study of elderly patients who were bedridden and whose prognosis was for more of the same. When started on a slow but steadily more challenging exercise regimen, many regained a remarkable self-sufficiency and were able to get around unassisted for the first time in years. Our inner resources, no matter how frail they may seem at times, are amazingly strong and capable of rejuvenation.

The medical profession can do remarkable things. They have an ever-growing arsenal of tools to treat both the body and the mind. But no physician has the power to heal. He or she can offer a cure and assist in the process, but healing comes only from within. So although I reach out for professional help when I need it, I'm a great believer in self-help, too. Deep inside every one of us resides a tremendous reservoir of will, insight, and resourcefulness just waiting to be unleashed. It's up to us to help ourselves.

We all possess this self-healing power. It is part of the human spirit. It's the same power that drives us to find beauty in the starkest landscape, joy in the darkest night, and love anytime, anywhere.

Where does one start to rejuvenate the spirit? Spas and retreats are environments specifically designed to help us slow down, catch our breath, and be in the moment. They are ideal places to begin our self-healing journey.

The most important decision we have to make is that we're worth it. And we are. We are all born to soar. Fear and doubt, pain and anger are meant to be temporary—not permanent—states of mind.

Know this, too: When it comes to self-healing, whether it is the body, the mind, or the spirit, there are no dumb questions. The greatest discoveries come when we are ready to abandon our preconceived notions and to start at the beginning again. Eastern philosophers call it "beginner's mind." You may feel like a beginner—but in fact you're now ready to face life's most fundamental and important questions. So, follow your heart. Read this book. And let the journey begin.

Frank van Putten, President, Spa Finder

Spa Finder, established in 1986, is the largest spa travel and reservation company in the world, creating and booking spa vacation packages for travel professionals, consumers, spa professionals, and the media. Additionally, Spa Finder publishes a quarterly four-color magazine that features timely articles on health, fitness, New Age topics, and more, as well as lengthy spa directories. *The Spa Finder Show,* a weekly half-hour television series, airs starting in 1999 and will introduce leading spas all around the world. In addition, Spa Finder radio show can be heard on WEVD radio in New York. To plan your spa vacation, or find the latest information on programs and prices, contact Spa Finder Reservations at 800-ALL-SPAS or 800-255-7727. In New York City, call 212-924-6800. Check out Spa Finder on the Web at spafinders.com.

Introduction

Wouldn't it be wonderful to have a grip on life every day? (Well, most of the time, anyway.) Then the search would be over for the perfect job; the highest spiritual attainment; the absence of stress, tension, anxiety, and worry; *the* relationship; and lots of free time to develop yourself and enjoy it all. It wouldn't hurt if you also discovered you had a scintillating mind, a perfectly curved body, and a spirit that was plugged in to the number one energy source.

Don't get so excited. Your life won't magically morph just by opening these pages. You have to work at it. But this book will certainly help. To begin, you'll get information on:

➤ How to choose the spa and retreat that's right for you.

➤ Why spas and retreats are good for you.

➤ What services spas provide.

➤ What to expect and how to act when you get to a spa or retreat.

➤ How to keep your glow when you return home.

For those times when you can't get away, you'll also learn how to duplicate the spa or retreat experience at home.

And there's more, much more. This potentially life-changing book goes beyond facts and figures (pun intended). It will lead you to new understandings about your life:

➤ What values you hold

➤ How to translate these values into daily attitudes and activities

➤ Discovering your inner beauty

➤ How to have a little quiet time every day

➤ Experiencing real peace

➤ Working with your energy

➤ Finding and singing your soul's sounds

➤ Understanding what real self-healing means and how to achieve it

Health and renewal are more than the absence of pain, stress, and worry. They are the positive results of knowing your place in the universe and coming to terms with that. How gratifying and exciting!

My purpose in this book is to help you open your entire self to the possibilities around you. Even though I'm the sole author of this book, I am not the only one helping you with this journey. Many people have, in one way or another, helped me with the material in this book. As I wrote every chapter, I have been much aware of the teachers, people, and retreat experiences that have formed me into who I am at this stage in my life. I cannot separate myself from them. We are one.

More than these people and events, I am profoundly aware of the spiritual dimension of this work. Whether you use traditional religious terminology or speak in terms of "being in the groove" or "going with the flow," I believe that I have been used to offer some simple words of encouragement and direction to those who are ready to listen. It's reminiscent of the time I stepped back from a silkscreen print I completed and thought, "Whoa! I didn't do this." I, alone, did not do this book, either.

How to Use This Book

As you read along in the pages that follow, find yourself, at this time in your life, and take from this book what you need.

Part 1, "Give Me a Break, Please!" convinces (hopefully) the unbelievers among you that you need a break—and a regular one at that. Your spirit knows it, and your health demands it. Besides, you'll be in great company when you take the time for rest and renewal at a spa or retreat.

Part 2, "Finding the Time You Need," gives you tips for doing just that. It helps you examine your day at home and on the job and squeeze out precious minutes. I'll give you some steps to take hold of your life to create a more satisfying and fulfilling one.

Part 3, "Taking Care of Busy-ness," is about slowing down, using stillness and silence for self-healing, and finding the way to peace, love, and joy. If you have children, don't neglect Chapter 9, "The Children's Corner," which focuses on helping children get a head start on mastering their bodies and connecting with their spirits.

Part 4, "Self-Healing Advice Your Mother Didn't Teach You," provides unique advice on how you can improve three key areas of your life: sleeping, exercising, and eating. Chapter 11, "Let's Get Physical," for example, stresses attitude, affirmations, and reverence toward your body instead of heavy exercise.

Part 5, "Getaways for Homebodies," is for when you want something between the spa and retreat visits to keep you going in your normal, everyday environment. I explain ways you can turn your home into a spa or retreat and how to draw on nature, music, and other creative outlets for self-healing and vitality.

Part 6, "Take Me Away from Here!" is for the time when you are ready to leave and have a complete getaway experience. It takes you through the ins and outs of spas, retreats, and pilgrimages and describes sample destinations. (Who would have thought you could get all this information in one place!)

Part 7, "Following the Spirit," helps you settle in without stress and trepidation when you arrive at your ultimate spa or retreat experience. Just as important is the guidance in the very last chapter, which helps you adjust once you get back home and incorporate what you've learned into your daily life for a lifetime of physical, mental, and emotional good health.

Further Enlightenment

Throughout this book, you'll notice a variety of sidebars that offer extra tidbits of interesting information and valuable advice:

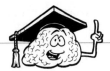

Mindful Moment

Whether wise words by an expert or additional background information, these notes are sure to make you stop and think.

Chill Out

As I tell my children when they need to settle down, "Calm down; chill out." These cautions and warnings are designed to help you avoid pitfalls.

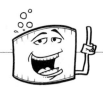

Jacuzzi Jive

You will find no jive here, just straightforward explanations about words and terms you need to know.

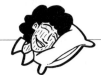

Take 5

Go ahead and take a mini break to read the helpful tips here.

Acknowledgments

I am grateful to many people who support and cheer me in my life. My special friends Deanna, Debbie, Mary, and Ron are available whenever I need them. Then there's my family. It's one thing to have a work-at-home mom, but it's something else when she's working on a project of this scope. Special thank yous to my children, Michael, Elisabeth, Kathleen, and Rebecca. I wish to express my tremendous gratitude and love for my husband, Lloyd, who solved my computer problems and accepted my crazy work hours to get this finished. (Where are we going now that this book is done? On retreat or to a spa, I hope.)

Special thanks to all who provided me with names of their favorite retreat houses and to those of you who accompanied me on my journey through the years and gave me so much, especially Windy and Jennifer. And for Ray, *in memorium*.

Finally, I'd like to offer particular kudos to the exceptionally talented folks who helped get the words to print—the team at Macmillan, including Carol Hupping, Christy Wagner, Heather Stith, Gary Krebs, and all others who helped along the way, and to Spa Finders for providing spa listings.

Special Thanks to the Technical Reviewer

The Complete Idiot's Guide to Self-Healing with Spas and Retreats was reviewed by experts who double-checked the accuracy of what you'll learn here, to help us ensure that this book gives you everything you need to know about how spas and retreats can enhance your well-being. Special thanks are extended to Spa Finder and Bambi Ward.

Spa Finder, the largest spa travel and reservation company in the world, also publishes a magazine that features timely articles on health, fitness, New Age topics, and more, as well as spa directories. Its television series *The Spa Finder Show* features spas from around the world, and the Spa Finder radio show can be heard on WEVD radio in New York.

Bambi Ward, M.B.B.S., F.R.A.C.G.P., Grad Dip Fam Med., is a medical practitioner who integrates complementary therapies with Western medicine in a holistic health practice in Victoria, Australia. Dr. Ward is also a part-time senior lecturer at Monash University, Australia, and facilitates educational workshops for doctors on the Internet.

Trademarks

All terms mentioned in this book that are known to be or are suspected of being trademarks or service marks have been appropriately capitalized. Alpha Books and Macmillan USA, Inc. cannot attest to the accuracy of this information. Use of a term in this book should not be regarded as affecting the validity of any trademark or service mark.

Part 1
Give Me a Break, Please!

Congratulations! By picking up this book you're listening to your unconscious telling you to slow down and take a break. I know, you have all kinds of excuses and all kinds of reasons why you couldn't possibly sit down and put your feet up, but listen for just 10 seconds to your body. How do you feel right now? Wouldn't a rest, even for 15 minutes, feel wonderful? You could handle 15 minutes: You use that much time looking for your keys, glasses, and the portable phone that seems to walk off by itself.

If you still have a doubting bone in your body, I'll do my best to convince you that a regular break is a healthy, reasonable, necessary, and even spiritual thing to do. Your head will clear, your creativity will improve, and your disposition will calm and brighten. You'll be good company and in good company when you give yourself the gift of rest and renewal.

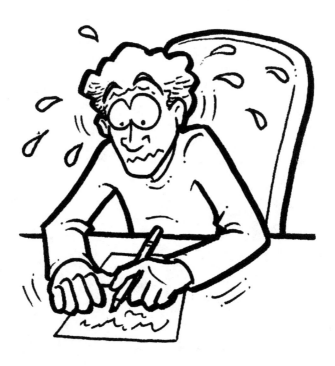

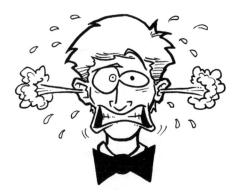

Chapter 1

Are You Going Crazy?

In This Chapter

➤ Deciding if you're going loony

➤ Remembering famous rest-takers

➤ Considering retreats and spas

➤ Taking a rest from excuses

Does any of this sound familiar: Your deadline (presentation, meeting—fill in with whatever) is tomorrow, so you decide to get to work earlier, but your car won't start, your pet just puked on the carpet, and your children walk in the front door because they missed the school bus and want to know how they're getting to school. You're getting a headache, and you begin to wonder if maybe you should just call in sick or go back to bed and pretend this morning never happened.

Listen. Do you hear your voice join all the others in a cosmic yell for help? The sound is so desperate. Listen. It says, "Maybe we're all going crazy." "Hold on," other voices yell back. "Help is on the way. We'll take you to someplace where you'll find peace and can begin to heal yourself: a spa or retreat!" But wait. Do you hear wailing? Listen. The wailing is saying, "We don't deserve a break; we have responsibilities; we can't shirk our obligations."

Do you sometimes long for a break? If you do, you've come to the right place. This book will lead you to the promised land of milk baths and honey. If you don't think you need a break, you're plain crazy (and probably need it even more)!

Where Are We Going?

The world has changed enormously in the last 100 years. As we race ever faster toward the future, perhaps we ought to take time out to look backward, to assess the amazing differences between life in 1900 and life in the year 2000. My mother-in-law was born January 1, 1900. Consider all the inventions and conveniences we take for granted that didn't exist when she was born.

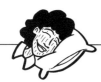

Take 5

Some would say it was a slower, more peaceful life without all our modern-day gadgets. Why not take part of a day and revisit that earlier time? Walk instead of ride. Visit or write instead of using the telephone or e-mail. Write your own story instead of watching television or a movie. Refrain from using your microwave, juicer, or espresso maker. Light candles and enjoy the stars after dark.

More than things, the industrial revolution and then the computer and information revolution reshaped how we live and work and even, to a great extent, how we relate to others. Our attitudes, expectations, and outlooks shifted. We went from a slow-paced lifestyle where our basic needs were met often by the toil of our own hands or with the help of our neighbors to a fast-paced, more solitary crusade of discovery and acquisition.

The busy-ness and hurry surround all of us. We are not alone in struggling with working and parenting, striving to meet goals (our own and those imposed upon us), and reconciling our values and morals with the realities of the day-to-day. But we don't like to ask for help. Our national pride is built on rugged individualism and independence. We hesitate to seek out or don't know how to find others who are in situations similar to ours. But lots of other people just like you are using spas and retreats. You're not alone here, and you won't be alone there, as you'll discover as you read this book.

Spin to a Halt

You hardly ever rest, you say? That macho stuff or that independence-at-all-costs mindset will get you into trouble. Consider a top—you know, that kid's toy. A top spins very fast and must continue to do so to maintain its momentum, but eventually it gets slower and slower until it stops spinning. Even a top, whose nature is to spin fast, doesn't do so forever.

For us humans, each day is followed by evening, a natural cycle that allows us to cease spinning in our routines. Do you get the connection? It's okay to put your feet up, to rest your body, and to stop thinking to rest your mind.

Rest in Good Company

If the real problem is that you're afraid of how others will label you if you take some rest and relaxation, then take heart and get some support from famous rest-takers. You can blame it on them when some unconverted soul wants to know why you're loafing around. These folks also offer us life lessons.

Goldilocks and the Three Bears

Goldilocks stumbles upon a retreat house while she is out hiking through the woods on a warm, sunny day. She samples the food, which is healthy and unlike her ordinary fare. She tries the cozy comforts of the retreat and finds a corner chair to her liking.

After some time, the nourishing food and a satisfied spirit lead her to seek some deeper relaxation. Initially thinking that she won't find any bed as snuggly as her own, she finds she is wrong and settles in. Unfortunately, she rudely discovers the bed is reserved for someone else.

What lessons can be learned from this?

> ➤ **Lesson 1:** Healthy food, physical activity, and relaxation prior to bed help create a deep, peaceful sleep.

> ➤ **Lesson 2:** Be sure you call ahead for retreat or spa reservations!

The Princess and the Pea

The princess's unlimited expense account allowed her the luxury of procuring an abundance of mattresses. There were mattresses covered in silk, mattresses covered in flannel, mattresses covered in 100 percent cotton, and mattresses covered in wool. She was sure she'd get a super night's rest. After all, she was a princess.

She piled the mattresses high to make a wonderfully comfy bed. Alas, she couldn't sleep. She piled on more wonderful mattresses. Still no sleep. Oh, what she wouldn't give for some common shut-eye!

What have we learned from this princess?

> ➤ **Lesson 1:** Until she emptied her pea-brained head of what ailed her, she would not enjoy the rest she sought, despite the care she took in creating a restful external environment.

> ➤ **Lesson 2:** If you cannot sleep, the reason may be your bed or bedding; then again, it may not be.

> ➤ **Lesson 3:** Wealth alone cannot buy a good night's rest. You can, however, use some of it on a spa or retreat experience.

The Tortoise and the Hare

Mr. Tortoise and Mr. Hare often disagreed. They might not do it openly, you understand, but each had his own way of dealing with work and the world. Mr. Tortoise was a Type B personality (see Chapter 3, "Let's Get Personal"), so he was told. He was patient and easy-going. He often took his time walking to work, stopping to say hello to others or noticing the changes in Mrs. Green's garden.

Mr. Hare was just the opposite, it seemed. He didn't notice people or places outside because he always jumped over them, darting here and there and hurrying to his next appointment. Sometimes he'd hit someone with his back paws when he didn't judge distances quite right. "They should be lucky I don't land on them entirely," he'd think. "Besides, I'm making things happen, I'm a mover and a shaker," he'd explain. "My way is better than old Mr. Tortoise's."

As it happened, someone overheard Mr. Hare's last remark and thought he'd start something by teasing Mr. Hare. "I bet Mr. Tortoise could beat you. If I set up a race, will you agree to participate?" How could Mr. Hare say no? He'd be humiliated if he backed out.

The day came and the race began. As was his nature, Mr. Tortoise plodded along, slow and steady. Mr. Hare, as was his custom, took off as though he were shot out of a cannon. About halfway through the race, Mr. Hare became very tired. Because he was so far ahead of Mr. Tortoise, Mr. Hare decided to curl up under a tree and take a short nap. While Mr. Hare was sleeping, Mr. Tortoise passed him and won the race. Mr. Hare lost the race, but all was not lost. He had been considering the advisability of making a retreat and decided that now was the perfect time.

This tale teaches the following lessons:

➤ **Lesson 1:** Retreats are a good bet, perhaps even more so when you've had a major setback in your life.

➤ **Lesson 2:** Be sure you get sufficient rest when you have a big day ahead.

➤ **Lesson 3:** Naps are great, but make sure you don't take them at inopportune times.

➤ **Lesson 4:** Know something about your personality type. It might help keep you from backing yourself into a corner you'd rather not be in.

➤ **Lesson 5:** Slow, steady, determined individuals get the job done at least as well as hurry-up-and-stop types and cause a lot less stress to themselves and those around them.

Snow White

What a life! How much more back to nature can you get? Snow White spends her time relaxing out in the deep woods, enjoying the wonderful fragrances, and perhaps finding a hot mineral or mud bath here or there. Taking care of seven little eccentric guys might be a lot of work some days, but they play music, sing, and dance, which gives a lift to the soul.

Then there was the pilgrim who happened by with foodstuffs from another part of the world. Snow White took a bite, dreaming of adventure and romance. Her dreaming continued, until she found romance with a handsome prince and adventures on the other side of the sunset.

Lessons learned:

> ➤ **Lesson 1:** Don't be afraid of enjoying a deep sleep. You, too, will come out of it alive.

> ➤ **Lesson 2:** If you don't have your own woods, a sensual spa experience will supply the fragrances, relaxation, and bath and beauty treatments.

> ➤ **Lesson 3:** Even goody-goodies who seem to like what they're doing need a blissful break.

> ➤ **Lesson 4:** Music chases away the cares of the world.

> ➤ **Lesson 5:** Believe, and your thoughts and dreams may indeed come true.

Sleeping Beauty

She had it all—beauty, position, and wealth, or so she thought. Then came a catastrophe. In an effort to escape, she went into exile, away from her family, friends, and social circle. A heaviness descended upon those left behind, and time seemed to stand still.

As for Sleeping Beauty, a tender trio sustained her throughout her ordeal and eventually guided her back home. Unhappily, what Sleeping Beauty tried to avoid was waiting for her, and because she was unprepared, it overcame her. Even so, her loyal ladies stood by her, and a special friend pulled her through. With the crisis over, the future looked brighter than it had in many a year.

Lessons learned:

> ➤ **Lesson 1:** Even one caring individual will help get you through the bleakest day.

> ➤ **Lesson 2:** Going on retreat or escaping to a spa won't help your problems if you don't use the time to address them.

> ➤ **Lesson 3:** The sun *does* come out tomorrow.

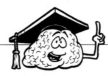

Mindful Moment

I don't recall the name of the children's book; it's been too many years ago. I remember the lesson, however, because I created a watercolor collage to remind me: The sun always shines somewhere, even when we can't see it.

Rip van Winkle

Rip's ideas of work were different. He preferred public relations: helping others, playing with the children, and swapping stories. But his wife preferred he pursue domestic relations: tending his own farm, helping with housework, and doing chores.

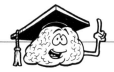

Mindful Moment

Scientists have found a biological reason for what all do-gooders knew anyway: Helping others makes for personal happiness. Researchers note that your level of endorphin (a hormone that makes you feel good) increases when you think of others first. This "helpers' high" may lead to longer and healthier lives for those who offer their services regularly.

One day, Rip decided he needed to visit the mountains, where he had spent many fine previous outings. While wandering new and different paths, his mind and body relaxed, and his spirit soared. He never knew what to expect on these visits, but he appreciated whatever came his way.

On this trip, Rip van Winkle had a particularly spectacular experience. Indeed, it would change his life forever. Rip met a stranger, who silently guided him to a new place and level of understanding he hadn't reached before.

In due time after a refreshing, deep sleep, Rip wandered back to his village and to his home. Everything had changed. Nothing looked the same. He didn't feel the same. People didn't act the same. He felt out of sorts, disoriented, lost almost.

Slowly, very slowly, Rip regained his balance. People understood him and accepted him again. Best of all, Rip found a new place for himself in the community, in public relations.

Take 5

Some retreats use periods of silence, as religious orders often do, for as long as 30 days, to provoke an intense interior experience.

Lessons learned:

➤ **Lesson 1:** Maintaining silence is a powerful prescription.

➤ **Lesson 2:** Be open to guidance you may receive from others.

➤ **Lesson 3:** You will be changed, and other people will notice a change, after a retreat or spa experience.

➤ **Lesson 4:** Go slowly as you re-enter your daily routines after returning from a retreat or spa.

The Highest Authority

The Holy One, Allah, Lord, God, Adonai, the Absolute, a Higher Power, the Creator, the Source—use whatever name is most meaningful to you. If even the Creator rested on the seventh day, who are we to say no? So be it.

Lesson to end all lessons: Take a break. You've heard it from the Highest Authority.

Get Yourself Spa- and Retreat-Ready

Maybe your idea of self-healing is a long sleep or walk in the woods (if you can find the time) to ease your troubled mind and aching back most of the time. On a daily basis, you may be right. Then again, there are also day spas. So sit back and listen up.

Spas, wellness retreats, and stress are definitely hot topics. You know something's hot when you see it on the cover of almost every magazine at the check-out counters and in the living and travel sections of the newspapers. Hot or not, the practice of taking some special time to contemplate your inner and outer person is ancient. The attraction of spas and retreats today also reflects the growing recognition of the need to find balance in a busy lifestyle. Besides, spas and retreats must be doing somebody some good to be around for so long.

A retreat or spa is also a great avenue for getting a new perspective on life. Does every molehill seem like a mountain to you now? (Or perhaps you have only molehills and yearn for a mountain?) Get away, relax, think, reflect, and come back ready to make the changes you want.

Jacuzzi Jive

In common usage today, **spas** conjure up images of mineral springs or baths, and of places offering a variety of beauty and body treatments, although additional services may be available. **Retreats** offer a withdrawal from the world of your regular routines, for a time of safe and quiet reflection to connect with something more profound that is both within and outside yourself. **Wellness centers** are a recent mix of spa services and retreat services focusing on total wellness.

From Spa to Retreat and in Between

I won't go into all the details and services of the different facilities here; you'll find this information in Part 6, "Take Me Away from Here!" This section is only an introduction to explain just what spas and retreats are.

Spas

As someone said to me recently, spas are more than just hot tubs, even though that's about what they were when they began. Of course, the spa hot tubs were soothing baths in hot springs. Today, spas offer many more services. They are places to de-stress, get fit, lose weight, and enjoy body treatments.

Enjoying a simple manicure at a spa gives you a relaxing moment and helps you feel good about yourself. Don't be surprised when others notice your calm, joyful attitude afterward.
(Photo © Artemis Picture Research)

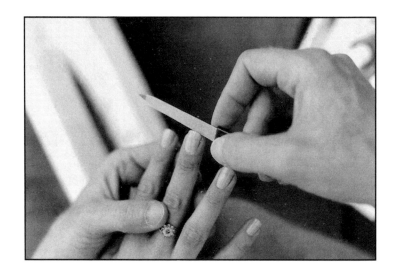

Spas are known by many names. They may be called day spas, destination spas, resort spas, vacation spas, adventure spas, even spa retreats. Whatever the label, it is the services and treatments that are important.

For this book, I divide spas into two main flavors: the day spa and the vacation spa. These terms give a hint as to the length of stay and quantity of available services. Both offer body care and beautifying treatments such as facials, manicures, pedicures, a variety of massage techniques, aromatherapy, perhaps reflexology, and sometimes more.

The *day spa* is a facility located near you, where you'll usually spend a few hours. The *vacation spa* requires a longer stay—it's more like a vacation. These spas often round out their program with nutrition and exercise programs, mind-body programs, and lots more time for pampering.

Retreats

There's such a variety of retreats: silent retreats, active retreats, centers that offer lectures and workshops, secular or religious retreats. Retreat centers also may offer some spa-type services such as massage and healthy meals. The emphasis in retreats is on interior beauty and understanding, leading some to connect with something more profound that is both within and outside themselves.

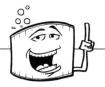

Jacuzzi Jive

Vacation spas are ones which often offer services such as nutrition and exercise programs, mind-body programs or workshops, and more time for pampering. They may be connected with a resort, and guests stay a week or more to enjoy the range of services. A **day spa** is a drop-in facility near home where you'll spend a few hours, and where fewer services are available.

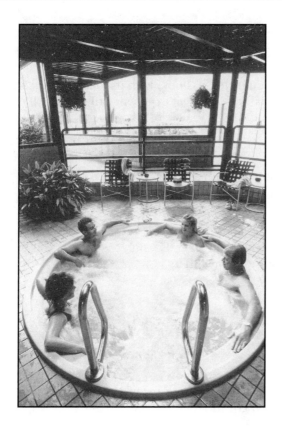

Get thee to a spa and soak up the rejuvenating bubbles and atmosphere. You might even make some friends along the way.
(Image © Camerique Stock Photography)

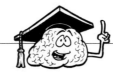

Mindful Moment

Pets now have their own resorts, spas, and daycare centers. One doggie (and cat) spa in Pennsylvania has hot tubs, swimming pools, massage, hydrotherapy, and field trips. Contact them at Cozy Inn Pet Resort and Spa, RR #1, Box 256-A, Stahlstown, PA 15687, 724-593-6133. As this is a new trend, listings are not located conveniently. Check out the Web site www.dogfancy.com as well as local sources for other possibilities.

Wellness Centers

The first wellness center was opened in the 1970s, as you will discover in Chapter 13, "Heal Thyself." Today, wellness centers are promoted as a holistic approach to wellness: soothing both body and mind. One magazine described these facilities as "more than the typical spa, [offering] everything from yoga to meditation to stress control." Look carefully, however, and you will find spas that also offer these kinds of programs.

You have so many choices! And you have this book, with its ideas, advice, and many listings to help you find that special spa or retreat experience that makes life more than manageable, perhaps even magnificent!

No More Excuses

So are you ready to go yet? If you're still not sure, let's get those flimsy excuses on the table.

I'm too busy.

Read on, and I'll show you ways to slow down and evaluate what it is you're so busy about. Maybe you need a time out to do just that.

It takes too much time.

Go to a day spa. Attend an evening or weekend retreat. They're only a few hours long, but you still get a refreshing rest.

It costs too much.

You are misinformed. Rates vary widely, and some are even downright cheap. It just depends what you want, where you go, and for how long.

What about my job?

What about it? It will be there when you come back, assuming you still want the job when you come back. Go when things are sort of slow at work. If you can stay away when you're sick, you can stay away to keep from getting sick (see what I mean in Chapter 2, "Simon Says Sit Down"). Besides, a rested employee works better. You're doing your boss a favor by visiting a spa or retreat.

Real men don't use spas and retreats.

On the contrary. Corporations long have used retreat experiences for their mostly male executives. Today, nearly 7 in 10 men feel stressed at work, says a Wirthlin Worldwide survey, and a growing number are de-stressing at spas. Spa clientele is now 25 percent men, according to the International Spa Association. Indeed, there are spas and retreats for men only.

What about my family?

They will manage, believe me. I have four children, ages 8 to 16. I've gone on retreats since before they were born. Your partner (or family, or friends, or neighbors, or a trusted sitter) will get it done in your absence, even if it's not the way you would do it.

If you must, write down everything and leave a detailed daily schedule. If this still sounds like too much, remember, you can also opt to go for a weekend or even a day.

I don't know what to expect.

No problem. Read on and I'll prepare you.

I won't know anyone.

So take a friend. Or decide you'll enjoy meeting new people. Remember, a stranger is only someone you haven't met yet.

I'll feel out of place.

Why? Because it's your first time? Spas and retreats are great places with good people. Besides, you'll only feel this way once. After that, you'll be an alum, taking others by the hand.

I'm scared.

It's good to be careful, but rest assured, the places listed in this book have been checked out to be clean and safe. It's just your adrenaline running, a natural stress reaction you'll learn about in Chapter 2.

After my son was born, I made a week-long retreat at a place called The Ashram in California. One evening, the speaker related this story:

"Lions roar to scare their prey. What the prey doesn't know is that the old lions without teeth do the roaring. If instead of running away scared, the lions' prey faces its fears and goes into the roar, it'll escape the danger. Only when the prey turns and runs away from the roar does it run into the strong hunters who attack and devour it."

Moral: Go into the roar. Face your fears.

I've never done anything like this.

As the saying goes, there's a first time for everything. What would have happened if you hadn't tried eating for the first time, or walking, or breathing on your own?

I can't afford new clothes.

Who said anything about a formal affair? Pick a casual place and take what you have. Besides, some places provide you with clothes, so all guests look the same.

What about germs?

Strict health codes apply. The facilities are inspected and must pass. Of course, if a guest has a cold or the flu, you have about the same odds of getting sick as if you were at work, at home, or in the grocery store.

Aren't people who go to these places weird?

Heck no. They're folks like you. Some guests are more stressed than others, true, but they're harmless. If you don't want company, you can always pick a place where you have lots of alone time.

My neighbors will think I'm weird.

Just stare them straight in the eye, and with a smile, inform them that *they're* the ones who are weird for not knowing what's in and beneficial besides.

Isn't the food there strange?

If the type of food served is a genuine concern, ask before you go. Many spots offer a health-conscious menu, but it's usually delicious and well prepared. I don't think you'll miss your junk food after the first day or two of withdrawal.

I just can't give up my high-tech toys.

If you're this much of a techno-junkie, you're long overdue to be unplugged. What are you hiding from? If your stress is this bad that you're escaping into an electronic world, or your stress is so great *because* you're escaping into an electronic world, I suggest you check out of your artificial world and get real. Humans (you still are, right?) need human contact.

I'm out of shape.

You're just the person that spa or wellness center is looking for. Their mission is to make you healthy and satisfied with your body. If you don't want to deal with, say, massage, just say so. You choose your services.

It's too hard.

This depends what you mean by hard. There are very active retreats, as well as active wellness centers, which do have a demanding physical program. During my time at The Ashram, a call came in while I was in the office. The owner answered and laughed. She held the phone in the air and said, "This caller wants to know if she should come. She's interested in manicures, facials, relaxing—that sort of thing." Our answer: a collective "no way." On the other hand, in the movie, *A League of Their Own,* the coach tells Dottie when she quits, "It's the hard that makes it great."

If you don't want challenging physical activity, no problem. Choose a facility that offers easier exercise or none at all. Go for 100 percent pampering, if that's what sounds good. Remember, *you're* choosing what you want to do.

I meant that it's too hard to face myself.

Yup. That's what I thought. So don't, if you're not ready. Just go, get pampered, and have everyone else do everything for you. Melt under the attention. Enjoy it, and come back fabulously radiant and relaxed. When you're ready, you'll look yourself in the eyes and deal with what you see.

I'll hate it.

How do you know unless you try it? So many people have missed so many glorious experiences because they prejudge rather than participate. Don't be one of them. Don't let this be an "I wish" experience. (You'll understand that better after you read Chapter 3.)

I'm a recluse.

So are the members of certain religious orders. Pick one of the spots run by them, and you'll feel right at home.

And furthermore ...

I lost my job. I just moved here. I just broke up with someone. I'm very ill. Someone I loved just died. These life situations create major stress. Check retreats or wellness centers for specialized programs—lectures, workshops, activities—that address your concerns. Now might be just the time to take some time to sort it out alone or with the support and help of trained staff.

I don't think you have any additional legitimate excuses, and I've answered the others. So take a vacation, long weekend, or even a day. A spa or retreat is a simple yet effective way to slow down, lower your stress level, put your life in perspective, and feel great.

The Least You Need to Know

➤ You may be going crazy like everyone else, but thankfully you're not there yet.

➤ Taking breaks to rest and renew yourself is natural and necessary. Lots of folks from the Highest Authority on down say so.

➤ Whether it's a spa, a retreat house, or a wellness center, there's a getaway just right for you.

➤ I have an answer for any excuse you have, so go and get out of here!

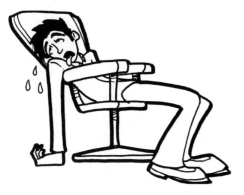

Chapter 2

Simon Says Sit Down

In This Chapter

➤ Understanding what stress is

➤ Recognizing where stress lurks

➤ Reviewing the harmful effects of stress

➤ Using your head to control stress

Stress follows you everywhere. Even when you come back from your retreat or spa, you'll step back into your life and whatever stresses go with it.

In this chapter, I'll familiarize you with good stress (yes, there *is* good stress), as well as the effects of bad stress. I'll help you see the physical and mental side effects of stress and how you can deal with them. I'll give you a nonmedical look at the body's response to tension and anxiety. You decide whether the side effects are worth the risk.

What Is Stress, Anyway?

It's probably easier for you to look at the effects of stress in your life than to describe exactly what it is. When I am so unfocused, agitated, and hurried that I back the car out of the garage through the garage door, I know for sure I am exhibiting the signs of major stress. (Yes, I really did this.) For you, it might be forgetting about a pot on the stove until it boils over because you're trying to do 40 million other tasks simultaneously. Or you find yourself yelling at a blameless co-worker when you discover you've misplaced your report, forgotten an appointment, or spilled coffee on your new slacks.

Signs of Stress

These are some signs of stress:

➤ Overeating or undereating

➤ Increased use of alcohol, tobacco, caffeine, tranquilizers, or drugs

➤ Withdrawing from friends

➤ Rushing

➤ Fidgeting

➤ Blaming, criticizing, or arguing

➤ Easily irritated

➤ Increased spending

➤ Trouble meeting commitments

➤ Poor work performance

➤ Lateness or absenteeism

➤ Being accident-prone (does the garage door fit here?)

➤ Staring endlessly at the TV

Stress is such a common part of our lives that most people can find themselves in this list somewhere.

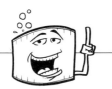

Jacuzzi Jive

Stress is the sum total of normal and abnormal pressures of living that test the individual's ability to cope and change a person's mental, emotional, or physical state. The **stress response** releases hormones that initiate a series of changes in the functioning of the body.

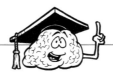

Mindful Moment

Credit Austrian-born physician Hans Selye (1907–1982) for identifying stress for what it is. He borrowed the term from physics and used it to describe what you're feeling. Unlike most of us, however, Selye believed stress could be positive or negative. Positive stress results from our doing something we enjoy, whether that is athletic competition or organizing a surprise party.

For me, stress is a feeling of pressure that makes life seem difficult and out of control. I have two common reactions: being angry and yelling, which is my way of fighting back, or crying, which is my way of hiding or running away from the pressure. What do you do?

You Can Run, but You Can't Hide from Stress

My natural reactions to stress demonstrate the "fight-or-flight" response. This response goes back to caveman days. When there was trouble, something happened in our bodies to release hormones that helped us find the strength to either fight back and save ourselves or our families or flee before harm came to us. This response is also called the *stress response.*

Good or Bad Stress

Selye called bad stress *distress.* Just imagine how you feel when you are distressed. You may feel frustration, worry, guilt, and/or anxiety. When you are distressed, you are unable to handle the many demands facing you. When distress becomes excessive and extended, your health and well-being suffer.

But good stress? Selye called this type of stress *eustress.* This feeling is enjoyable because eustress helps you

➤ Meet deadlines.

➤ Be more creative.

➤ Experience adrenaline rushes that allow some people to perform beyond their natural capacities during emergencies.

Exercise is a good stressor, as long as you enjoy how you're exercising. You need a certain level of stimulation to perform your daily tasks and to achieve your goals.

Interestingly, your body doesn't know the difference between eustress and distress. Your body exhibits the same changes whether you love or hate the stress you're under. It's how we perceive the stress that's important.

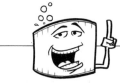

Jacuzzi Jive

Distress is excessive and extended stress that may cause bodily or psychological harm. **Eustress** is good stress that may result from creative endeavors, heroic acts, or enjoyable activities, such as athletic competitions.

Stress, Stress Everywhere

Events that create stress fall into four basic categories:

➤ Major changes in your life situation that have long-term results

➤ Pressures you feel that come from daily activities, including lack of activity

➤ Time pressures, including trying to squeeze too many activities into a given amount of time

➤ Lack of personal satisfaction

Let's look at each category and see how healthy you are.

Life Ain't What It Used to Be

Common sense tells you that any major change in your life creates disruption. For example, if you need to move, you are starting all over again in a new area: new schools, new medical services, new place of worship, new neighborhood. You probably no longer have the structures and people—the friends, family, social ties to activities, clubs, networks—you counted on in the past to support you in your new, current situation.

Marriage also creates major stress. In addition to learning about the habits and idiosyncrasies of your partner, there are issues such as location and purchase of a residence and finding time for just the two of you while responding to the demands of dual careers and a combined network of friends and family. In a changing corporate climate, when one partner faces a job change, there is concern for the relationship and for the other's career path.

One final example is from today's changing pattern of children caring for aging or ailing parents. Think of your life today. You're holding it together pretty well. But what if a parent became ill and couldn't function alone? Even if you find a residence for your parent outside your home, you'd still feel the burden. The additional worries and stresses include how often to visit, to what extent to include your parent in your regular activities, how well your parent is faring in his new environment, arranging for and coordinating therapy, medical treatments, doctor visits, and medications, not to mention taking care of his finances.

Thankfully, major changes such as these occur occasionally. Nevertheless, they are stressors that affect our health daily.

What a Day This Has Been!

Daily or recurring pressures also create havoc. Maybe your child is sick but you must be at your job. Or you anxiously await word whether you have a job after the latest corporate takeover. Or you can't stand your neighbor's loud music. Or you just got the new puppy that the kids wanted but you end up cleaning up after it and taking care of it.

Physicians point out that stress may also come from "hanging out." (Is *nothing* immune to it?) Boredom is tough. You may begin to think, "I shouldn't just be sitting here. Why don't I have something to do or someone to do it with? Poor me." If you escape with TV or chemicals, your mind is on hold or worse, and your body suffers as well.

Time pressures of daily living are nothing new. They are aggravated when you bring work home or fill up every waking minute of your family's schedule with "meaningful experiences" such as music, sports, clubs, and enrichment activities. Leave some time unstructured. Give yourself and others time to just rest and regroup.

Stress and the knowledge of its detrimental effects on each one of us have spawned all kinds of questionnaires, scales, and instruments to measure how stressed you are. Questions regarding personal pressures may include whether you worry about

➤ Having enough money.

➤ Conflicts with a partner.

➤ Conflicts about house and family responsibilities.

➤ Problems with children, in-laws, family, or friends.

➤ Having enough time.

➤ Work-family conflicts.

Whatever your source of stress and dissatisfaction, taking time for reflection, either at home or away on retreat, is a wonderful way to get a new perspective on your life and your goals.

Are We There Yet?

Do you like your life? Even if you do, there's probably something you'd like to have that you don't have now. Maybe it's something quite serious, or maybe it's just some fantasy, like a dishwasher that loads itself, weeds that walk out of your planting beds, or the perfect house on a mountain by the ocean with a view.

You've heard the saying that life is a journey. If so, are you enjoying the ride? Are you basically satisfied? If your life were somebody else's, would you be envious? Would you want to switch? Interestingly, the experts say that your life satisfaction stems from the number or kinds of support people you have in your life.

How many close friends do you have? We are so mobile today and so busy. Many of us move away from our main support system, our family. We make friends, but how close are they? We replace family with neighbors, whom we usually don't know very well. (When was the last time you dropped in on someone to chat, have a cup of coffee, munch a muffin?)

We need support and encouragement from somewhere. We need to know there is someone who cares about us and on whom we can depend. It's the friend we can call for advice, the partner who encourages us, the gang that goes out for lunch or a beer to just be together. If we believe we have even one person who will be there for us regardless of anything that happens, then our anxiety is likely to be lessened. Some people look to their faith for such support. Wherever you find your special relationships, it's the caring that makes everything else more manageable.

You Don't Look So Good: System Failure!

Stress creates changes. Some changes are immediately recognizable, like the look on your face. Other internal stress-related changes like high blood pressure may prove deadly over time if unchecked and untreated.

You Seem Nervous

Stress produces definite changes in your body. Some noticeable reactions include:

➤ Sweaty palms or underarms.

➤ Increased rate of breathing.

➤ Muscle tension.

➤ Increased heart rate.

➤ Dry mouth.

You may even get that kind of wild, crazy look in your eyes and face. These reactions are all holdovers from that old fight-or-flight response. They probably saved lives back then. But what about today?

Okay, this is not a test, so don't get stressed, but do you remember some of that stuff you learned in grade school about your body? One part is called the nervous system, and it looks something like this picture. Think of it as a complex road system throughout your body, bringing messages to and from your organs, muscles, brain, and spinal cord. You are a mass of nerves, and it's a good thing, because you need them!

The brain and spinal cord make up the central part of the nervous system and receive messages from the network of nerves.

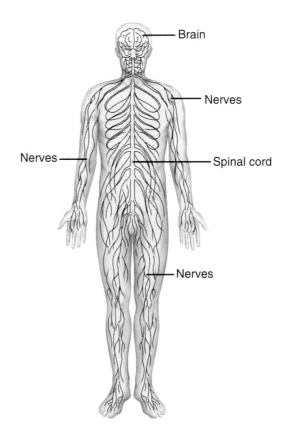

Brain

Nerves

Nerves

Spinal cord

Nerves

When you think you are in danger, the stress response begins in the nervous system. There are three stages:

1. Ready! You get pumped up. Your breathing becomes more rapid, your heart rate increases, your muscles tense, and your blood pressure rises.

2. Steady! To keep you pumped, hormones, including adrenaline, are released into your bloodstream.

3. Charge! Your hormonal system is fully engaged, producing more hormones, including one that produces glucose (sugar) to increase your energy levels so you can meet the threat.

The problem comes when you don't take action in the face of stress. Remember, the purpose of the fight-or-flight response was to help you take action: either fight or run away. You don't usually have physical threats today, so you don't respond physically. Yet your body reacts the same, and over time, the effects of all this unused nervous energy may create exhaustion or disease.

Take 5

Physical activity or exercise is recommended to relieve stress. Your body expects a physical release. When you oblige, your bodily systems balance again, and you feel better.

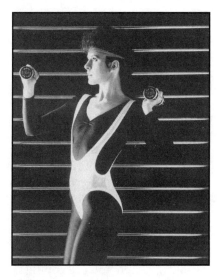

When doing your workout at home, keep activity within safe limits considering your level of fitness. Don't add to your stress response.
(Image © H. Armstrong Roberts)

You Are Not Immune

Research shows that a stressful situation, whether it is a move or keeping emotions locked inside, can weaken a person's immune system. Continuous stressful conditions may significantly suppress your immune system. Translation? Calm down, or you'll get sick. Count on it.

The job of your immune system is to keep you well. It uses two kinds of special cells to help fight off bacterial and fungal infections, some viral infections, cancer cells, and foreign agents. These cells are blocked or damaged by some of the hormones produced during the stress response, which means they can't do their job properly.

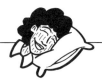

Take 5

Be happy and don't worry! Studies over the years (Grace, 1952; Graham, 1962; Kimball, 1969; and Carnegie Mellon, 1999) indicate that positive attitudes increase your chances of avoiding disease and surviving surgery. In 1989, researchers at Ohio State University found that the immune systems of people who changed their thinking and eliminated negative, self-defeating ideas made more disease-fighting cells.

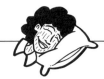

Take 5

Research in 1989 by American psychiatrist David Spiegel shows just how important relationships are. In a study conducted with women whose breast cancer had spread to other parts of their bodies, the women who attended group support sessions lived an average of twice as long as the group who did not have the group support sessions. Dr. Spiegel observed that social support is important in how individuals cope with stress.

The result? You're likely to get more bouts of common ailments like colds or flu. In addition, you're lowering your resistance and increasing the possibility of getting more serious maladies.

On the other hand, a positive outlook and other practices, such as meditation, visualization, and relaxation, can make our bodies release good hormones and reduce stress and strengthen our immune system. Even with cancer, Simonton in 1978 and Chopra in 1989 report case studies of patients whose disease went into remission after using these techniques. These and other self-healing methods used in combination with conventional treatments offer hope in fighting disease.

The results of stress may also cause your immune system to misread signals emitted by other triggers in your body and make mistakes. For example, your immune system may sense something—like dust and pollen—as harmful when it isn't, causing an allergic reaction.

Oh, My Aching Back

Remember, the first stage of the stress response includes tightening your muscles. If you stay in a state of stress long enough, your muscles will have a hard time relaxing. Continued muscle tension may bring on headaches, backaches, ulcers, and digestive tract problems. If you think you're falling apart now, there's still more, and the worst is yet to come. (Are you beginning to understand how important relaxing experiences and regular use of calming techniques are?)

One Thing Leads to Another

Problems pile up when you use coping mechanisms that are detrimental. For example

➤ Increased sweets may lead to obesity and diabetes.

➤ Increased alcohol may lead to liver disease.

➤ Increased coffee and salty products (chips, snacks) may lead to high blood pressure.

➤ Increased fatty foods may lead to obesity and heart disease.

➤ Increased tobacco use may lead to heart disease, lung disorders, high blood pressure, higher levels of blood cholesterol, ulcers, miscarriages, premature labor, and low birth-weight babies.

Taking time out, even for a mini retreat at home, in the office, or at a day spa, is much healthier way to cope.

Doctor, It's My Heart!

Of all the medical problems related to stress, the most problematic are those affecting the blood and heart system (the cardiovascular system). Stress can cause changes in heart rhythms. You may experience *arrhythmia, tachycardia,* stroke, or heart attack as a result of extreme stress.

What About Your Brain?

Stress effects your brain, too. Do you regularly find yourself

➤ Anxious, nervous.

➤ Depressed, feeling hopeless or lonely.

➤ Moody, angry, frustrated, or harboring negative thoughts.

➤ Feeling trapped or emotionally drained.

➤ Having trouble sleeping or concentrating.

➤ Forgetful, confused, disorganized, overwhelmed.

➤ Indecisive, doubting yourself, using poor judgment.

I'm sure you can think of other reasons, like dementia or Alzheimer's, for these symptoms, but they are also signs of mental fatigue created by stress.

Good Thoughts Help

Now that I've thoroughly depressed you (hopefully not causing you *extra* stress!), I'll give you some good news: You can think yourself into lower stress. That's one aspect of self-healing. Your mind, body, and emotions are linked together and influence each other. This connection means you can use your mind to train your body to not get so worked up.

Chill Out

Hans Selye said, "Don't be afraid to enjoy the stress of a full life."

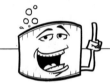

Jacuzzi Jive

Both **arrhythmia** and **tachycardia** are conditions of the heart. In arrhythmia, the heart does not beat in a regular rhythm. It may skip a beat or two. A racing heart, one that beats faster than normal, is a sign of tachycardia.

Remember that the fight-or-flight response happens when you *think* you are in danger. If you change how you see what's happening to you, you can change the result. Even one retreat experience may be enough to give you a life-changing insight. Then you can cope with stress, rather than let pressures trigger a harmful response. Talk about taking control of your life!

The Least You Need to Know

➤ Stress (both good and bad) is all around, and there's no getting away from it.

➤ Having people in your life who care about and encourage you helps lessen stress.

➤ Stress may cause many physical problems, including heart conditions.

➤ Dealing with stress by excessive eating, drinking, and smoking increases your health risks.

➤ Coping with stress with techniques such as quiet time and reflection helps you.

➤ You can use your mind to change how you see and understand stress in your life and to control your body's response to it.

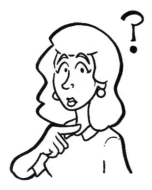

Chapter 3

Let's Get Personal

In This Chapter

➤ How your family matters

➤ Understanding personality traits

➤ How your environment influences you

➤ Deciding what's important

If you can't help how you react to stressful situations or people, you'd better get out your owner's manual and read the instructions. What? No manual? No wonder you don't know how your parts work!

Okay, take a deep breath. Let's use some common sense to try and figure this out. It's true you can't change your genes. (I hope they came with a warranty. Do you still have it?) But what about your environment and your personality? Let's see if we can't track down the missing manual pages and get a handle on why you are the way you are.

Who Are You?

What do you do in difficult situations? Do you tough it out or slow down? Do you suck it up or cave in? Are you able to make difficult choices to maintain a healthy lifestyle? Or are you afraid of being called a wimp, an underachiever, a complainer?

There are some genetic-based reasons for reacting to stress the way you do. For example, you may be among the 8 percent of the population whose autonomic nervous system develops severe stress responses. You can't change the genes—not yet, anyway. More likely, however, other factors are responsible for how you handle stress.

Are You at a Critical Age?

Carl Jung, Gail Sheehy and her passages, Erik Erikson and his eight stages, Anita Spencer's seasons, and Daniel Levinson's eras all recognize periods of increased stress and turmoil during normal psychological growth and development. These more stressful periods are transition times. Generally, they occur at the following ages:

➤ Ages 12–17: early adult transition

➤ Ages 28–33: adulthood transition

➤ Ages 35–40: mid-life transition

➤ Ages 50–55: middle adult transition

➤ Ages 60–65: late adult transition

Each stage is an opportunity for re-evaluation and renewal or a lament for what could have been and an uncertainty about what is to come. (It would be wonderful to visit a retreat or spa once during each transition phase, at least.)

Chill Out

If it's been a while since you were active, you may want your physician to give you the once-over.

Another way age may be a culprit is if you're not in good physical shape. Older individuals who are not physically fit do not react as well to stress as younger persons might. The older you get, the more susceptible you may be to infectious illnesses and stress. Your general physical condition and immune system may be weaker than a younger person's. However, if you don't let age slow you down too much and you keep fit and active, your body's stress reactions will be healthier, despite your advancing age. A spa or active retreat may be your ally here.

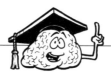

Mindful Moment

There are 35 million Americans aged 65 and over. A 1994 survey by the American Association of Retired Persons showed that travelers aged 50 and older spent more than $30 billion on vacation travel. While estimates vary, this group contributes to the estimated $8 billion a year (and growing fast) adventure travel business. That's a lot of people, travel, and money. Even kid-oriented places like Walt Disney World are aiming at this group of travelers, enticing them with new facilities, including two spas.

Male or Female?

Although I'd like to believe that men and women are equal, I have to admit there is a difference between my daughters and my son when it comes to stress. One writer in particular, Dr. Georgia Witkin-Lanoil, has written two books exploring the gender differences. In her book *The Female Stress Syndrome* (Newmarket Press, 1984), she suggests that women experience the same potential dangers of stress as men, such as increased risk of infection, depression, accidents, heart attacks, and so on. But in addition, women experience biological and psychological stressors specific to females, as well as what I call the "of course it's *her* job" syndrome.

Biological stressors include those related to menstruation, pregnancy, motherhood, and menopause. Psychological stressors include those related to body image such as anorexia; societal norms like motherhood and career; and the workplace norms concerning sexism and aging.

It's All in Your Head!

You store different information in each half of your brain. Depending on what information is stored and which half of your brain gets activated, different responses are triggered.

Your brain is a wonderful and necessary part of you. But it can cause a lot of trouble! It stores everything. What your family and society put inside your head could account for many dollars of counseling. You should be this; you should act like that. You must do both; you must not do either. What values, consciously or unconsciously, did you learn? What anxiety-heightening guilt do you harbor for not conforming to someone else's "shoulds"? (If you have children, see if you can recognize what attitudes you may be passing on to them.)

You have only one brain, but at least you can dip into either or both of its two sides. Maybe you'll find some relief (and some memory of where those owner's manual instructions went) in one or the other. Each side controls different functions. If you are right-handed, the left side of your brain is rational, logical, mathematical, whereas the right side is emotional, creative, holistic. If you are left-handed, it's just the opposite.

Maybe we can change our reactions by getting into the other half of our brains more often. In our logical, work mode (whether that's at home or away), we are too wrapped up in left-brain activities (right, for lefties). Right-brain activity predominates in calm yogis and meditative folks, allowing them to better cope with stress and stay more relaxed. Go to a spa or retreat to see if acting more right-brained works for you, too.

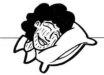

Take 5

If you are curious about developing your right brain, consider attending workshops or retreats that include art, music, or writing activities. The retreat listings in Appendix A offer suggestions.

Use the rhythmic, hypnotic action of waves to give you focus and allow yourself to become introspective. Take a closer look at yourself and see who you are. (Image © H. Armstrong Roberts)

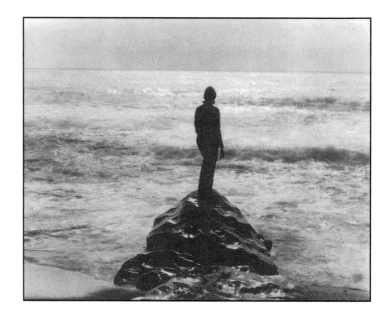

What Goes Around Comes Around

To everything, there is a season and a time for every purpose under heaven. The stars move in predictable paths. The moon exerts its influence on the tides. The seasons flow in a seamless circle. The changes in the amount of daylight affect your moods. Your universe and your body go through cycles. Perhaps being more aware of your cycles will show when you are prone to bad moods and more stress and when you are more relaxed and joyful.

Your genes are unchangeable. You are the gender you are. You are the age and race and nationality you are. But you can be aware of how you think and react. Knowing that, you can control your attitudes and behavior and modify your responses to lessen your anxiety levels.

Type A or Type B?

I laugh at my son when he eats a piece of hard candy. He can't let it dissolve in his mouth; he has to bite it, finish it, and get on to the next one. It describes his way of moving, too. It's called "ants in the pants."

How do you move through life? Do you push, push, push? Do you find it difficult to sit still? Researchers love to study people, and they do it from all different angles. They've grouped us according to body type, bodily fluids (called humors), behavior, and the well-known Type A and Type B. I'm not talking about blood type here, but personality type. Cardiologists Meyer Friedman and Ray Roseman developed the labels *Type A personality* and *Type B personality*.

Research has linked the Type A behavior pattern with heart disease and stroke. Think of it this way: If you regularly react strongly to almost any stimulus, or perceived stimulus, regardless of how minor it might be, then your body constantly goes into the fight-or-flight response, which raises your adrenaline and triggers other stress factors. Keeping your body at this level, without rest, eventually tires it out, wears it out, and collapses it. In the end, you lose. (Hopefully, it's only a temporary loss, and you're able to get up and try again.)

On the other hand, the Type B person constantly has a bet with the world to see whether someone or something can get an angry or violent response from him. Put your money on Type B. He usually wins.

What type are you? How, honestly, would you respond in these situations?

➤ Your guest knocks over a bottle of expensive red wine that works its way across your beautifully decorated table and onto the floor.

➤ Your boss (or a co-worker) takes credit for your idea or work product.

➤ Your child breaks a china heirloom.

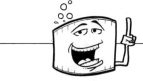

Jacuzzi Jive

A person with a strong **Type A personality** experiences high levels of stress. He's hard-driving, competitive, verbally aggressive, easily angered, time-conscious, and unable to relax. He needs to be in control and hates delay. In contrast, a strong **Type B personality** is easy-going, relaxed, and restrained.

You are probably Type A if your first, strong reaction is one of yelling, fuming, getting angry and upset, calling people names (even if it's only in your head), or otherwise going berserk; or if you can't let go of the situation, and you keep turning it over in your head during the day and at night when you're trying to sleep.

If, however, you generally remain calm, find the good in the situation (at least it wasn't my grandmother's handmade tablecloth), or see the important values (friendship over wine; integrity over dishonesty; forgiveness over shame), then you're more likely a Type B.

An In-y or an Out-y?

No, this question doesn't refer to bellybuttons. Rather, are you an introvert or an extrovert? Carl Jung developed this method of personality typing.

Introverts react to stress by withdrawing into themselves, like a turtle retreating into its shell. These personality types keep their anger, sadness, and distress to themselves, where it can build up and finally explode like a volcano. (I'll show you how to get rid of some of your pent-up emotions by creating distressed furniture, a hot trend these days, in a later chapter.)

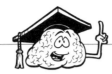

Mindful Moment

Carl Jung (1875–1961) was a Swiss-born psychologist who initially studied with Freud. Later, he developed his own theories apart from Freud. Jung believed that human behavior was not random, but predictable, and was a result of preferences about people, tasks, and events.

Extroverts are at the other extreme. They may escape from their troubles by getting lost in other endeavors or with other people. (Remember Rip van Winkle from Chapter 1?) They may "fly off the handle" or "blow up" as their first, rather than delayed, reaction to stress.

Which type are you? Do you

➤ Dance or watch people dance?

➤ Climb into a bottle or climb a mountain?

➤ Read a book or live the book?

Introverts watch, ruminate, and suffer in silence. But watch out for extroverts, who let you know what they're thinking and feeling. Fortunately, spas and retreats don't care which you are; everyone's welcome.

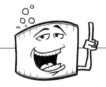

Jacuzzi Jive

The **Myers-Briggs Type Indicator** (**MBTI**) is a test that is used to establish individual preferences in daily behavior. The MBTI is one of the most widely used psychological tests today.

Four-Part Typing

Another means of describing people is by using the *Myers-Briggs* personality test. The Myers-Briggs test uses a series of multiple-choice questions to identify which one of their 16 personality type combinations best describes you. One of the four pairs of indicators is extroverted (E) or introverted (I). The other three pairs are sensing/intuitive, thinking/feeling, and judging/perceiving.

Remember as you go through these pairings, they are not absolute. Just as you may *prefer* to squeeze the toothpaste from the bottom, you may on occasion do so from the top. So, too, you may resemble one category sometimes and a different one another time. But there is usually one category that best describes you most often.

1. Extrovert (E) or Introvert (I)

This first pairing concerns how you observe and make decisions about your surroundings. An Extrovert

➤ Uses words; talks.

➤ Is energized by people and action.

➤ Likes things lively.

In contrast, an Introvert

➤ Keeps things inside.

➤ Prefers quiet and solitude.

➤ Thinks and listens rather than talks.

Do you act more like an Extrovert or an Introvert?

2. Sensor (S) or Intuitive (N)

The Sensor (S) versus Intuitive (N) assessment looks at how a person prefers to collect information. Someone who is an S type is more

➤ Realistic and practical.

➤ Interested in hands-on experience.

➤ Focused on facts and details.

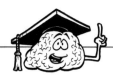

Mindful Moment

Does your body chemistry dictate your personality? Or does your personality dictate your body chemistry? A study by psychiatrist Michael McGuire, noted in *It's All in Your Head* (Prentice Hall, 1994), found that Type A leaders had higher levels of the hormone serotonin in their blood. When removed and isolated, however, the levels halved. When the leaders rejoined the group, they again became leaders, and their serotonin level rose to normal. When given to passive monkeys, serotonin changed timid, insecure males into strutting, authoritative animals. McGuire concluded that our bodies and minds interact to determine what we are and how we feel, and that changes as our surroundings change.

In contrast, an N type uses his intuition with the data he has collected. An N type

➤ Accepts approximations; doesn't require exactitude.

➤ Looks for possibilities, meanings, and relationships.

➤ Looks at an overall framework or grand scheme of things.

Do you behave more like a Sensor or an Intuitive?

3. Thinker (T) or Feeler (F)

Once you have gathered information, you often use it in some way to make decisions or take action. This pair looks at how we make judgments and specific decisions. A Thinker

➤ Is logical and analytical.

➤ Seeks justice and clarity.

➤ Tries not to get personally involved.

The opposite of a Thinker is a Feeler, who

➤ Uses subjective values like harmony and circumstances.

➤ Looks at the impact of any decision.

➤ Identifies with people's emotional states.

How do you prefer to make decisions? Are you a Thinker or a Feeler?

4. Judger (J) or Perceiver (P)

The fourth and final pair of personality types describes how you function in the world. If you prefer making decisions, you are a Judger. But if you prefer gathering information, you're a Perceiver.

A Judger prefers an environment that

➤ Is structured, organized, planned.

➤ Lets her make decisions.

➤ Lets her judge things independent of new information.

A Perceiver prefers

➤ Flexibility and spontaneity.

➤ To wait and see what happens with most issues.

➤ To keep collecting more information.

Do you sound more like a Judger or a Perceiver?

When you put all four categories together, you have your four-letter personality type, according to Myers-Briggs. (What am I, you ask? An ESTJ, but only weakly in some pairings.)

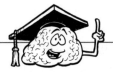

Mindful Moment

The MBTI is named for two women, Katharine Briggs and her daughter Isabel Briggs Myers. Katharine Briggs began classifying people's behavior early in this century before Carl Jung's work became known. After English translations of Jung's studies appeared, she supported and, with her daughter, further developed these ideas. As World War II began, Briggs realized that many people were holding jobs for which they were not suited. The two women developed the MBTI to help employers recognize the differences between workers and find ways to promote harmonious relationships to the benefit of both employee and employer.

Which Sign Are You?

Astrologers believe the stars tell us about ourselves. As *The Complete Idiot's Guide to Astrology* (Alpha Books, 1997) and many other such books point out, the heavens don't make us behave in certain ways, but they do describe who we are. The various signs indicate personality traits and needs, physical characteristics, and how we use our personal energy in relationships.

Many people believe in astrology. No, I don't plan my life by a daily horoscope and only on rare occasions do I even read it. But I do accept that persons born under a particular sign share character traits. I remember Nancy Reagan's turning to astrology to plan President Reagan's schedule after the failed assassination attempt. Then there was the late J. Pierpont Morgan, a billionaire, who used astrology to plan his business investments.

Yes, there are unbelievers, but consider this: I'm a scientific type myself, yet I also recall a statement Carl Jung made that rings true for me: "We are born at a given moment, in a given place, and like

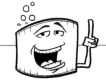

Jacuzzi Jive

Consider comes from *con*, or "with," and *sider*, from the word *sidereal*, which means "to look to the stars." So when you *consider* anything, you may be making your decision based on the stars without even realizing it!

vintage years of wine, we have the qualities of the year and of the season in which we were born."

Whether you believe or not, here in one word is a description of each sign:

➤ Capricorn (December 22–January 19): achiever

➤ Aquarius (January 20–February 18): innovative

➤ Pisces (February 19–March 20): compassionate

➤ Aries (March 21–April 19): pioneer

➤ Taurus (April 20–May 20): dependable

➤ Gemini (May 21–June 21): quick-thinker

➤ Cancer (June 22–July 22): nurturer

➤ Leo (July 23–August 22): big-hearted

➤ Virgo (August 23–September 22): servant

➤ Libra (September 23–October 23): harmonious

➤ Scorpio (October 24–November 21): powerful

➤ Sagittarius (November 22–December 21): explorer

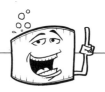

Jacuzzi Jive

In *The Enneagram: A Journey of Self Discovery*, by Maria Beesing, O.P.; Robert Nogosek, C.S.C.; and Patrick O'Leary, S.J. (Dimension Books, 1984), **compulsion** is explained as a basic driving force in one's personality. The compulsion is hidden or unknown to the individual and causes them to be blind to the real motives for their actions.

What's Your Compulsion?

The Enneagram is another method of determining personality type. In this method, each type is identified in a negative way by naming a person's particular *compulsion*. The compulsion is the strong need to avoid some feeling, behavior, or situation. Each personality type has its own specific avoidance. Knowledge of the avoidance explains why that personality type reacts as it does to people and situations.

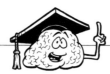

Mindful Moment

The Enneagram (from the Greek word *enneas* for "nine") outlines nine personality distortions and is thought to have originated about 2,000 years ago. Until the present century, it was an oral tradition known only to Sufi masters. Through a series of encounters, the Enneagram became known, was taught, and put into written form. Enneagram workshops address three stages of self-discovery: discovering one's compulsion, understanding its causes, and overcoming the compulsion.

The Enneagram method assigns a number to each personality type. The following table matches each type with its corresponding compulsion.

The Enneagram Types and Their Compulsions

If You Are Type	Then You Try to Avoid
1	Anger
2	Need
3	Failure
4	Ordinariness
5	Emptiness
6	Deviance
7	Pain
8	Weakness
9	Conflict

When you identify your type, use it to consider your reactions in different situations. If you are type nine, for example, you may avoid confrontation and give in despite your better judgment to avoid conflict. Your actions, or lack of action, will be directed toward avoiding conflict. Enneagram workshops or retreats are available for further study. Check the retreat listings in Appendix A, as well as notices of workshops in your area.

Becoming aware of your natural reaction is the first step in changing. Time away at a retreat or spa can offer an opportunity to see who you are, accept who you are, and grow. If you're too hot-tempered, try the old "count to 10" or take a walk approach. If you keep everything inside and stew over it, try journaling (writing your thoughts and feelings in a journal or notebook). It's a non-threatening way to release some of the stressful emotions you're feeling. Flip through this book, and you'll find even more suggestions. Your personality doesn't have to get you in trouble. You can work with it to adjust your responses to potentially stressful situations.

What's Your Answer?

If this is just another book you'll skim through and then put aside, go ahead and skip this section. But if you are serious about self-healing and motivated to get your life under control, then you must answer this question: What is important to you? Retreats are a great time away to contemplate an answer.

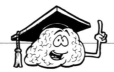

Mindful Moment

Remember what question Alice asked the Cheshire cat in *Alice in Wonderland?* She asked, "Which road shall I take, Mr. Cheshire Cat?" "Where are you going, Alice?" he asked. "I don't know," she said. "Then it doesn't make any difference," he replied.

What is most important to you? Note that I didn't ask what's important to your family, your partner, your children, your neighbors, your co-workers, or your friends. What is important to *you,* now, at this time in your life? Realize that your priorities change, and that's natural, because your abilities, goals, and values change. You need to look at what you want to do and at what you spend your time doing. The following sections describe several approaches you can take to help you find your answer.

Funeral Test

A minister once asked, "If people were filing by your grave today, what would you want to hear them saying about you?" What adjectives would you want them using to describe how you lived your life? The kind of person you were? How you acted? What accomplishments would you want them to remember? Taken together, it describes how you see your purpose in life, your reason for being.

Take 5

Use your time effectively by working with your ultradian cycles. During the first 75 minutes of these 90-minute cycles that wash through our minds, we feel energized, in tune with the universe, and seem more able to cope with problems effortlessly, according to Dr. Ernest Rossi, psychobiology researcher. Then, for the next 15 to 20 minutes, the body sends our minds into a low, to repair stress and strain and recharge our energy for renewed work.

Not-Long-to-Live Test

If you knew you would have only three or six months to live, how would you spend the time? What would you *not* do? How do you decide? Look at what you *like* to do and what you *have* to do. Forget about what you don't like and don't have to do. If you have answers for this test, then you may decide to live your life this way, only doing what you have to do and like to do.

A friend told me that his goal, his "have to do," is to make enough telephone calls each day to book two sales appointments. When he has his two, he does what he likes for the rest of the day. That may not be your answer, but it's one approach to doing what you have to do and then using the rest of your time to do what you want to do.

Time Test

Write down how you spend your time each day. Do this for at least one week. Notice how your activities match up with your answers to the other questions here. (Look for more on this test in Chapter 4, "Time Won't Let Me.")

Money Test

How do you spend your money? It may be very different from what you think. Take out your budget, your checkbook, your credit card statements, and your savings account statement. List your recurring monthly expenses. List the extras. Do you use some of your money in pursuit of what you value most?

Legacy Test

What do you want to accomplish? What are you most proud of? What do you want to be able to leave behind? If you have children, the question becomes what do you want to teach them about values, work, service to others, and their place in their community?

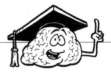

Mindful Moment

Don't let this verse be true of you: "The song that I came to sing remains unsung to this day. I have spent my days in stringing and unstringing my instrument."
—"Gitanjali" by Rabindranath Tagore (1861–1941) in *A Tagore Reader* (Macmillan, 1913)

"I Wish" Test

How often, and in what circumstances, have you thought, "I wish I had done such and such," or "I wish I hadn't done that"? How would you need to live your life so you won't say, "I wish," in the future? Begin to say, "I will," instead. Turn the things you wish to do into things you've done or have made definite plans to do.

You may want to try more than one of these tests or create others. The objective is the same: Take a serious look at your values and goals and then re-align your daily activities and attitudes to reflect them.

So, Who Are You?

Even without that owner's manual, you might now have a pretty good idea of who you are. By working your way through this chapter and taking my little tests, you should have a basic picture of yourself. So far, you've thought more about

➤ Your gene pool.

➤ Your personality type.

➤ Your value system.

I'd say that's progress—and you're only up to Chapter 3! But remember, your picture keeps changing. Chin up, I'm sure your warranty hasn't expired yet.

The Least You Need to Know

➤ Some aspects of yourself are unchangeable, such as your genes, your gender, and your age.

➤ Taking one of any number of the personality tests available will give you a better handle on who you are.

➤ The reflective part of self-discovery is deciding what's important to you: your values and goals.

➤ Taken all together, you now have a foundation for looking at your lifestyle and deciding whether changes are appropriate. Going away on retreat or even to a spa helps in the decision-making process.

➤ If you decide to make changes, you'll need courage and determination to jump in. But jump you must; you'll never know the temperature of the water until you do.

Part 2

Finding the Time You Need

You have appointments listed on your home calendar, your date book, and your office calendar. If you don't have enough to do, there's always today's mail and yesterday's phone messages to respond to. You have more lists than you'd like. Some days (only some? aren't you lucky!) are a blur from one scheduled crisis to the next.

Enough already. It's time for you to slow down, look at all your running, and decide whether you need to do everything. I'll help you find some time for yourself at home (wouldn't that be a welcome change?). I also have some suggestions to keep your work life from spinning out of control.

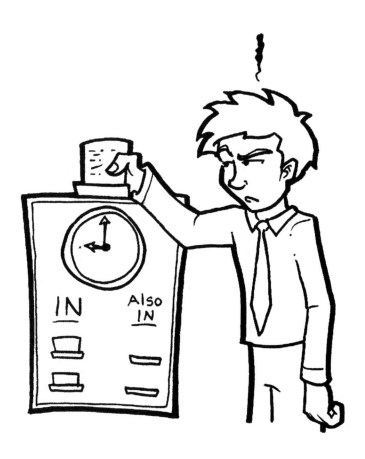

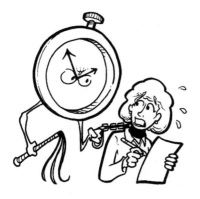

Chapter 4

Time Won't Let Me

In This Chapter

➤ Learning how to beat the clock

➤ Finding 25-hour days

➤ Understanding that every minute counts

➤ Believing that you deserve a break

You've gone through Part 1, "Give Me a Break, Please!" and you're convinced. You agree that you need a break for your physical and mental (and I would add spiritual) health. But you have a problem: You just don't have the time. Hang on to your second hand, we're going to find some extra time. In this chapter, I'll show you how to beat the clock at home. In Chapter 5, "Dealing with Your Job," you can read about stress, time tricks, and relaxation at the office.

Do you remember the game show *Beat the Clock?* (I'm dating myself here.) Contestants rushed to accomplish a variety of tasks before their time was up. The idea has been repeated in other shows, including the children's show *Where in the World Is Carmen Sandiego?* where a contestant runs around on a floor map of the world, placing identification markers in their proper places before the buzzer sounds. Such games are fun, but nobody should live their lives that way. If you have children, don't forget they need down time, too. So let's see if you can find some time for all of you.

Beat the Clock: Then and Now

I have this wonderful image of taking a heavy bat or other blunt object and, after having placed a beautiful clock ceremoniously on the floor, using the bat to smash that timepiece to smithereens. Unfortunately, getting time to stand still isn't that simple.

There are better ways to "beat" the clock. Here are just a few:

➤ Hiding clocks and pretending not to know the time

➤ Designating each room as a different time zone

➤ Running faster than your watch's or clock's second hand can turn

➤ Using a universal time watch and forgetting where in the world you are

➤ Cloning yourself

If you've had a laugh, great, but I know you're thinking, "Get real. Even if I don't know the time, everyone else will, and I'll be left behind in the dust." That's your serious, tense side coming through now. Dust yourself off, pick yourself up, and let's try again.

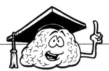

Mindful Moment

With so many people around the world using the World Wide Web, someone thought there might be interest in a universal time clock. People at the Swatch Group, the world's largest watch maker, developed something they call "Internet time." Their plan divides the day into 1,000 "swatch beats" equivalent to 1 minute and 26.4 seconds each. The time's meridian, or zero line, is Biel, Switzerland, where the company is located. Frankly, I'm not interested in knowing what time it is in cyberspace. I'll use my trusty, 12-hour watch or look out my window to know if I should be awake or asleep in my corner of the universe.

Three o'clock P.M. on a standard clock is @625 in universal time.

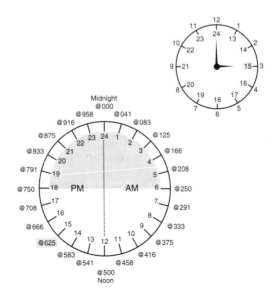

Time Management in a Minute

Library and bookstore shelves are full of time-management books. (I just discovered *The Complete Idiot's Guide to Managing Your Time* [Alpha Books, 1999].) In case you haven't had time to check out or buy any of these books or have yet to read the ones you have checked out or bought, the following sections outline some basic time-management principles to help you out.

Log Your Time

What do you do all day, anyhow? The boss wants to know, and your spouse wants to know. I even had one of my children ask me this question now that I work mostly from home. Do you know the answer?

One way to know is to keep a log. Whether it's losing weight, attacking bad habits, or examining priorities, you cannot make changes until you know what it is you are currently doing. In other words, you have to establish a baseline. People wanting to lose weight are advised to keep a list of what they eat during the day. If you want to change the use of your time, you first need to know how you spend your day.

Take 5

Therapists suggest taking an object, such as a tennis racket, and using it to strike a pillow or your bed as a way to relieve tension or anger. Allow your feelings to surface. Yell, scream, or cry as you need. But do it while you're alone—no one needs to see you so emotional, especially children.

Include All You Do

Be specific about what you record. Include waiting time, interruptions, whether phone calls were for pleasure or business, and who called whom. Record what you did, who helped, who benefited from your work, and what breaks you took. Everything. Your memory can't hold all this info. You need to write as you go.

Keep your log for one week. Make a form on paper or in a notebook and carry it with you as you go about your day. Use the sample daily time log shown on the following page, if you wish. If you forget your log, begin from where you are. Note what you are doing, how long it takes, how you are feeling, and how energetic you are while completing that activity.

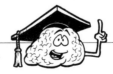

Mindful Moment

Time as we know it began on my birthday (well, not in the same year). The date was November 10, 1883. A schoolteacher and railroad engineer persisted until the United States adopted four time zones so trains could be scheduled. Before then, each community could adopt its own time. The 24 worldwide time zones we use today were created a year later.

Time Log

Tasks	Time		Emotional State	Energy Level	Priority
	Start	End			

Review Your Tasks

After the week is over, although you'll no doubt see patterns before then, take time to review the log. Go back and review one day at a time. Don't jump back and forth between days. That's the scattered approach. Stay with one day at a time and concentrate on it alone.

Look at each activity listed on your sheet. Rate each activity: Is it a high-, medium-, or low-priority item? A high-priority item is one that absolutely must be done that day. A medium-priority item needs to be done, but perhaps not right away. A low-priority task is something routine, something that doesn't need to be done, or something that doesn't need to be done by you.

Next, total up the time spent on each kind of activity. How many minutes each day do you spend in high-priority tasks? In low-priority tasks? No matter what you may say about how important your work is, a close look at your actions may reveal a very different, even disturbing, picture.

How Are You Feeling?

Knowing how you feel when you engage in each activity is also important. Look at the words or phrases you used. Were you half asleep, bored, tense, enthusiastic, worried? Which words or phrases show up most often under Emotional State? The answer tells you how happy you are with your work. If you're not very pleased with it, you can begin to understand why you feel so crummy during the day.

Your Energy Level column helps you understand your natural rhythms and how in sync you are with them. Some people are night people; some are morning people. Some seem to have an inexhaustible supply of energy all the time. Others are either in bed or look like they should be.

When is your energy level at its peak? Review your log to see. Next, look at when you work at your high-priority tasks. If you are not working on those important projects when your energy is at its highest, you're probably not able to give the tasks your best effort, and it's probably taking longer to finish them. That's time wasted.

Keeping a log is a tedious process, but the results are invaluable. Remember, the log is only for you. No one else will see it. Include everything. Don't second-guess yourself and leave out items you think are silly or unimportant. Be absolutely honest. It may seem like drudgery now, but such a log, once you review it, will provide you with a wealth of information to begin your program of taking back control of your time and of your life.

Why Do *I* Have to Do It?

You now have a better idea of how you spend your time. You also know whether you are spending time on high- or low-priority tasks. Even if the item is high-priority, the next question is: Are you the best person to complete this activity, or could someone else handle it?

Keep This, Toss That

Look at each activity on your log. Note as well those activities that, although they don't reappear on your log, you know to be regular, repeating tasks. Recall the household chores, the volunteer activities, the memos. Must they all be done by you? If you possess a particular skill or talent specifically needed, then you are certainly the person for that job. But what about other tasks? Could a co-worker or child or even hired help complete it just as well? If so, delegate!

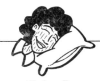

Take 5

Have a family gathering to review and list household jobs and identify which ones others could do. Talk about consequences when tasks are not completed. Make copies of the list. Have someone, not necessarily a parent, assign a person to each job for the week, and rotate this job. Post the task list. Consider offering small rewards for cooperative behavior. A new routine needs time to become a habit. Stick to it.

I recall a time when I was so angry at all the stuff I was doing at home that I called a family meeting. I put sheets of paper on the walls (can you tell I have a history of running workshops?) and asked the family members to begin naming all the large and small tasks of running a home. You may take this approach at the office as well. Perhaps you need to review how your product is manufactured, or the addition or subtraction of employees necessitates a reevaluation of job roles. Involving everyone offers a more complete picture of the operation and promises more helpful suggestions to restructure your organization. Reward yourself (or your employees) with time out at a spa.

The lists are the equivalent of your daily activity log. The exercise opens eyes and perhaps creates a new appreciation among all the staff or the family to the important roles each member has. It may also indicate tasks which might be shared or rotated, thereby teaching others a new skill.

New Routines Take Time

Will other people complain when tasks are shifted? Sure. That's one reason some of us don't like to delegate. We don't know how to handle this natural resistance. Most people don't like change; they like what's familiar, what's predictable.

What's important is how you handle the complaints you will most certainly receive. When someone complains that they need to take a written test before they get their driver's permit, do you say okay, forget it? Meet their complaints head on, calmly, matter-of-factly. This needs to be done, and you're the person for the job. If it's a group project, like taking inventory, tell them it's okay to complain to each other (but not to you), if that makes them feel better.

But I Don't Want to Share

You are your own worst enemy if you won't give up a task because you think no one else can do the job exactly like you can, for of course no one can. Nobody else is you.

If you insist that the job be completed in a specified number of steps in a specified order, then you're also insisting that you must be the one, always and only, to complete that job.

Lighten up. (Get thee to a spa or retreat and learn how to lighten up if you've forgotten.) Children won't fold and put away their laundry as neatly as if you do it. If you call clients first and do your paperwork later, ignore the employee who does paperwork as he goes. Despite the order, or lack of it, the task is being completed and you have more time to do what you must do.

Every Minute Counts

If you can find just 60 minutes every week, you have time for a day spa or retreat workshop, lecture, or quiet time every week. That means finding less than 10 minutes a day. When you think in those terms, it's doable.

Chill Out

It takes more time initially to help someone learn a new skill. Explain the task, and be clear about the desired result. Also, don't use I-do-it-this-way statements. Instead, ask in what ways someone might do the job. If the person needs ideas, offer one, which happens to be the way you do it. Bottom line: Don't hover. Praise a completed job.

Here are some suggestions, in no particular order, to get you started. (I'll bet you can find 60 minutes a week even without changing anything you do now.) They will help you and your family get organized, make your day run smoother, and find those few minutes—which are all you need—to put your feet up (pedicure, anyone?):

➤ Lay out clothes and make lunches the night before.

➤ Delegate! Others can help with simple chores like making beds, vacuuming, dusting, taking out the trash, helping with dinner, tidying up rooms, and many other possibilities. (Remember my family's four-page list? What's on yours?)

➤ Have children read together or help each other with homework sometimes, or set up a homework club (a group of families whose children study together and whose parents, on a rotating basis, offer space and help). Rotate supervision responsibility.

Take 5

Line trash containers in bedrooms and bath with recycled plastic bags from the grocery store. The bags' handles enable even young children to grab hold and deposit the bag and trash wherever you want.

➤ Have a place for everything—use containers, boxes, shelves, drawers—so everything can be put in its place and found easily next time.

➤ Hire a cleaning service if you can (even once a month helps); find someone else to do the yard work if you don't enjoy it.

Chill Out

If you intend to trade meals with another person or family, plan the menus together to avoid a let's-see-what-I-can-make-that-is-better-than-what-they-made frame of mind. Remember, this arrangement is intended to reduce stress, not increase it!

➤ Put a list on the refrigerator and add to it as each food item is finished or diminished so that you'll know most of what you need next time you go shopping.

➤ Cook larger quantities of food and freeze or store for future meals, or organize a meal pool: persons or families cook for each other.

➤ Have stairs? Don't always run up and down. Put items that need to go upstairs on the steps. Anyone going up should make sure their hands are full.

➤ Shop alone: You won't have others begging to add unneeded items to the cart. Shop during the less-busy times of the day to avoid long waits at the check-out counter.

➤ Sit down once a week and plan menus; it beats the hassle of last-minute "what's for dinner" ideas, saves money, increases variety, and makes shopping more efficient.

➤ Throw all that paper that comes into your home in the guise of mail in a basket or drawer to find it easily later. Do the same for bills, but separate them out as they arrive. Then when you're ready, handle paper only once, if possible: Use it, file it, or toss it.

➤ Animals? If you can't spend the time to take care of yours, get someone else to help, or think seriously about why you have that pet you don't spend time petting.

➤ Be positive: You positively will find the time!

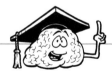

Mindful Moment

Now that you're saving time here and there and everywhere, reward yourself with a breather and recall songs (my preference), movies, or books that refer to sitting or resting or include the word *time* in a title or lyric.

A Day of Rest

Whatever happened to the seventh day? Or to nights and weekends, for that matter? We try to scratch out a few extra minutes here, an hour there. Whatever happened to entire days we were given for rest? Weekends were created to provide rest and recovery time. What a glorious chunk of sweet, unscheduled time a weekend could be. (A weekend is also time you could use at a retreat center or spa.)

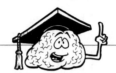

Mindful Moment

A week wasn't always seven days long. In 1792, France experimented with a 10-day week with 10-hour days. In 1929, Russia tried a five-day week, naming the days after colors. (Do you suppose Monday was blue?)

Don't Fill Every Minute

What do we do with our days of rest? Pack them with work, most often, thanks to overtime, telecommuting, home businesses, and the availability of fax, pagers, modems, and online services. Or we use the time to engage in heavy, unpaid work around the house like painting, building, lawn maintenance, and repair. Or we moonlight as unpaid chauffeurs.

We need that day—or preferably days—of rest. We have it for good reason, not because we are out of shape and can't keep going, but to keep us from getting that way. Superperson is a myth. If you pile on enough stress, even the best will crack or erupt. That's what volcanoes and earthquakes are about.

Observe a Sabbath

Even if you cannot put aside an entire weekend, try to find a day, your "seventh day," sometime during the week. Take this day to pause, to think, to be refreshed, and to be nourished so as to bring a constantly renewed sense of commitment and joy—yes, joy!—to your life.

A *Sabbath* day shouldn't be used for errands or going to the mall or to the movies. The Bible tells

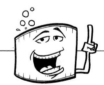

Jacuzzi Jive

The name of the seventh day of the week in the Hebrew calendar, the **Sabbath,** is derived from the root *sbt,* which means "to cease from" or "rest." It evokes the most characteristic trait of the Sabbath, which is the cessation of all activity that fills ordinary, everyday life.

us God rested on the seventh day. Perhaps we, too, need to work at resting. It seems so simple, taking time to rest. Parents make "play dates" for their children to reserve time in their calendars for play with friends. Why not make "rest dates" for yourself? Schedule rest time; put it on the calendar. And you're not allowed to cancel this appointment!

Take 5

Keeping flowers in your house is an easy way to add beauty and bring the refreshing scents of nature into your home year round. Flowers lift your spirit. Small bouquets are available today in almost any grocery store. Next time you shop for food, shop for flowers as well.

What Will I Do on Rest Day?

When we rest, we appreciate life and what it has to offer. We don't miss out on life—just the opposite. Set this time apart by doing something very different from the other hours of the week. It might be spiritual reading or prayer. (More on this in Chapter 8, "The Sounds of Silence.") It might be turning your home into your castle and pampering yourself with fine linens, china and crystal, fresh flowers, good food, and good company. (There's a chapter on this, too: Chapter 12, "Restful Repasts.")

Time Out

Stop your usual rush. Do the following:

➤ Turn off the telephone. (Okay, so have your answering machine take calls if you must.)

➤ Hide the car keys.

➤ Stop channel surfing just because you're bored.

➤ Don't spend any money.

➤ Avoid the technology.

In my home, my family enjoys activities other than TV, videos, and computer games on our "seventh day." It's a time to enjoy each other and others. Isn't there someone better than a machine to keep you company? Try one of the following activities:

➤ Invite people over.

➤ Play games.

➤ Visit someone.

➤ Telephone someone you haven't heard from in a while.

➤ Whip up a new recipe. Don't cook? Try.

➤ Rediscover the lost art of letter writing.

➤ Read something just for fun.

➤ Lie around and listen to some good music.

➤ Watch some old Marx Brothers movies. Laughter is life-giving.

➤ Soak, sigh, sleep.

➤ Find free and freeing ways to enjoy nature, beauty, and spirit.

This change of pace will work wonders. (That's the idea of spas and retreats, folks.) You will handle disturbances better during the week knowing that this sacred time awaits you. The days afterward are calm and serene, as you carry with you a changed attitude and outlook. As you continue to honor this special time of rest, you create a cycle of reflection and renewal that brings some peace, joy, and hope to your life. Go for it. You deserve it. You need it.

The Least You Need to Know

➤ You can beat the clock and find more time in your day by using principles of time management.

➤ Enlist the help of others; you're not in this alone.

➤ Rest is necessary for reflection and renewal; make a "rest date" with yourself every week.

➤ Experience the peace, joy, and hope that comes from observing regular, special times of rest, at home or away at a spa or retreat.

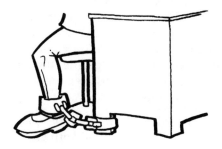

Chapter 5

Dealing with Your Job

In This Chapter

➤ Beating stress on the job

➤ Putting work in perspective

➤ Finding the time you need

➤ Understanding how to relax

Everyone has a job, in the broader sense of the term. Children's jobs are to learn the best they can. Parents' jobs are both to be good teachers to their children and to realize their children's own unique talents. Everyone engaged in trading services and skills for financial gain or quiet recognition has a series of tasks or duties that they complete, hopefully to the best of their ability.

Much of our stress is job-related. A recent study found that people are working, on average, 158 hours more each year than people worked 20 years ago. (So explain to me how technology is saving us time?) For good or ill, your job, whatever it is, takes a big chunk of your time. In this chapter, you'll read about ways to reduce your stress and feel better about your job, despite it all. I'll also let you in on some quick relaxation tips that will help keep you focused and able to do your best at whatever work you do. (If and when you're ready to make changes in your life or work, turn to Chapter 6, "On the Road to Happiness.")

Attitude Is All

Your attitude about your job, and not the job itself, is what matters. Every job is needed. Every job is important, whether it's a homemaker or pilot, artist or delivery man, auto mechanic or accountant.

Jobs and Joy

Your attitude also determines whether your job embarrasses or elevates you. Although the opinions of others are sometimes hard to ignore, they ought to be of no importance. If you want to save the rainforest and your parents or spouse think you ought be logging the forest instead, you need to take time, perhaps even on a retreat, to examine what is important to you.

Whatever you do in your daily life, whether for financial reward or not, you can choose to do it with great purpose, gratitude, and joy. For example, St. Theresa, a Catholic contemplative nun, had her "Little Way." She paid attention to the little things she did every day to see the beauty and spirituality, in every piece of her life. You could do that as well.

Take 5

Like ripples moving out into the rest of the pond, one person's cheerful, positive disposition will be noticed, and in time perhaps even emulated, by others working with that person. Be a ripple and spread joy among those who can't find theirs.

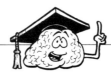

Mindful Moment

The "Little Way" of St. Theresa refers to the attitude with which she approached everything in her daily life. She believed that each task, no matter how small or seemingly insignificant, was a part of and contributed to the harmony of the universe. As such, and to honor the one who created the universe, each task ought be done with love and total concentration and with the sense that at this moment, this task is the most important thing that needs to be done.

No Labels, Please

Work is a big part of our identity. Some people don't have any identity outside of work; that's why work is so stressful. We desperately need to succeed, continuously. We must never fail. If we fail even once, we feel humiliated and inadequate.

We use work to label others. What assumptions do you make when someone says he's a gastrointestinal doctor? A plumber? They both fix plumbing if you think about it. I once had a neighbor who, after her husband told her I had worked as a lawyer and lobbyist, felt compelled to tell me she had thought I stayed home with my children because I didn't have anything going for me. I suppose that was some kind of an apology.

Be Challenged, Not Crazed

The next time you're confronted with people or situations at work that drive you crazy, try to approach them differently. See every situation as an opportunity to do the following:

➤ Learn a new skill

➤ Manage your time better

➤ Deal with and understand other personality types

➤ Showcase your talents

➤ Review your value system

➤ Learn about yourself, your needs, and your goals

In this way, change is normal and an opportunity, rather than a threat to your status or job security.

When you view stressful situations as challenges you look at them in a different way and can project a sense of

➤ Adventure.

➤ Interest.

➤ Curiosity.

➤ Flexibility.

➤ Energy.

➤ Joyful anticipation.

Your spirit is brighter, twists and turns are exciting rather than excruciating, and your efforts are rewarded with eustress, or positive stress (see Chapter 2, "Simon Says Sit Down"), rather than distress. All it takes is a different frame of mind.

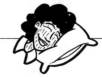

Take 5

I have a rule when I meet new people. I don't ask what they do for a living, and I avoid answering that question when asked. Instead, I use books, movies, music, or adventures as conversation starters. It's my way of saying, "You are more than what you do."

Take 5

Gandhi said, "What you do may seem insignificant, but it's very important that you do it." Thomas Jefferson said, "It is neither wealth nor splendor, but tranquility and occupation, which give happiness."

Whom Do You Serve?

Regardless of whether you are in a recognized helping profession, you serve others in your work. How would you prefer offering and receiving that service? Would you want service with a smile or with a grunt? It's back to attitude again.

When you help others, you also help yourself. Remember that helper's high I mentioned in Chapter 1, "Are You Going Crazy?" You don't need scientific studies to tell you how good you feel after a job well done. You feel bright, confident, and perhaps exhausted, but wonderfully so. You are experiencing what spiritual teachers have long taught: You receive when you give.

Check Your Attitudes

Try some of these activities to take a closer look at, and make the best of, your situation:

1. Make a list of all the reasons your job is important to you and to others.

2. List what you like about the people you work with.

3. Make a list of what you like about everything else related to your work.

4. List the skills and lessons that you could take with you to another workplace.

5. Try for one day to follow St. Theresa's "Little Way."

6. Hold on to your answers, and in times of doubt or distress, read all the positive aspects of your job that you listed.

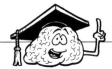

Mindful Moment

Regardless of whether you consider yourself spiritual, Ignatius of Loyola's life offers two lessons for workers. First, he founded the Order of the Society of Jesus, commonly called the Jesuits, at the age of 50. You, too, can begin a new career at a later age and flourish. He also taught and practiced what he called **detachment,** which in simple terms means exerting your best efforts to the task at hand and then moving to the next task. Once you have done your best, there is nothing more to do. You leave the completed task without investing your personal integrity or worth in the eventual outcome.

People Problems

A new, more positive attitude helps wherever your employment takes you. You might be among those who decide to work at a home-based business, or you might find yourself moving to a new state for employment reasons. You may need to adapt to a new organizational structure after a corporate merger. New work situations bring new co-workers. Although you cannot change them, you can treat them with respect and protect yourself from undue stress. They may take getting used to, but the more open-minded you are, probably the easier the transition for you and the lower your stress level.

Provoking Personnel

You can't always get along with everyone, even when you try. Everyone has his own problems and bad days, and on occasion you may have to deal with bosses or co-workers who think their purpose in life is to sharpen everyone's nose on the grind-stone. They don't seem to respect your talents or responsibilities. They may prefer hierarchy to collegiality.

If you have difficulties with people who don't respond to any way of getting along, you might follow this suggestion from Dr. Robert Eliot. In his book, *Is it Worth Dying For?* (Bantam, 1984), he advises that you pretend the person has a brain tumor and is not responsible for his behavior. I think the idea can be phrased in a more generous way, but you get the picture. Maybe the person's compulsion (remember this from the Enneagram in Chapter 3, "Let's Get Personal"?) is driving him or her. Perhaps the person's Myers-Briggs type (also in Chapter 3) is the complete opposite of yours. Keep in mind that it's not your place to figure them out or to twist yourself into knots trying to remake yourself to their liking.

You do need to protect yourself from unnecessary stress, however, and you do need to do your best work. Remember

> ➤ Relaxation exercises.
> ➤ Your talents.
> ➤ To avoid, change, or deal with stressful situations.

Do you feel secure in your talents? Do you know what an asset you are to your employer? Do you realize what an asset you could be to another employer? If the answer is no, then you might want to take some time out to think about the answers to these questions. Going on a retreat or to a wellness center will help give you the physical and mental space you need to think about them.

If you are confident about your talents, then you don't need to be consumed with pleasing your boss at the expense of your physical and emotional limits. You can rest in doing your best and then move on to the next task. You can take comfort in your competence in other areas of your life—family and friends, hobbies, volunteer activities—and bring that to your workplace.

Managers and Managing

Being "just an employee" has stresses associated with it, like having little or no control over the required tasks, perhaps putting up with the routine nature of the job, and feeling less than important, as in "only a worker." If there comes a time to decide whether to attempt or accept a managerial position, the decision-making process itself is stressful. Perhaps you'll decide to go on retreat or visit a spa for a few days to relax and sort things out.

If you move to a management position, you have new challenges. You may have more control, but you also have more responsibility for making correct decisions. You may have more variety in your job, but this variety also includes more personalities to deal with, including a new tier of bosses (after you finally figured out how your former boss operated!) and maybe even clients. You also may have more visibility, as in the proverbial fishbowl, with everyone second-guessing you.

If your product depends on creativity, you might also have to anticipate fads and trends, be original but not too original, and grow and change, but remain identifiable to consumers or clients. A changing market or one unsuccessful decision may result in a substantial economic loss, including your own position.

Chill Out

High job insecurity is always a condition for high stress. In one study, Melvin Glasser noted that worrying about their employment termination led to a 700 percent increase in heart attacks and stress illnesses among ground controllers for the Apollo space project toward the end of that project in 1969.

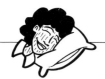

Take 5

Get your office to bring in someone to do 10-minute upper back and neck massages. Some companies do this on a regular basis. These massages sure help get out the kinks from all those hours bent over desk or computer!

Delegating Involves Others

If you are in a position to delegate work, you have a marvelous opportunity to help other workers hone or expand their skills. Be sure you

➤ Explain the task.

➤ Offer aid if requested.

➤ Review to see whether your needs were understood.

➤ Refrain from dictating the exact steps of the process, unless it must be done in one way only.

You can avoid anxiety for yourself and your co-workers if you are clear about your expectations and courteous.

Some folks are afraid to delegate because they don't want a boss to think they're unnecessary because other people are doing the tasks. If you have this fear, feel better. Remind yourself you

➤ Are overqualified for the tasks you're delegating.

➤ Have your other tasks to do well.

➤ Are acting as a competent executive.

➤ Recognize the talent and strengths of others.

➤ Can use the time saved for creative endeavors, breaks, or planning.

Both employees and their organizations benefit from good delegation and management.

My Office Is Killing Me!

If you don't have people stresses at work, you might have stressors caused by the space itself. I remember living next to the furnace in a dark basement whose only window opened on a parking lot. It was hard to be happy in such a dreary, stressful, carbon monoxide-filled space!

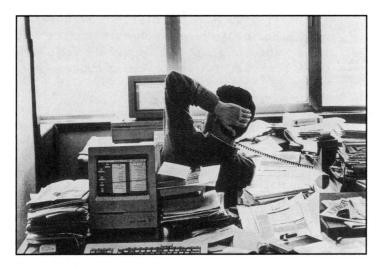

The ubiquitous computer helps as well as hurts us. Just look at the ways in which we contort our bodies in the office. No wonder we have aches and pains in addition to our stress and worry. (Image © Stock Imagery NY)

Workplace Worries

Where you work can hurt you. Does your space suffer from poor lighting, foul odor, excessive noise, constant computer use, or asbestos and fiber dust?

Dress, and Other Styles

Your workplace includes a psychological environment. Each company's psychological environment is different. Dress-down days have become commonplace, but does the casual tone carry over into employee-manager relations? Would you feel free to approach your boss with an opinion that is contrary to hers? Some executives encourage this kind of exchange; others do not. You know where your supervisor fits.

What is your work environment like? Do you have one or more persons who don't manage well, court the approval of the higher-ups at the expense of the lower-downs, compete rather than cooperate, or promote personal gain at the expense of company goals? Perhaps your organization is in limbo as it sorts out mergers and sales. That environment increases stress and job dissatisfaction and may

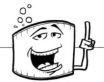

Jacuzzi Jive

Ions are small, charged (either positive or negative) particles found in the air that are produced by radioactivity, cosmic rays, the movement of hot, dry winds, and waterfalls.

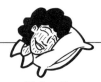

Take 5

Debra Dadd, in her book *Home Safe Home,* offers these recommendations for making your computer use safer: Block electrical fields with a grounded screen. Unplug unused computers to eliminate magnetic fields. Consider using a negative-ion generator to balance the buildup of positive ions. Finally, take regular breaks to prevent eye and muscle strain.

Chill Out

Dr. Eliot's *Is It Worth Dying For?* notes a North Carolina Industry Commission study of 2,000 textile workers over a two-year period. The study found that 75 percent of on-the-job accidents involved workers who had not eaten breakfast.

lead to your doing less than your best as you struggle with how to cope. If you can't deal with your workplace environment, consider a break at a spa or retreat to help you sort out your thoughts and plans.

Employee Edibles

You're late for the train, and you have a meeting to make, so like most other mornings, you rush out of the house without breakfast. Food, or lack of it, has a lot to do with your anxiety levels or peace of mind.

Morning Munchies

Your mommy was right: Breakfast is the most important meal of the day. Can't you hear your tummy grumbling for breakfast? Your brain is yelling for an energy boost. After all, it's been a number of hours since you last ate, and your body is hungering for some attention. Lack of food may leave you

➤ Feeling edgy.

➤ With poor coordination.

➤ With low blood sugar levels.

➤ At a greater risk of having an accident.

Rushing to work adds to your already poor start.

If you eat breakfast, are you one of those donut-and-coffee types? Sugar ain't where it's at. It does give you a temporary rush, with the emphasis on *temporary*. But then what? Your body reacts to balance it out. The after-effects of sugar are tiredness and an even lower dip into blah-land. This kind of feeling is not good when you need to be fresh and alert.

What are some better morning alternatives? Try

➤ A whole-grain English muffin or bagel.

➤ Fresh fruit.

➤ Juice.

➤ Yogurt.

➤ Oatmeal or whole-grain cereal.

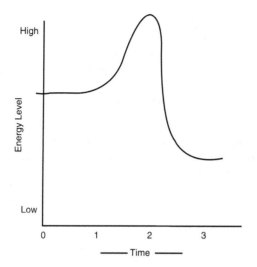

It's unscientific, but you get the idea. See where you started off? Where did you end up after your sugar snack? The high you briefly enjoyed is balanced by the low you don't want.

Working Lunches and Afternoons

You made it through the morning, now you have a long afternoon ahead. Why can it sometimes be so hard making it to five (or six or seven) o'clock?

Your body is in a down cycle from about noon to about 4 P.M. Notice what you're eating or drinking in the afternoon to counter your cycle. Is that the time you reach for caffeine or sugar to rev you up a bit and get you through? Reach instead for

➤ Veggies.

➤ Fruits.

➤ Protein.

➤ Whole grains.

These foods give you energy without the peaks and valleys that stimulants such as caffeine and sugar are notorious for.

If you have a lunch meeting that's more work than enjoyment, you may not get that afternoon off to such a good start. Eating and meeting don't always mix. Meetings may be very stressful. Remember the fight-or-flight response from Chapter 2? The anxiety of a meeting sets up the stress response, and the body reacts accordingly, including causing changes in your digestion.

Take 5

Reaching for that sugar because you're anxious about what you're reading? Don't. Instead, read *Lick the Sugar Habit* (Avery Publishing Group, 1996) by Nancy Appleton. After reading this eye-opening book, I didn't touch a drop of sugar for eight whole days afterward. (More on anxiety-causing or calming foods in Chapter 12, "Restful Repasts.")

Take 5

To be at your best, schedule meetings at the beginning or end of the afternoon slump cycle (12 to 4 P.M.).

Your stomach stops digesting food so that more energy can be moved elsewhere to fight the cause of the stress. As long as the stress reaction is temporary, the body will correct this is normal reaction by digesting food again. But if you continue to meet with stressful people or experience stress in any meeting, watch out. The tension between your body's reactions might just lead to ulcers and other problems.

Of course, if Mylanta is one of your favorite snacks, you already know this. How do you wean yourself off medicines like this? Go to the cause of your distress. Consider these changes:

➤ Cut down or eliminate coffee, a known stomach irritant.

➤ Watch your diet, especially heavy and spicy meals.

➤ Do breathing exercises for relaxation.

➤ Build up a noncompetitive exercise routine, such as walking, biking, or swimming.

You don't have to do this all at once. Taking it step by step will slowly but surely improve your disposition.

When you don't have to use your lunchtime for a meeting, consider having your lunch

➤ Outside: get some air, stretch, and sit in the sun.

➤ With friends.

➤ While listening to Mozart.

Fresh air, companionship, and beauty are healing influences.

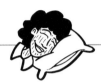

Take 5

Have your meeting, and then eat. Trying to do both at the same time is like trying to mix oil and water: It doesn't work well.

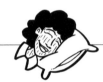

Take 5

Sunlight works on the pineal gland, deep in the skull, to counteract depression. Not enough sunlight upsets pineal secretions, giving rise to too much melatonin, a cause of depression.

More Than Money

A task done well offers you more satisfaction and happiness than money ever could. Don't spoil your bright outlook with tension-filled days. Try these additional suggestions to keep your mood optimistic, hopeful, and productive:

➤ Listen to others.

➤ Learn to work (it out) with others.

➤ Put balance in your life: The harder you work, the harder you should play.

➤ Smile and laugh more.

➤ Find a sounding board: Talk it out.

➤ Enjoy time with friends.

➤ Rest alone for about 15 minutes when you get home.

➤ Take short breaks throughout the day and stretch.

➤ Check your posture: Sit and walk tall.

➤ Walk, eat, talk, and drive more slowly.

➤ Check your face in a mirror to catch signs of stress, tiredness, and irritation.

➤ Remember your values, your goals in life, and your spirituality.

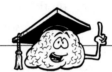

Mindful Moment

One of the trendy new words might just be *resilience*. It means being challenged but not breaking down and finding ways to thrive in the face of life's stresses. An executive quoted in *USA Weekend* magazine (March 5 to 7, 1999) observed that corporate training in resiliency and relationship-building skills helped employees bounce back faster after a major personal disruption such as illness or divorce. The company's productivity is up, and sick leave is down.

Relaxation in a Minute

It takes just one minute to try these relaxation exercises. Instead of taking another walk to the coffee station or water cooler, shut your door and breathe.

1. Sit comfortably in a chair, feet on the floor, hands resting gently on your lap.

2. Close your eyes (doing so makes it easier to cut out distractions). If the phone rings, ignore it—better yet, take it off the hook.

3. Take in a deep breath through your nose, inhaling to a count of four.

4. Let the air escape, just as slowly, through your mouth, emptying your lungs completely.

5. As you inhale, think of a calming word like peace, joy, or serenity.

6. As you exhale, think of one word that describes what you want to get rid of, such as stress, tension, anxiety, or frustration.

7. Rest quietly with an empty mind for about 15 seconds. Slowly open your eyes and come back into your space.

If you inhale and exhale slowly, you can do about five of these breathing cycles per minute. Repeat steps 3 to 6 for each cycle. After this calm minute, you will notice your breathing and heart rate are slower, your energy is more controlled, and your voice is softer and less edgy. Take one more deep breath and open your door to serenity in the midst of a storm.

Visualize Your Way to Vitality

Here is another quick refresher:

1. Sit comfortably in a chair, feet on the floor, hands resting gently on your lap.

2. Think of a place you love to be or a person you love to be with.

3. Imagine a relaxing, beautiful scene. You can be wherever you want: on a beach, on a mountaintop, by a river, lying under a tree, or on your back looking up at the clouds.

4. Put yourself into the scene. Notice what you are doing and the smells, sounds, and sights.

5. Enjoy the moment.

6. When you feel peaceful, slowly bring yourself back into the room. Notice that you're in your chair.

7. Open your eyes. Rise slowly and stretch.

Squeeze out the Stress

You might be tense and not even know it. Here's a fast way to slow down and find out if your muscles need to relax:

1. Sit in a relaxed position.

2. Scrunch up your face. Hold for a count of three. Relax it completely.

3. Bring your shoulders to your ears. Hold. Relax.

4. Make a fist and tighten your right arm. Hold. Relax.

5. Repeat step 4 with your left arm.

6. Tighten your right leg. Hold. Relax.

7. Repeat step 6 with your left leg.

8. Bend over and tighten all 10 toes. Hold. Relax.

Over time, your body will recognize when it is tense, and with just a mental scan of your body, you'll be able to relax.

Dream Breaks

Every organization needs dreamers. They're individuals with vision; they're people who can look ahead and create new product lines, better ways to improve cooperation among departments and to do business, better recognition of individual efforts, and new business strategies. You might be sitting there, looking as though you're doing nothing, but what wisdom might be whirling around inside and unseen.

Dreaming needs unstructured time. Just think about the last time you wanted to remember something but couldn't. You thought hard, and harder, and—nothing. Then, when you were doing something else entirely, the answer surfaced because your mind was unpressured and free!

Take a dream break. Maybe you can even get an office-wide dream time, or brainstorm together. Take time to shut your door or put up a "Do Not Disturb" sign, even if it's only for 15 minutes.

The Least You Need to Know

➤ Your attitude about your work and workplace make a world of difference.

➤ Treat all pains in the neck—people as well as physical pains—with respect.

➤ Eat smart to keep your energy high and your stress low.

➤ Take relaxation and dream breaks throughout the day to keep you fresh, alert, and calm.

➤ Take time to clarify and remind yourself of your values and your goals in life.

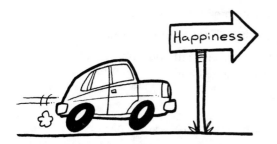

Chapter 6

On the Road to Happiness

In This Chapter

➤ Reviewing your life until now

➤ Recognizing the possibilities

➤ Listening to your heart

➤ Taking the first steps toward the future

Every year, my husband and I sit down and ask each other, "So, where do you want to be in one year, five years, 10 years?" None of us ask ourselves this question often enough. Making a happy life is a lifetime adventure (just getting people to agree on what happy means could take all day), but you should take time to consider some possibilities and how to make them realities. And that's just what you're going to do in this chapter. Where do you want to be next year?

Get Ready for Some Reflecting

You may very well have a happy life, whatever that means to you, just by drifting through each day (and taking great vacations). But if you long for a full life that makes a meaningful difference, a life that you can look back on and be proud of for many reasons, then you need to take some time on a regular basis to see where you've been, where you need to go, and how you're going to get there.

There are a number of good ways to examine your life, as you'll soon see. But first, let me get you warmed up for your little excursion. If you're getting a little tense about grading your life, take a few minutes to relax and calm down. You can use one of the techniques mentioned in Chapter 5, "Dealing with Your Job," or use the following one:

Chill Out

Don't criticize yourself for being lazy or stupid or afraid to change what you've wanted to change for so long, and don't think that making changes means your life is a mess. No one is perfect. That's good news because it means that even happy, successful people will want to change, to improve, or to try out new or neglected talents.

Take 5

In Alexandra Stoddard's *Tea Celebrations: The Way to Serenity* (Avon Books, 1995), she shows readers how to make this ancient, calming practice a part of daily life.

1. Sit down (you probably are), get comfortable, put your feet on the floor, and close your eyes.

2. Take a deep breath through your nostrils.

3. Hold the breath for a count of three.

4. Slowly exhale through your mouth; take at least a count of six to exhale.

5. Repeat.

While your body is doing this, your mind is active, too. On the inhale, think "Peace in" or "Calm in." On the exhale, think "Tension out" or "Worry out."

If you like tea, brew yourself a cup of one of the soothing herbal blends. Even if it is daytime, consider lighting a candle as a symbol of the holiness within and around you or just to symbolically light your way. Have a paper and pen handy in case you want to jot down some notes.

Those Were the Days

Even if you would like to go back to earlier days, you know you can't. You can't go "home." Home won't be the same, and even if it seems like it *is* the same, you aren't. Heraclitus, an ancient Greek philosopher, put it this way: "You cannot step twice into the same river, for new water is always flowing in."

Fortunately, you don't need to journey back home to discover the lessons waiting for you in your past. The following sections offer three ways to make those discoveries right now. Take your pick—or try them all!

Chapter and Verse

One way to organize your thoughts is to look at your life as a book:

➤ Divide your life into chapters.

➤ Give a title to each chapter.

➤ List your five greatest achievements for each chapter.

The chapters needn't be the same length. Look to events that appear to end one segment (chapter) of your life and begin another. The title is a way to summarize how you feel about the years in each segment. The achievement exercise is to accent the positive things you learned or did during those years. You have done good things. Applaud yourself by recognizing them.

However you feel about the earlier times of your life, they are over. You cannot change what happened or didn't happen. But you can come to terms with events in your past and make peace with them. Do that now.

➤ Express thanksgiving for the gifts you received during that part of your life. By gifts I don't mean material presents, although include those, too, if you think that is appropriate. Rather, I mean all the wonderful people, events, and lessons that were part of your earlier life.

➤ Express sorrow for what you didn't do and what you did that you regret.

➤ Offer a prayer or request or make a declaration out loud of anything you wish you could change from that part of your life.

If this process is one you would like to spend more time with, perhaps a directed retreat with a spiritual advisor would be beneficial for you.

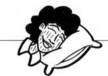

Take 5

Choose someone from history whom you admire or wish to emulate. Read their biography or autobiography. Notice the similarities and differences in your lives.

Crossroads and Detours

If you're a visual person, you might like this approach: Take a big sheet of paper and draw a road leaving from the place you were born. Along the way, mark significant events. Especially notice the crossroads, the points that marked major consequences one way or another, depending upon the choices you made at that time. Write a description or draw a symbol for the road not taken. When you are finished, you will have a line drawing of your life's journey so far, noting the major events and people and forks in the main road when you chose one path and ignored others.

Sometimes we lose our way but are fortunate to encounter people and situations that bring us back on the main road. In this case, our path at that point was only a detour. Mark your detours. Name the incident or person who brought you back. For example, I might examine my writing path. I would indicate writing stories as a child, then note women's rights law reporter in law school, writing workshop materials, legal education materials, religious materials, and finally this book. I would recall and add how and with whom I came to be involved in each of these endeavors.

If you engage in this activity with any degree of emotional attachment, you will need to grieve at the crossroads and detours. Take time to do that. Just as you grieve, so also must you rejoice. Remember and celebrate the moments of clarity, purpose, and peaceful communion. If you draw your map with others, you might join in a ritual to put closure on those times.

The Inner Journey

These two methods help you see and understand the outer part of your life. You looked at the people, places, and events that influenced you and upon whom you left your mark. What was going on inside you during those years? Where was your center?

For this exercise, make either a timeline or a list noting anything that relates to your spiritual life. This list could include formal or informal associations, traditional or nontraditional relationships. I don't want to be more specific because I don't want to limit what you include. Whatever it is, if you consider it a piece of religious or spiritual experience, then name it.

Where are you now in your spiritual life? Do you have any yearnings or desires in this regard? If so, write them down.

Life Is ...

If you had to describe life in just one word, what would it be? I'm not talking about your life in particular, although you can label it as well. I mean your sense of what life *is*.

Several years ago, I began collecting "Life is ..." descriptions. Here's a sampling of them. See whether any make sense to you.

Life is ...

... a journey	... a puzzle
... an adventure	... a painting
... a river	... confusing
... a symphony	... a sport
... short	... a story
... but a dream	... glorious
... a blast	... never ending

During the time that I was a member of a liturgical dance company (meaning that the group used dance as a prayer form), it occurred to me that "Life is ... a dance." I wrote a poem with that title and produced it in poster form. You may find it useful in your own reflections. It may also lift your spirits in preparation for the next part of your journey.

LIFE IS A DANCE

Feel it. Accept the aches and pains. Do your best.

Put your whole self into it. **Have fun.** Meditate.

REFRESH YOURSELF. **Learn new steps.** Practice.

Don't be afraid to fall. BE OPEN TO NEW IDEAS. Express yourself.

Change the tempo. Solo sometimes. *Bless yourself.*

Appreciate the talents of others. Take care of your body.

Stay in touch with the Spirit. Be at peace. Show emotion.

Take *leaps* of faith. **Dream.** *Savor the memories.* ImProViSe.

Be graceful. **FLY.** Land gently. *Trust your intuition.* **SMILE**

Learn from others. Repeat what's good. Don't forget to breathe.

Teach children. **Be a child.** Keep your balance. **Be centered.**

Shine even as an understudy. Expect no applause.

Accept roses graciously. **Respect your limits.** *Be prayerful.*

Stand TALL. **SHARE YOUR GIFTS.** Do it because it's right.

Expect magical moments and miracles.

© Linda Short 1994

It's Seven o'Clock: Where Am I?

At the moment, it's safe to assume that you're sitting down, reading this book. But how do you use the rest of your free time? Why do you spend your free time as you do?

All Booked Up

Some people fill up free time with committee or volunteer work. If you are one of these people, how many committees are you on? How much of your free time is taken up by them? Are you satisfied with the groups' purposes and goals? Do you find the meetings focused and productive? Even if you answered yes to these questions and believe the causes are worthy, are you the only one available? Must you continue, or can you step back from one or two?

Take a few moments to list all your associations:

➤ Clubs

➤ Professional organizations

➤ Neighborhood commitments

➤ Volunteer duties

➤ Religious activities

➤ Study groups

If I missed a few of your commitments, just add everything that keeps you away from your family and home.

Look at your list and mark those that

➤ You enjoy.

➤ Promote your career or vocation.

➤ Are personally satisfying.

➤ You do because "someone has to."

Must you continue with everything? When you are selective, you will increase the quality and effectiveness of your commitment and have more time for yourself and your family.

There's Nothing Different I Want to Do

Did I hear right? Isn't there anything you like to do? You want to do? Making time for yourself and using that time for self-healing and rejuvenation is more than escape and more than the absence of stress. Sure, television and such is relaxing and passes the time, but it doesn't regenerate you to better meet life's responsibilities. Remember, you're choosing your course, not drifting away.

If you choose to just be, that's positive and satisfying and gives you peace of mind. Did you choose:

➤ To be with others or alone?

➤ A variety of activities?

➤ To listen to your body's signals for rest or activity?

➤ To be comfortable not producing or accomplishing?

If you have no ideas about what to do, the organizations who are losing folks because they are overcommitted would love you to stop by. If you don't want to go it alone, maybe you could ask friends or co-workers about their activities. If something sounds interesting, tag along. If you're overwhelmed by all there is to do, figure it out at a spa or retreat or stick around for the next section.

This is an exercise I did once upon a time:

➤ List everything you enjoy doing.

➤ Mark your top 10 activities.

➤ Mark your second 10.

Your list should include everything you enjoy, from building models to shopping and from intimacy to deep-sea diving. Don't forget the little moments that bring you peace and joy, moments you may overlook.

When you have your top 10 activities, see whether you can enjoy one of them each day. Of course you can't take a vacation every day or even every week. Depending upon the items on your lists, work them into your life weekly or monthly. Perhaps once each season is more appropriate. Whatever you decide, choose to include joyful moments regularly.

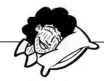

Take 5

A number of books help you follow your heart in your job. For starters, try *The Complete Idiot's Guide to Making Money Through Intuition; Is It Too Late to Run Away and Join the Circus?: A Guide to Your Second Life; What Color Is Your Parachute?: A Practical Manual for Job-Hunters and Career Changes;* and *Do What You Love, the Money Will Follow: Discovering Your Right Livelihood.* (See Appendix C, "Further Reading," for more.)

Be True to Your Heart

Staying true to your heart is the way to make sure your body won't go into knots when you walk through the office door. When you follow your heart, your center, your soul is likely leading you on your right path.

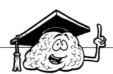

Mindful Moment

A recent newspaper article described a man who decided it was more important to leave an ethical will for his children than mere material possessions. The purpose of an ethical will is to commit to writing a statement of beliefs, values, and guidelines for living right. Certainly, not many people write down such a statement. Yet every business has a mission statement, a focus, a purpose for its being. Perhaps it makes some sense to write a personal statement for yourself and for your family. Regardless of whether you write it down, you follow a code of conduct. This code says a lot about you and the fulfilling life you want to lead.

Be true to your heart, not someone else's. Look at what you want, not what you think you should want as a result of societal or other influences. If you continue to draw from your well without replenishing it, you will dry up and have nothing to give to others or to yourself. Be brave. Be honest. Go into the roar (remember the story from Chapter 1?).

Who do you want to be? Notice, I did not ask, what you want to do. Define yourself beyond a list of tasks. What kind of person do you want to be? Set your vision and your standards high. You may not reach the goal every time, but you will always have something to aim for.

Remember Chapter 3, "Let's Get Personal," when I told you to make the things you wish to do into things you've done? If you have that list of wishes, keep it handy. If you didn't make one, you'll need it. After all, you want to make your wishes come true.

Chill Out

When you go looking for your life's purpose, realize you might not have to save the entire world (although you might), just contribute to your piece of it.

Take 5

The late Sister Thea Bowman said: "You have a gift; you have a talent; find your gift, find your talent, and use it. You can make life better in this world just by letting your light shine and by doing your part. You can help somebody just by caring, just by loving somebody. Then, sometime, tell them, 'I love you.'"

Decisions, Decisions

If you've come this far with me, you have a lot of information about yourself. You have a clear sense of your

➤ Past decisions and their consequences, whether you regret them or celebrate them.

➤ Spiritual journey to date.

➤ Secret heartfelt desires.

➤ Wishes.

➤ Pleasurable activities.

➤ Talents, independent of job titles.

➤ Values, mission, and purpose (maybe).

But information isn't of much value unless it's used. It's like buying a good book and putting it on your shelf, unread. So use what you have.

Circle of Life

In all the people and events of your life, find the similarities. Find circles in your life, movements ahead that brought you back to some physical, emotional, psychological, or spiritual place you've been before, that have brought you "full circle." Maybe a circle is a talent or a skill that you continue to use. Certainly, a circle is work that energizes and excites you and encourages you to rise each morning and eagerly greet the dawn.

Everyone has a gift, a special purpose that no one else can give to the world. When you discover it, or part of it, life is full of joy and easy. You feel you have a purpose, and life has meaning. If you have some inkling of your place in the sun, then live each day with it in mind. If not, it's time to figure out what your purpose is.

Darts, Anyone?

You could live your life by throwing darts at random and seeing where they land, or like an ostrich, you could stick your head in the sand and make no decisions. There has to be a better way to live your life. One way is to take a look at that personal mission statement, if you have one, or the road map that gave you clues to your destination. Where do you want to go? What are your gifts that might get you there?

When you take a conscious look at what you intend to do with your life, you choose your purpose or *goals*. It is a broad statement that does not include details. When you are ready, choose no more than three goals. Then look at each: Are they manageable? Achievable?

Setting too many goals gives you more opportunities for problems. Do you have enough energy, money, skills? Do you need to break the goal into smaller pieces? Give yourself sufficient time to accomplish your goal and to account for delays and problems.

One Day at a Time

Now it's time to start making your dreams come true. For each purpose you have, note

➤ What you want to achieve or change.

➤ The steps you'll need to take.

➤ A realistic time frame.

➤ Some way to know whether you've achieved your dream.

Remind yourself of your intentions often. Post your objectives on the mirror, fridge, and in your date book. You need to see them and be reminded of them. Use your gifts in pursuit of your new life.

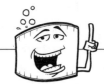

Jacuzzi Jive

Your personal **goal** is not about football or soccer, but it is similar in that it is your desired end result. This goal is a broad statement, similar to a mission statement, of what you intend to do, be, and achieve. Your **objectives** are the details, the steps you need to take to make your goal become reality.

Chill Out

Change your goals or objectives if necessary. Be open to suggestions from others. Acknowledge and use their gifts, too, when they point the way to achieve your purpose.

Making It Happen

Don't those goals and objectives look great on paper? Guess what? You won't accomplish any of your dreams reading and re-reading the paper. If all those lists and ideas and dreams seem overwhelming, then pick what you're most excited about and start there.

Start right now; not later, which sometimes never comes. Just one step now will get you going. The first step is the hardest. Then one thing follows another, and you're feeling good about getting closer (okay, so you're only inching at the moment) to the finish line. Before you know it, you have a full head of steam, and you're chugging along the track.

So Get Started

You're ready to take the first step. You've

➤ Identified the goal you're going for.

➤ Looked at the list of objectives.

➤ Picked the objective you'll accomplish.

Now you get to work backward. (Isn't this fun?) Ask yourself, "To achieve this goal, what must I do first? To achieve that, what must I do before it?"

Chill Out

Sometimes feelings of being dreadfully overwhelmed or deeply disappointed are not momentary. If there are no recent changes in your life (becoming a new parent, starting a new job, or recently moving) that might explain your feelings, there may be another cause. You may have a problem that needs professional attention.

For example, if my goal is to be a master gardener, one objective might be to obtain the appropriate education. Working backward, the answers to my questions might go like this:

➤ To get an education, I need to receive training.

➤ To receive training, I need to attend a training program.

➤ To attend a training program, I need to find out where one is and what its requirements are.

➤ To do that, I need to look in the library, look in the phone book, and so on.

Your first step is to go to the library or take out your phone book. That's quite manageable, isn't it? What are you waiting for?

Keep on Keepin' On

You are on your way. Continue to remind yourself of your goal. Be gentle with yourself when you forget and revert to former patterns.

The new you will relate to people differently. You'll be more confident and centered in your new purpose. You've changed the rules of the game of life. In a real sense, the reactions of people to the new you are tests of your resolve. The universe is asking whether you are serious about your new direction.

Keep your purpose uppermost. It takes a couple of months for new behaviors to become habit. See yourself satisfied and enjoying your new role. If you must, change your timetable or your objectives to point you toward the person you want to be, not the tasks you need to accomplish.

Help Is Waiting

You are not alone in finding your perfect purpose. Help is out there. Don't think so? If the universe wants you to move in a certain way, and you are interested in moving in that direction, don't you think there will be a few signs along the way to help you out? These signs are called *synchronicity*.

I'll give you a true instance. A friend comes to my home to drop off something I ordered. While we're talking, I feel a need to speak about a personal situation I had a few years back. As I finish, I notice she is staring at me with her mouth open. When she speaks, she asks whether I had invited her there to tell her what I just did. (Never mind I didn't do any inviting; she came to deliver something, remember?) Turns out, she's going through the same situation in her life. We talk a bit more, and I suggest a few books. She leaves, and forgets the list. The next day she goes to the library. Of all the thousands of books on the shelves, the one book that is lying out on the table is the one I recommended.

In any aspect of life, if you put your mind and attention to something, it will grow. The more you become aware of meaningful coincidences, the more they'll occur. They appreciate being noticed! In Indian (as in India) tradition, the two characteristics of a person on the right path are

➤ Far fewer worries.

➤ Awareness of far more synchronicities.

Celebrate coincidences. They show you you're on the right track.

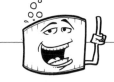

Jacuzzi Jive

The Swiss psychologist Carl Jung created the word **synchronicity** to describe moments of meaningful coincidence, a coming together of seemingly unconnected events.

Peace Be with You

You're on your way. May you go in peace. There's the door. It's time to fly.

we, like butterfly:
lifting sacred wings, trusting,
soaring to unknowns

(© Linda Short, 1992)

The Least You Need to Know

➤ Before you know where you're going, you need to find where you've been.

➤ Notice the threads that are weaving the tapestry that is you.

➤ When you choose goals, look to the kind of person you want to be, not the tasks you wish to achieve.

➤ Be alert to synchronicities that help you know you're on your soul's right path.

Part 3

Taking Care of Busy-ness

You spend the entire day running around, or so it seems. You're like the White Rabbit in Alice in Wonderland, *always scurrying somewhere. What is it that keeps you so busy? Hopefully, you've been able to use some of the suggestions in Part 2 to adjust your attitude and your day to free up some minutes or even hours. If so, congratulations! You've begun to get some control over the busy-ness of your life.*

Here in Part 3 you'll discover ways to make the most of the stillness of your life. What do you do with the quiet you've found? Not all of us are comfortable, at least at first, with "time on our hands." Some of us never adjust to feeling completely at ease with even a few free hours. I'll show you how to free your body and mind to experience feelings of peace and joy throughout your day. I'll also suggest ways you can lead children to master their bodies and connect with their spirits.

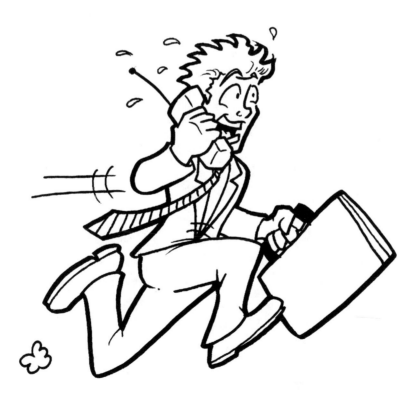

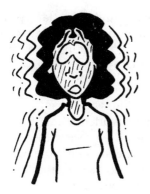

Chapter 7

Keep Still!

In This Chapter

➤ Appreciating silence

➤ Practicing meditation

➤ Understanding the body's energy

➤ Learning how to heal the world

A while back, people used porches to just sit, ruminate about life, and reflect on their surroundings. It's a hopeful sign that porches are coming back, because they are symbols of people's desire to enjoy quiet, stillness, and contemplation.

For millennia, meditation has been an avenue for stillness without and connection within. In this chapter, I'll drag you to a chair and explain how to stop fidgeting and even enjoy the absence of sound. You'll understand why quieting your body and mind connects you with your spirit and with the spirits of others. To help you practice, I've included a sampling of meditations.

Sittin' on the Dock of the Bay

The singer Otis Redding had the right idea, and not just for lazy summer days, either. Maybe you like to watch the tide roll away or the waves undulate toward shore on an eternal dance. Maybe you fish to get away and enjoy the solitude, to just be. Or you may sometimes stare into fires or candle flames. In such moments, you experience some of the stillness and inner peace that you feel when you practice *meditation*.

Whether you meditate in the privacy of your home or outside under the stars, you have no goals to achieve and no expectations to meet. You become aware only of your feelings and interior space at that moment. When you practice meditation, you simply exist. Indeed, meditation is also known as *sitting*, because that is what you do, nothing more and nothing less.

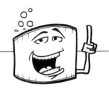

Jacuzzi Jive

Meditation is an altered state of awareness during which the meditating person is in a type of trance state, experiences relaxation, is able to tune out all external activity, and goes within herself.

Take 5

Hermann Hesse wrote in *Siddhartha* (Bantam, reissued 1982), "Within you there is a stillness and a sanctuary to which you can retreat at any time and be yourself." Go there regularly.

Anyone may practice meditation, without regard to religious beliefs or philosophical orientation. It is a process that allows you to practice peace within you. However, you may associate the method more with hermits and religious persons because meditation is a way to understand our soul purpose and to just be with the Holy One. If that is not your reason, so be it. You can still benefit from and use meditation.

Meditation may be difficult for you if you can't sit still. Otherwise, the meditation process is easy to learn. If there is a key to meditation, it is to not try too hard. Be effortless while being still. Remember, you don't have to do anything.

Some people aren't just fidgety; they have another reason to avoid meditation, and you see it in meditation classes. The reason is that they are unable or unwilling to face themselves at that particular moment. It isn't unusual for a large group of people to begin meditation classes, for example, and then to drop out after the first session. In one series of classes I completed, about 60 people started the six-week beginning meditation sessions. By the time we reached the fourth and final phase of the program almost a year later, there were six of us left.

All kinds of medical research has documented tremendous physical and psychological benefits from meditation. These benefits include:

➤ Deep relaxation and inner calm and tranquility

➤ Decreased muscle tension

➤ Slower breathing

➤ Drop in blood pressure and heart rate

➤ Change in brain waves from busy beta waves to the calm, joyful alpha waves

➤ Spontaneous reduction in use of alcohol, cigarettes, and drugs

➤ Increased creativity

➤ Enhanced problem-solving and learning abilities

➤ Reversal of the aging process

These effects begin with the very first meditation and become cumulative as you continue the practice. During meditation, the body may go into a state of relaxation that is deeper than that found in deep sleep.

As for meditation being too much sitting, you may have something there. Think how much sitting you do throughout your day. It's almost as though you go from one seat to the next. What your body needs is movement, which you'll read about in Chapter 11, "Let's Get Physical." At least meditation is sitting for a higher purpose. If you still won't sit, then do a walking meditation, which is described in Chapter 15, "Nature Calls!"

Our marvelous central nervous system is at work, or at rest, during meditation. With regular use, meditation rids the nervous system of stress and trains the body to enter the meditative state. Meditation can become a powerful habit that allows you to maintain your relaxed and aware state throughout the day and fill yourself with energy and joy. For more on meditation, read *The Complete Idiot's Guide to Meditation* (Alpha Books, 1999).

Energized Stillness

No, being energized and still is not a contradiction in terms, as you'll see in just a moment. To understand how energized stillness is possible, you'll need to review your body's energy systems and how they work and learn how meditation affects them.

A Body of Energy

Back in school, you learned that all matter is made up of atoms. Each *atom* is made up of *electrons*, *protons*, and *neutrons*. These particles have electrical charges.

Even when you think you are still, as when you are sitting, you have billions of atoms moving about inside you. Even more, those billions are charged with electricity. You are a constant bundle of moving energy.

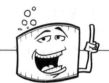

Jacuzzi Jive

The basic unit of all matter is the **atom.** Each atom is made up of three main particles: **electrons,** which have a negative electric charge; **neutrons,** which have no charge; and **protons,** which have positive electric charges. The neutrons and protons are located in the nucleus, or center, of the atom, and the electrons orbit, or circle, the nucleus.

Take 5

You can learn how to activate your energy centers through meditation. Look in your community for classes you can take. Better yet, begin at a retreat or spa that offers meditation sessions.

Running Your Energy

You may have no clue what "running your energy" means. In fact, you may be unaware that your body can feel any different from the way it normally feels to you.

Here's a simple demonstration to experience the difference: Stand up and lift one arm and shake it for a count of 30. Stop shaking your arm and then stand quietly. Focus on the sensations in this arm and compare them to the feelings in your other arm. What you ought to feel in the arm you have shaken is a kind of tingling or pulsating sensation. Your other arm feels still. In the shaken arm, you are feeling your energy flowing.

When you run your energy, you have your energy flowing throughout your body. You know it is happening because you can feel it. Your body is alive, awake, and active. Eastern medical tradition believes that this energy both vitalizes the body and protects it from disease. In the expanding field of mind-body research in this country, Western scientists are beginning to understand how this energy works.

As you continue your meditation practice, your mind trains your body in the way it is to behave, and your body converts these individual acts into a habit. Then one day you discover, as I did, that you don't need to be seated at all. You can turn on your energy at will, just by thinking it.

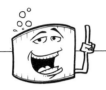

Jacuzzi Jive

Although the dictionary definition describes an **aura** as a subtle quality or atmosphere that emanates from a person, place, or thing (yes, trees and flowers have auras), I think of an aura as a vibrating field of energy that totally engulfs the body. It is over, under, around, and through each of us.

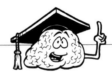

Mindful Moment

In ancient Chinese medicine, **chi** is the body's vital life force, which also protects the body from disease. The Japanese call it **ki.** In the Indian yogic tradition, **prana** is the energy that animates all physical matter, including the body.

Aura: More Than Just Flesh

Kirlian photography was used as early as the 1890s to record the unseen fields of energy that surround living organisms. The fields change according to your health and your moods. The name given to this energy field that pulses around and through the body at all times is called your *aura*. In 1975 in the United States, the University of California at Los Angeles used Kirlian photography to measure auras.

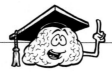

Mindful Moment

Your aura fits you best when it is about 12 to 18 inches from your center. If it's closer than that, it's constricting. If it's farther out than that, it's uncontrolled and being compromised by the energy of others. So how can you get your aura under control? Just think it, know it, and it is. If you are a visual person, close your eyes and visualize your aura positioning itself at a proper distance. If you are auditory, hear it move; if you are kinesthetic, feel it move. If you are sentient, sense your aura at its proper distance.

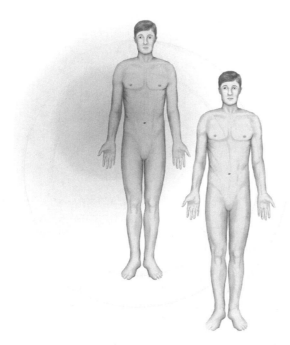

The aura of the figure on the left is so extended outward from the body that the other figure moves through it, disturbing the energy field and the individual's peace.

Healing Your Energy Body

In Eastern belief, the energy that flows within and around you emanates from seven major centers in your body, called *chakras*. As long as the energy flows freely, there is health. When the energy system is blocked, for example, by holding in tension or upsetting emotions, then the physical body is unhealthy.

That your emotions are stored in your body may be a new concept for you. It means your emotional baggage—your anger, distress, unforgiveness toward yourself or others, fear, and hopelessness—is trapped in your energy body. I will never forget watching the segment of Bill Moyers's public television series, *Healing and the Mind,* in the early '90s, when he responded to the scientist he was interviewing at the time with "It sounds as though you're saying our emotions are stored in our bodies." The scientist, with a look of incredulity on her face, answered, "Of course! Didn't you know that?"

The seven chakras are numbered from the base, as one, up through the crown chakra, as seven. In order, they are called the base, the sacral, the solar plexus, the heart, the throat, the forehead or third eye, and the crown chakras.

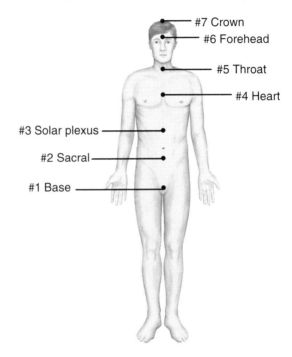

#7 Crown
#6 Forehead
#5 Throat
#4 Heart
#3 Solar plexus
#2 Sacral
#1 Base

One of the great reasons for using a practice like meditation is that it moves your energy, connects you to the source, and gets rid of that junk inside you. It helps you to be the glorious being you are meant to be.

Your negative emotions can block the natural, vital flow of life-giving energy throughout your system. If you continue to hold these hurtful feelings in and allow them to fester, you create a climate of *dis-ease* in your body.

Here's what meditation will do for you:

➤ Bring you in touch with your energy.
➤ Identify where blockages are to clear them.
➤ Help you receive spiritual guidance.
➤ Bring you peace and relaxation.

You can use meditation to clear your chakras for optimum health.

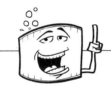

Jacuzzi Jive

According to Eastern belief, **chakras** (wheels) are centers of energy from which rays of life-giving light and energy radiate. They are located between the base of the spinal column and the top of the head. Even Western medicine accepts them, but calls them the nerve plexus. During meditation, the soul rises upward through the seven centers to connect with the Infinite.

Cosmic Consciousness

When you are aware of the energy that flows through you, you realize it flows through all of creation. You receive your energy from an all-encompassing source. Each of us receives life from this same sacred flow of energy. When you reflect on a deeper level, when you meditate or pray, you may experience this realization as an interconnectedness of all life.

We Are One

Years ago B.C. (before children), my husband and I canoed through the Boundary Waters Canoe Area in northern Minnesota. On one trip we discovered a place we named Blueberry Island. Half the island was covered by wild blueberry bushes in full fruit, and we enjoyed the luscious bounty until we wished for no more. For the rest of the afternoon, we found our own ways to bask in the warm sun that nourished our spirits.

I found a place on the edge that rose perhaps six inches above the water line. I used a tree to support my back as I gazed out at sparkling sapphires. Then I noticed movement on the earth beside me. My focus shifted as I studied first one ant, and then others, in their pursuit of survival. One larger ant was trying to invade the smaller colony. I spent most of the afternoon sitting still, contemplating this scene and wondering about their lives.

During that time, the ants and I were connected. In the terminology of psychologist Abraham Maslow, Blueberry Island was a "transcendental" peak experience. It was a time when "the whole universe is perceived as an integrated and unified whole."

Take a moment to stop and consider your life up to now. What is one peak experience you have had? Now go into the experience more fully. Remember how you felt, both during and after. You can recapture that deep sense of peace and tranquility for your daily life by remembering that moment.

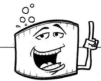

Jacuzzi Jive

The natural, healthy state of your body is when it is entirely at ease and at peace. Any condition that affects your body so as to cause pain, discomfort, or ill health is causing a state that is in **dis-ease**, or separation from, negation of, or a reversal of, that healthy, vital state.

Chill Out

We carry many hurtful emotions inside because we don't practice forgiveness. Do you want to be right or in a blissful state of peace? Look at how much energy you use defending positions that make you feel right for a short time. Practice forgiveness by recognizing the perfect inner core of yourself and of other people.

Shhh

Sitting meditation is not easy for some people, especially those who are impatient, busy, and rushing around or who are simply new to the practice. I remember a time in college when an advisor led a small group of us in a discussion. There was a pause in the flow of words. Silence. Those few minutes were too much for one student who began squirming and laughing uncomfortably; he finally said something stupid just to break the silence.

With practice, sitting in stillness becomes more comfortable. Your body adjusts. Your attitude adjusts. Begin with just five minutes. See how you do. If that is too short of a time, try 10 minutes, and then 15. Some retreats are conducted in silence. If you choose, you can be introduced to stillness by attending a retreat that uses silence for all or part of the sessions.

Although the lotus position is associated with meditation, it isn't the only position possible. You may meditate sitting in a chair (preferably straight-backed), which is my favorite, or even walking. (Image © Index Stock Photography, Inc.)

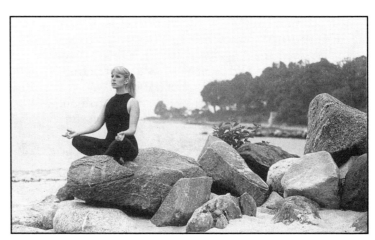

Practicing the Practice: Once

There are various schools of meditation, so you may notice differences between what I'm describing here and classes that you take. If you pray regularly, meditation won't be as unfamiliar as you might expect. Sometimes, it's just the terminology we use that sets us apart.

This exercise is an easy type of meditation where you simply focus on your breath:

1. Many people sit on the floor on cushions. I don't. I use a straight-backed chair, with my feet on the floor, hands comfortably on my thighs, palms up. (You can also stand, walk, or lie down, although you may fall asleep if you do the latter.)

2. Close your eyes. Take a few deep breaths. Quiet yourself.

3. Imagine that you are entirely surrounded by brilliant white light.

4. Focus on your breath. Breathe in through your nostrils. Keep your breathing as even as possible.

5. If thoughts come to mind, acknowledge them, but let them go by. It's almost like watching a movie, where the images drift by. Don't hold onto any thought.

6. The longer you sit and give yourself to just being there, the less you will pay attention to your thoughts. On occasion, you will experience a flow of pure sensation or emotion that has no thought or mental picture associated with it. It might even feel as though you are being held in the palm of the Holy One's hand.

7. End by saying a prayer, a thank you or amen, or sending the healing light to a person or situation that could use its help.

Whatever you choose to do, relax and be effortless. There is no right or wrong way to meditate. It is a personal process. Whatever works for you is just great!

Twice

You can also meditate on a single word or phrase, called a *mantra*. The book of Psalms contains a verse that directs us to "Be still and know that I am God."

You may use each line of this passage as a mantra. Do not meditate on all these words at one sitting. This one passage is sufficient for five meditation sessions.

➤ Be still and know that I am God.

➤ Be still and know that I am.

➤ Be still and know.

➤ Be still.

➤ Be.

This last idea, to just *be*, is the essence of meditation.

Take 5

The more you practice, the more you will rely on your inner experience. You will have less reason to become anxious, angry, or depressed.

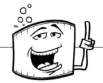

Jacuzzi Jive

The word **mantra** is Hindu for a word or phrase that is said or chanted repeatedly. The sound vibrates in the body (each chakra has its own sound) and facilitates meditation.

Thrice

You can also meditate by focusing upon an object. This is called contemplation. I began this chapter referring to the trance-like, or meditative, state you go into when you stare at candles, or fires, or waves. Let's end this chapter where it began:

1. Light a candle.

2. Darken every other place.

3. Focus on the flame, and quiet yourself.

Continue as before.

Meditation is another avenue to self-healing. However you choose to practice meditation, you will reap the benefits.

The Least You Need to Know

➤ Within you is a river of energy from the Source, waiting for you to discover and use it for healing, vitality, and spiritual guidance.

➤ Meditation, also called sitting, is one practice you may use to go within.

➤ With meditation, you can heal yourself, and perhaps others as well.

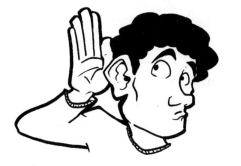

Chapter 8

The Sounds of Silence

In This Chapter

➤ Understanding the nature of prayer

➤ Discovering different prayer styles

➤ Examining the benefits of prayer

➤ Learning how faith can heal you

Whether you belong to a faith community or follow some spirituality of your own, prayer is probably part of your practice. Prayer has physical, mental, and spiritual benefits like meditation. But unlike meditation, which is used by some people as solely a relaxation practice, prayer is understood always as a way to experience or communicate with a divine presence.

This chapter looks more closely at prayer. Even if you already pray on a regular basis, you may learn different ways, such as using clay or dance, to pray. After all, prayer styles are as varied as people who use them.

Fold Your Hands, Bow Your Head

For many people, Albrecht Dürer's masterful praying hands drawing is the epitome of prayer. Indeed, one of my sixth-grade religious education students asked whether there was another way to pray—as though the only way to do it was to fold your hands and bow your head. (That's not true, of course, but I'll get to that later.)

For some people, prayer is the center of spirituality. Take this moment to reflect on what role prayer and spirituality play in your life. Ask yourself these questions:

➤ What does prayer mean to you, today?

➤ Have you ever prayed regularly?

➤ If you do pray, why do you do it?

➤ Have you ever fasted for a spiritual reason (not to lose weight)?

➤ Have you consciously tried to practice new behavior, like being more patient, or forgiving, or peaceful?

➤ Is prayer or spirituality what you do alone, or with others?

➤ Have you ever used or created ritual or ceremony for a special occasion?

➤ Are you aware of the sufferings of others? Do you help in any direct way?

➤ Do you feed your spirit like you feed your body?

Your answers to these questions give you a perspective from which to review this chapter.

These hands are reminiscent of the famous drawing by Albrecht Dürer. Although his masterpiece is known by most as The Praying Hands, *its actual title is* Hands of an Apostle. *Dürer's famous picture has been used on everything from postcards to bookends.*
(Image © H. Armstrong Roberts)

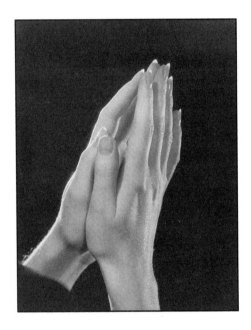

In the Beginning

When did people first begin praying? Is it possible to go back to the very beginning when man and woman first wondered about who they were, where they came from, and what they were to be? In searching for understanding, might they look to that which surrounded them?

People today ask the same questions and look for inspiration in the same things. They notice the cycles of nature: the movement of stars in the dark sky, the coming and going of the sun, the changes in temperature and in seasons. You can look at other people and see patterns repeated: Everyone lives and dies; everyone searches for nourishment and seeks out others for friendship or community. These patterns and cycles and similarities lead many people to wonder about the existence of something or someone much greater and grander than themselves.

There Must Be More

What is this human experience? The words *experiment* and *experience* have the same root, which means to try. Is living an experiment? In trying to feel, touch, taste, smell, and hear new foods, new attitudes, and new people, you experience life. You live through these experiences.

If you look outside yourself to those around you, to those who live on the other side of the mountain, you will notice that all peoples participate in similar experiences. In Thornton Wilder's play *Our Town,* the Stage Manager says, "I don't care what they say with their mouths, everybody knows in their bones that something is eternal, and that something has to do with human beings ..." The something that is eternal is way down deep in each and every one of us.

Forming a Relationship with the Mystery

When you meet someone, isn't the first question you ask, "What's your name?" So it is with this "other," this mystery that people know in their bones exists. Some speak directly to this mystery by name: God, Allah, Lord, Intelligence, a Higher Power, the Holy One, the Source, the Creator, Yahweh. Others feel uncomfortable with names, especially exclusively male names or any name for the One who is beyond all human naming. Still others are content to let this mystery approach on its own, in its own time.

In name and in attitude, people recognize this supernatural other as beyond words, beyond mind. Yet they feel they are, and want to be, connected to it. Lacking words, they turn to other ways of expressing their feelings, their moods, their questions. People act in many of the same patterns. When they are happy, they dance, move, or sing. When sad, they remain alone, cry, or cry out. They join with others who share their experiences. Their patterns of motions or words are continued in oral or written tradition, and ritual is born.

Talking to Whom?

Years ago, I took a book on prayer with me to a dental appointment. I figured it would give me something to read while I waited. My turn came, and I took the book with me. The dentist noticed it, and said he didn't pray because it's only talking to yourself, so why bother? Indeed, why bother if you're only talking to yourself?

I know lots of folks, including me, who talk to themselves on occasion, and it does help. But are you just talking to yourself when you pray? Some may answer yes, saying that if you believe that the Divine, however you name it, is within you, then you are in a sense talking to yourself.

But you can look at it another way, too. Prayer is a way of bridging the separation of the material and spiritual worlds, of experiencing unity, if only briefly. In a child's terms, prayer is talking to God from the depths of your heart. Or as a church bulletin once put it: "If God is your father, call home."

Is Anyone Listening?

I hope someone is listening. Isn't that the basis of prayer, hope? You hope that this greater and wiser someone can clean up your messes and guide your life. This someone won't desert you even if everyone else does and wants to see you live a joyful, peaceful, satisfied life—and may even help you get there.

The question, "Is anyone listening?" can be interpreted another way: Are *you* listening when God calls you? This might be one of those chicken-and-egg questions, except you know what the beginning is—God came first. In creating you, doesn't God call you to respond? So prayer is not only calling out to God, but also responding to God's first call to you. In that mysterious relationship of prayer, God gradually reveals himself, and you understand your place in the universe of his creation.

It's All Right

Is there a right way to pray? If you get caught up in praying the right way, you may not pray at all. Perhaps the only rules might be to

➤ Raise your heart and mind to God.

➤ Recognize that the one you address is eternal; be humble.

➤ Trust that you are praying the way you need to and that you are heard.

Take 5

If you feel distant from a personal God, or have some issues that create barriers from getting closer, you might try any number of books (or a retreat) to help. *Your God Is Too Small* (Collier Books, 1961), by J.B. Phillips, addresses stereotypes of God and then goes on to suggest ways you can find God for yourself. For women, I like *The Feminine Face of God* (Bantam, 1992) by Sherry Ruth Anderson and Patricia Hopkins or *Dance of the Spirit: The Seven Steps of Women's Spirituality* (Bantam, 1991) by Maria Harris.

Your intention to join with the Holy One in this experience is what is important.

In general, people offer prayers of

➤ Adoration: expressing love for the Holy One

➤ Blessing: dedicating themselves to God

➤ Contrition: being sorry, asking forgiveness

➤ Intercession: asking for help on behalf of another

➤ Petition: asking help for themselves

➤ Praise: giving glory to the Almighty

➤ Thanksgiving: being thankful for blessings received

Sometimes these prayers use a person's own words; sometimes they use the words of others.

Find Your Own Way

There is no preferred way to pray. God leads you according to your needs. If you have prayed often, you understand this. If you don't pray regularly, or have never prayed, here are some suggestions that may help you:

1. Prayer works best on your mind and body when it's cumulative. Pray every day, even if you think you have nothing to pray about.

2. Pray for others as well as for yourself. You will tighten the bonds between you and them, whether friend or stranger.

3. As in meditation, let the feelings flow; try not to think consciously. Say what your heart is feeling at that moment. It may be different from what you thought. Pay attention to what comes up for prayer. You may have needs you haven't acknowledged.

4. Feel free to change the location and style of prayer. Although sacred objects and sacred places help many people feel closer to the Creator, you don't need them all the time.

Pray All Ways

Pray always, and pray all ways. People pray without ceasing when they unite their prayerful words to good works and their good works to prayer. You also pray at all times when you see God's presence in each part of your daily life. Brother Lawrence, a seventeenth-century Frenchman who joined a monastery as a lay brother, learned how to practice the presence of God while working in the monastery's kitchen. Brother Lawrence described it this way:

> [T]hink often on God, by day, by night, in your business, and even in your diversions. He is always near you and with you; leave Him not alone. You would think it rude to leave a friend alone who came to visit you; why, then, must God be neglected?

Fortunately, we don't have to call home using the same phone. If you'd rather, there's smoke signals, banners trailing behind airplanes, and even letters (you remember them, right?). You can pray:

➤ With your mouth, out loud or silently

➤ Using formal prayers or your own words

➤ With actions, including song, dance, and even molding clay

➤ Using sacred writings, objects, or prayer books

➤ By writing in a journal

➤ By fasting

➤ By acts of service to others, alone or in community

➤ In a place of worship or in the kitchen

➤ Seated, standing, or walking

Actions Speak Louder Than Words

I recently taught a danced prayer to a group of religious educators. (We were exchanging samples of prayer.) By way of introduction, I reminded them of the expression "giving lip service" to something. It calls to mind how people can say one thing and do another or say something and not mean what they say.

In contrast, actions speak even when words fail you. You cannot hide what you mean. When you pray with actions, you pray with your whole self, your entire being. You bend, bow, kneel, or dance. You sit still, in total concentration. It is said, when you sing, you pray twice. A poem on my wall says, "For heights and depths no words can reach, music is the soul's own speech."

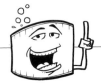

Jacuzzi Jive

In **inspired** writings, God guided the writers so that their words were God's words. God speaks to us through these writings.

Sacred Writings

Religious traditions have collections of sacred writings. These writings tell us of God and our relationship to each other. Often, the writings are believed to be *inspired*. More than just reading the words, you may use them for prayer.

To pray from sacred writings, begin by choosing a passage. Read the passage, and then put the book aside and recall what you read. Write down a word or words that made an impact on you. If you cannot remember the passage, read it again.

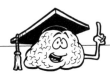

Mindful Moment

I was told of a corporate executive who keeps a poster of the Lord's Prayer in his office behind a panel in a kind of sacred space. When he is in a meeting that appears to be going nowhere, or he is having difficulty, he will excuse himself as though going to the restroom. Instead, he will enter his office, close his door, and gaze at and recite this prayer. When he goes back to his meeting, he's renewed and ready to deal with the impasse.

After you have the word or words that seemed important, reflect on them in turn. What did they make you remember? How do they affect you? How do you feel? Are you being called to change in some way, create a new habit, or develop a new attitude?

Close by reading the entire passage again. Offer a prayer in your own words, incorporating what you understood, or say a prayer from your tradition.

Using Sacramentals

You may also pray by using *sacramentals*, which are objects that are precious or important to you. Perhaps it's a bit of Earth you brought home from a pilgrimage or perhaps a cross or candles. There is an increasing interest in using objects for creating home altars (which you'll read about later in Chapter 14, "Creating Your Home Spa and Personal Retreat"). Collect, arrange, and display these objects to help you pray.

➤ Focus on them to become still.

➤ Use them to celebrate a physical connection with the divine being.

➤ Use them throughout the day as reminders to return to a peaceful stillness.

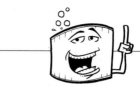

Jacuzzi Jive

A **sacramental** is a holy object that is infused with divine power. In the field of comparative religions, the word *sacramental* is sometimes used as a general term for anything that represents a hidden reality that is sacred or mysterious.

Good, too, is that these items are portable for moving around your living space or taking with you. Have sacred, will travel.

When you use an object as a focal point of your prayer, this is contemplation. Did you ever take a magnifying glass outside, and hold it so still, hoping the paper underneath would catch fire? In that experience, you became still within. You did nothing and waited. In prayer, you wait for God to find you, to reveal himself to you.

Journaling

Whether you go out and purchase a beautiful book with blank pages or use a spiral notebook, writing prayer is journaling. There are many ways to keep a journal. For some, it's like a diary but with an emphasis on the spiritual. Sometimes the writing takes the form of letters to Allah or poetry that seems to flow right through you and out your pen.

One exercise from a workshop I attended years ago was what I call continuous writing. The object is to write without stopping for 20 minutes. Set a timer or have someone tell you so you don't have to keep looking at the time. Put writing implement to paper and start writing the first thing that comes into your mind. And keep writing.

Don't censor, edit, or paraphrase. Write whatever presents itself. If you seem to get stuck, continue to write what you last wrote until a new thought occurs to you. When the time is up, look at where you began and where you ended. These points are the two important messages for further reflection and prayer.

Fasting

Although I'll address fasting more in connection with food in Chapter 12, "Restful Repasts," there are other possibilities for fasting. Rather than abstain from food or drink, you might abstain from a regular habit. By doing so, you can become aware of how that habit is affecting you and how you live. You can look at yourself and your world from a different perspective. You might consider giving up or fasting from television or the Internet, fasting from your car, or fasting from the telephone.

Many religious traditions include the practice of "giving up" or fasting. In Islam, during the month of Ramadan, devout Muslims fast from sunrise to sunset. Jews fast on Yom Kippur. Christians observe the 40 days of Lent by either giving up something or pursuing some form of positive action.

People don't fast to inflict pain on themselves, but to help them consider other and more active ways to be alive and to see life. Instead of relying on television and computers during your leisure time, you might, for example, visit friends or neighbors, write letters, play games with your family, or work in a garden. Instead of using the car, you might pedal a bicycle or walk. You might stay close to home and notice the trees, the sky, and the people. Think about how you would live if you had no car. You get the picture. These kinds of "fastings" will give you a new sense of time, of yourself, and of prayer-filled moments.

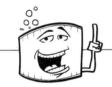

Jacuzzi Jive

Liturgy is the traditional name given to the service of people coming together to pray and worship. The word itself means the "work of the people" and reminds us that we praise our Creator together and carry into our lives this prayerful relationship to each other.

Apart or Together

You can't always pray with others, and you don't always want to. Some types of prayer require solitude. But being in community with others and worshipping together is an important part of spirituality. *Liturgy* offers opportunities to celebrate a common presence and common beliefs before and in the midst of the Holy.

You needn't think only in terms of formal worship. Folks who want to mix and match traditions can join together at their own place on a regular basis for communal sharing and prayer. You can begin your own traditions and your own rituals. When you join together, you support, strengthen, and help each other live more deeply.

Service to Others

Service is a spiritual discipline. The more you experience the love this Mystery has for you, the more that love impels you to reach out to others. Someone is ill. Do you send a card, call, bring a covered dish, or tell yourself that you're too busy and that the person will get help from someone else anyway? Do you walk or raise money for a charitable cause or decide you're too tired? I know you can't do everything that comes your way, and if you look closely, you will notice daily, perhaps even hourly, invitations. But do something, you must. If you do nothing, meditating and praying will not come easily.

The Beginning and the End

From ancient times, people have begun each day by greeting the sun. They pray, chant songs, play flutes, and ring a thousand golden bells. You, too, can offer your own words or a deeply grateful heart for the rest you received and the blessings you know will come. Make time each day for prayer. Make time each week for different forms of prayer. When you pray, don't just talk to Yahweh. Be sure to spend time waiting quietly and listening to hear what Yahweh has to say to you.

The Healing Power of Prayer

The power of prayer to heal is true. It made the cover of *Reader's Digest,* so you know it's mainstream. Faith can heal you. For people who read the works of Eastern religions and the ancient stories of the Bible, this knowledge is not new. What is new is that the medical establishment, in increasing degrees, accepts the link between faith and healing. Indeed, as of 1997, 30 medical schools in the United States were offering courses in faith and medicine. In addition, all American residency programs for new psychiatrists are required to address religious and spiritual issues in their formal training.

Whether it is Harvard Medical School associate professor Dr. Herbert Benson who has studied and written extensively on the subject of the beneficial health effects of a relaxed state brought on by prayer and meditation, or Dr. Larry Dossey's book *Healing Words: The Power of Prayer and the Practice of Medicine,* which discusses many additional studies, findings show that when you pray and meditate, your blood pressure drops, your heart and breathing rate slow, and anger vanishes. You are able to tap into your body's healing intelligence.

Chill Out

Most physicians caution that prayer isn't a panacea that should replace medication or conventional treatment.

Harold Koenig, an associate professor of psychiatry at Duke University School of Medicine, and a chief researcher in the scientific study of faith's healing potential, has led a team studying thousands of Americans since 1984 and compiled evidence that religious faith promotes overall good health and aids in recovery from serious illness. His findings include:

1. If a lifestyle change is needed, faith tends to encourage discipline so that the changes are followed.

2. The belief that the patient can get well again is transferred from mind to body, which does what it's told.

3. Faith calms and supports, which strengthens the immune system.

4. Prayer gives patients an indirect form of control over their illness. They believe they're not alone in their struggle, and that God is personally interested in them.

5. Patients receiving prayers from organized prayer groups have less mental and emotional distress (and greater rates of recovery). They are encouraged by the numbers of people who believe they may be able to heal and believe that God will be more responsive to so many requests.

One can only imagine what may be discovered in the next millenium!

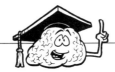

Mindful Moment

Apart from the studies focusing on faith, the investigation into mind-body medicine also continues. Certainly these two areas are related, because your faith determines what you hold in your mind. After reading Deepak Chopra's book *Quantum Healing* (Bantam, 1990), something clicked for me. I knew I could avoid further skin rashes from working outside, and headaches, and I have. If they appear, I think them away. Chopra offers numerous case studies of healing, including patients with cancer and brain tumors. He reminds us that the body knows how to heal a cut. Why not something more?

The Least You Need to Know

➤ Meditation can be a form of prayer, but prayer is more than meditation.

➤ Whether you have prayed your entire life or not at all, there is a prayer style that will help you experience a closer relationship with the Mystery many call God.

➤ Prayer can heal many ills.

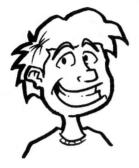

Chapter 9

The Children's Corner

I have four children. I know how difficult it can be to get them to see beyond the latest toy, fashion, or invention. I also know how rewarding it is and how joyful I feel inside when they have experienced a sacred moment.

In this chapter, I'll take you through a variety of ways to help children develop spiritual awareness. Some techniques are especially good for integrating mind and body. Some are activities you may do together as a family or in a group. All are ways that a child may continue to use throughout his entire life.

Keep in mind that each child needs her own way to reach her center. If you have children or are around them, you notice soon enough how very different they are and how they demand your attention in varying ways. Their age, both chronological and developmental, plays a role, as does their personality and interests. Use different techniques while your child grows so she can find the ones that work for her.

But I Don't Know What to Say

When asked to express gratitude or reflect on their lives, children commonly complain that they don't know what to say. Write a letter? What should I write? Talk on the phone? What would I say? (Definitely not a problem as the child hits the preteen years!) Formal prayers from your tradition, from other traditions, and from philosophies are a good starting point. Books that have valuable lessons and memorable characters are another. Pray those words as they are, or reflect on them to see hidden layers of meaning.

Take 5

Innumerable children's prayer books are available in stores. Find one your child likes. Let her pick it out. Use short, simple prayers for young children. Teach your child to memorize his favorites.

More than 200 children's prayer books are listed on Amazon.com alone. Visit the children's section of your bookstore to select one you like. Possible choices include:

➤ *Anytime Prayers* (Harold Shaw Publishing, 1997)

➤ *Blessed Are You: Traditional Everyday Hebrew Prayer* (Lothrop Lee and Shepard, 1993)

➤ *A Child's Book of Celtic Prayers* (Loyola Press, 1998)

➤ *Children's Prayers from Around the World* (Augsburg Fortress Publishing, 1995)

➤ *Could Someone Wake Me Up Before I Drool on the Desk?* (for teens) (Bethany House, 1996)

The following sections describe some fun ways to encourage prayer.

Children learn by doing and by example. Set an example for the child in your life by showing them you pray.
(Image © H. Armstrong Roberts)

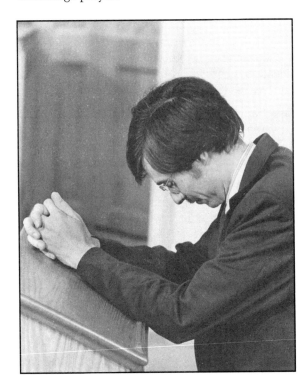

What Day Is It?

Each faith celebrates different holidays and events throughout the calendar year. Use these special times to continue family traditions from your childhood or begin your own customs. These books (and many others) offer suggestions:

➤ *Circle Round: Raising Children in Goddess Traditions* (Bantam, 1998)

➤ *Family Prayer for Family Times: Traditions, Celebrations, and Rituals* (Twenty Third Publishing, 1995)

➤ *The Heart of a Family: Searching America for New Traditions That Fulfill Us* (Random House, 1998)

➤ *Jewish Family and Life: Traditions, Holidays and Values for Today's Parents and Children* (Golden Books, 1997)

➤ *Nonviolence to Animals, Earth and Self in Asian Traditions* (State University of New York Press, 1993)

Use Food

Almost every minute of every day children seem ready for a snack. Use food as the incentive and the reward for saying a prayer. Here are some ideas:

➤ One prayer for each handful of popcorn

➤ One prayer for each piece of candy

➤ Pray for those who grew and harvested the food you're eating

I'm sure you'll discover even more ways to incorporate food into your child's prayers.

Play Ball

Have your family stand in a circle and throw a ball to each other. Whoever has the ball says a prayer and then passes the ball to someone else.

Only One Word Allowed

You or they pick a prayer topic, for instance, people who are sick or happy times you're thankful for. Older children might want to name qualities of a good person. Then take turns saying one-word prayers. For example, just say each sick person's first name.

Tell Stories

Children (and adults) love a good story. Set aside a half-hour each night instead of other activities, or use bedtime for stories. Read stories that teach a lesson or explain a value such as patience or kindness. Or make up your own story and invite your child's help. Better yet, take turns telling each other stories.

Go with the Flow

Children are a bundle of energy. Use that energy and help children harness it in new ways. Use clay and other art materials. Children also love singing, which wakes up your entire being from the base chakra (one of the body's seven energy points, according to Eastern belief), on up. Here are other possibilities.

Dance to the Music

Children love music and love to dance. Any crazy kind of nutty way to throw around their bodies is just fine, thank you. My son and his buddies slip and slide all over the place. A good beat will get anyone's toes tapping.

➤ Use quiet music to calm them down: Have them move to that beat.

➤ Use crazy music to "get their sillies out" before settling down for a quiet practice.

➤ Use music to get them in touch with how their bodies feel and how they work.

➤ Use words and let them move to express how the words feel.

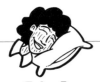

Take 5

Music is the soul's own speech.

This last suggestion is an introduction to danced prayer, or prayer through movement. I taught a series of danced prayer classes to children ages five through seven. In one class, I used a short, simple prayer they all knew: "God is great. God is good. Let us give thanks for this food." Then we went through the prayer line by line.

I asked, "How does your body want to move to show that God is great?" This is not a thought process. It's meant to evoke emotions and encourage kids (and adults) to express them through movement. It's a process to get in touch with the messages of the body. You can try this exercise, too, with or without children.

Chill Out

The kids in my prayer class were so excited that they couldn't wait to show their families their danced prayers. One mom complained to me that her family couldn't eat their dinner until the daughter danced the prayer for them. Don't be like this parent. Celebrate with your child. Don't stifle her blossoming spirituality. She may be more in touch with the spirit around her than you are.

Singing out Loud

Children love to sing. Teach them the songs of your faith, tradition, or others dealing with peace, joy, and love.

For older children, use contemporary music. Listen to the words yourself, and when something strikes you as a value you'd like to reinforce, mention it to your family. Listen to the song together and then talk about it.

Playing Around

The next time your child acts up, give him something to act about. The stage might be a chair covered with a sheet that he hides behind. The story line might be something he knows by heart, or if he is a reader, a shortened version of a story from sacred writings. As for the puppets, colored and cut paper plates taped to Popsicle sticks make fast and functional puppets. Be sure you set aside performance time.

More than 100 books of simple scripts are available on Amazon.com. The variety includes:

➤ *The Dramatized Old Testament* (Baker Book House, 1995)

➤ *Easiest Gospel Plays Ever* (Trudy Schommer, 1996)

➤ *I Witness: Dramatic Monologues from Hebrew Scriptures* (United Church Press, 1997)

➤ *My First Bible Verses: Finger Plays for God's Word* (Concordia, 1996)

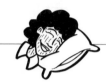

Take 5

For older children, have them rewrite a story from sacred writings so it has a contemporary setting and lesson.

Walking Quietly

Go outside with your child to walk and pray. Doing so will let your child know that the Higher Power may be found anywhere when you are open to receiving it.

➤ Use what you see—the animals, the trees, the water—and talk about what they are and how they came to be.

➤ Pick up a leaf, stone, or flower and examine it closely. Consider its beauty, its use, and its part of a whole.

➤ Talk about all the things your body has to do when walking and give thanks for it.

Don't always talk. Go quietly amidst the haste and let your spirit breathe in the goodness that surrounds you.

Another way to focus a child's (or your) mind and use his energy is to walk a maze or labyrinth pattern. Some churches have permanent ones or even portable ones on large sheets that are put down and taken up during different seasons of the year. They are walked in silence, going from the outer edge into the center, just as you leave the outside world and go inside yourself to find the Mystery.

This famous pattern from a French cathedral is copied on the floor of Grace Cathedral in San Francisco.

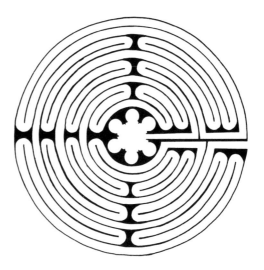

Yoga for Children

Changing poses in *yoga* is good for little and big people who can't stand being still. Practicing some form of yoga or meditation with some regularity can nurture a sense of security and order in children's lives. They learn discipline and control of their bodies. They also understand how peace feels and can recover the feeling whenever they need it. For lots more information on yoga check out *The Complete Idiot's Guide to Yoga* (Alpha Books, 1998) and *The Complete Idiot's Guide to Power Yoga* (Alpha Books, 1999).

Because children like animals and the outdoors, you may want to begin with a few of the poses named after animals or the mountain pose. While showing them the poses, remember to

➤ Keep directions simple and short; children want to *do,* not watch.

➤ Be sensitive to their moods; be flexible.

➤ Let them make up their own poses and teach you.

➤ Stay calm: Your calm presence is as much a part of the experience as the poses.

➤ Teach them to honor and care for their bodies and use them in cooperation, not competition.

➤ Have fun and be joyful.

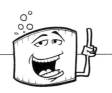

Jacuzzi Jive

The word **yoga** comes from the ancient Indian Sanskrit language and means "yoke," or that all is connected. Yoga is a form of meditation that lets you know that your individual self and the totality of the universe are no different. When you realize this, you experience unity with others and all of creation.

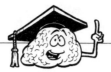

Mindful Moment

Every pose that the body takes has a feeling associated with it. You can experience this just by curling up the corners of your mouth into a smile the next time you feel down. Smiling is good for you. When you're angry, clench your fists and notice how your arms feel. Then unclench your fists and put your hands together in prayer. Feel the difference. You can't hold on to your anger for long with your body in this prayer position.

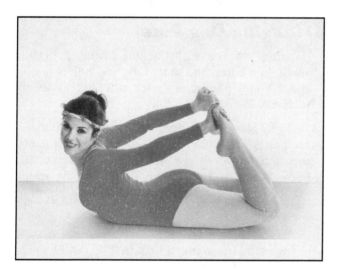

Doing yoga with your children is fun and provides a great stretch, too. Then ask children how their body feels and whether they want to create the next posture. (Image © H. Armstrong Roberts)

Mountain Pose

Mountain pose is a good pose for feeling self-confident and alert. Stand tall, feet parallel and pointing straight ahead. Very slowly raise your arms, palms up, over your head. Your hands do not touch, but remain parallel to each other, reaching for the sky. Stand very tall, as though someone were pulling you up by your fingers. Relax your shoulders. Relax your neck. Hold for a minute or more. Then lower your arms to your sides very slowly. You'll notice you carry yourself straighter and taller after doing mountain pose.

Cat Pose

Like mountain pose, cat pose helps your spine, but in a different way. Get down on the floor on your hands and knees, like you're playing horsy with a young child. Have your back parallel to the floor. Then arch your back, rounding it and lifting it high, and hang your neck and head down. Hold this pose for about 15 seconds. Balance out the movement by doing the opposite: Raise your neck and head and become a sway-back horse. Hold the pose. Repeat the cycle.

Cobra Pose

For cobra pose, lie on your stomach. Raise your head and chest. Hold. Release and lie flat. Cobra pose benefits your abdominal muscles and strengthens your back.

Lion Pose

For this pose, children can stick out their tongues and not get yelled at. Stick out your tongue. Roll your eyes all the way up. Now roar like a lion!

Hanging Dog Pose

Hanging dog pose is a little more advanced, meaning that you'll do it better and more fully the more you do yoga and as your leg muscles stretch out. But this description will serve as an introduction.

Begin by getting in cat pose. Curl your toes under. Then, keeping your weight on your hands and rolling off your toes onto your feet, raise your butt up into the air, so your body is in an inverted V. You'll look like the upside-down version of the V sit you do (or did!) in gym class.

Chill Out

Don't pull your Achilles tendon or a muscle in your calf doing hanging dog pose. If you're not flexible enough yet, don't force your foot flat. Stay on your toes or the ball of your foot.

Faith in Action

There are so many people who are asking for so much help that you will have no trouble finding ways to put your feeling of connectedness into practice. Children love helping, especially when Mom or Dad is doing it, too.

When our youngest was five years old, we found a 5K walk that was raising money for a good cause. With lots of encouragement and a little help, he finished the walk. Was he proud! Another idea is to go out in your neighborhood and pick up the trash along the street. Use the time to talk about pollution or the sacredness of creation. Children remember more and learn better by doing.

Quiet Time

Children need quiet time just as much as we adults do. After spending all day at school with noisy kids and with teachers, my daughter would come home and go directly to her room. As she said, she just needed some peace and quiet for a while.

You can both get some rest and soul nourishment. When I was pregnant with my second child, I would take a time-out every afternoon. I didn't want to tend to anyone else but me in that half hour. During that time, I asked my first child to go to her room for a half hour of quiet play. As I told her, I needed some quiet time.

Time-Out

If you use the discipline of time-out when children act inappropriately, you'll notice that my quiet time sounds a lot like time-out. I hope my daughter noticed the difference; I know I tried to make sure she did. I wasn't angry or upset, just calmly asking for peace. It was also a time she could do whatever she wanted (within reason) without my interference. It helped her discover her ability to occupy herself in satisfying and healthy ways.

Chill Out

Be sure your child is in a childproof environment if he is left unsupervised, even for short periods of time.

Stony Silence

When I use the word *stony* here I don't mean people who grit their teeth, look sullen, and won't speak when they are upset or angry. I'm talking about using stones for stillness and for prayer. Years ago, someone gave my husband a large oval rock that he still has. On it are painted the words: "The greatest architect, and the one most needed, is hope." It sits out in the open, an ever-present reminder both of its message and the caring of the one who gave it.

Children can use stones, too, by painting words on them. In Christian tradition, at Confirmation the Holy Spirit confers the seven gifts of

➤ Wisdom.

➤ Understanding.

➤ Knowledge.

➤ Right judgment.

➤ Courage.

➤ Reverence.

➤ Wonder and awe.

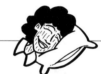

Take 5

Ever mindful of trends, someone has marketed a set of stones engraved with words like "sister," "love," and "peace."

In celebration of my daughter's receiving these gifts, I found seven stones similar in shape and size. I painted the name of one gift on each stone. When she cares to, she can hold that gift, reflect on its meaning, and pray about it. The stone is the physical connection between her and the Spirit.

You may also use this idea of stones when disciplining a child. Make (with your child, because he or she will love painting rocks) a set of stones, each bearing the name of a quality or important idea. If your child has been selfish, for example, you could ask him to sit with the "sharing" rock and think about what that means. If your child has

111

been fighting, use the "peace" or "family" or "love" rock. (Just hope he doesn't throw the rock through the window!)

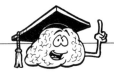

Mindful Moment

Here are some values or qualities that could be used for your sacred stones: loyalty, thankfulness, achievement, confidence, contentment, friendship, balance, learning, action, patience, ethics, faith, hope, courtesy, beauty, pride, love, truth, happiness, kindness, health, prayer, creativity, responsibility, goodness. Look to your faith's traditions for lists of virtues. For young children, be sure to use words they can understand, as well as ones that describe their world, such as share, play, laugh, work, help, sister, brother, family.

Inner Stillness

Sometimes you may appear calm on the outside but be a raving lunatic inside. Your thoughts and feelings are running a mile a minute—and not usually in the right direction! Meditation is a wonderful way for adults and children to quiet down inside.

Meditation works so well for children because it uses their imagination. Children are wonderful at fantasizing and pretending. In teaching them meditation, you can take advantage of this ability. The following are two simple meditations: one with a spiritual flavor and one plain. Take your pick, or use both.

Take 5

There are entire series of books with meditations for children of all ages, including *Children's Book of Poems, Prayer and Meditations* (Element, 1998), *Children's Meditations with Music* (Airplay, 1995), and *Radical Advice from the Ultimate Wiseguy: Solomon's Up-to-Date Insights for Young People* (Bethany House, 1990).

Meditation #1

This meditation uses a child's joy in pretending and settles his body and spirit.

1. Ask the child to sit down and get comfortable. (If he lies down in bed, he may fall asleep, but you can try and use the bed if he is not tired.)

2. Tell him to close his eyes and listen to his heart beating. He'll need to get quiet to do this.

3. Have him imagine a bright, sunny day.

4. Let him pretend where he is, what he is doing, and whether he is alone or with someone else.

5. Tell him he can stay there and enjoy the day for as long as he wishes.

6. When he is done, have him say good-bye if someone was with him.

7. Let him sit for a moment remembering how happy he feels. Then have him slowly open his eyes.

If he wants to share his experience with you, fine. If not, he may never, or he may just not want to at that moment. Older children may want to draw a picture or write about their experience in a journal.

Meditation #2

This second exercise introduces the child to the idea that help and comfort are within her. Self-healing is available throughout life.

1. Begin with steps 1 and 2 in meditation #1.

2. Have the child visualize a door in her heart.

3. Have her walk up to the door and open it.

4. Have her go inside and look around.

5. Ask her: "How does it smell? What do you hear?"

6. Say something like: "You are not afraid, and you are happy. You know that someone else is inside with you. That someone else is (supply a name for the Holy One). He says he loves you very much. See how he smiles at you and how happy he is. Sit next to him and see it raining smiles and hearts and balloons on you. He tells you he will be there whenever you need him or even if you just want to visit."

7. When she is ready, tell her to say good-bye, get up, walk out through the door, and slowly open her eyes.

The child might talk with the Almighty. She could relate sad and happy times she has experienced. Instead of being inside her heart, you could set up the meditation so she is on a beach or anywhere else she chooses and meets God there.

If the child is older when you begin using meditations, then allow time to adjust. He may be squirmy until he gets the idea of how the practice works. In any case, take your cue from him. If he's in the middle of a basketball game with his friends, it's not the time to call him inside for a meditation session! Catch him when he appears ready.

Take 5

Some retreat facilities welcome families with children. Try one on vacation some time.

The Least You Need to Know

➤ You can use a child's natural tendencies toward activity, imagination, and kindness to build lifelong habits of health and community.

➤ Introduce a variety of spiritual practices, from art and dance to meditation and yoga. Your child will remember them and use what seems right for him.

➤ Be models for the children around you. Be peaceful, compassionate, and loving. They will learn by example.

Part 4

Self-Healing Advice Your Mother Didn't Teach You

Mom knew to give you chicken soup for what ails you even before there was scientific proof that soup was helpful. She knew a hug or a kind word could sometimes be more effective than a doctor's prescription. She also knew you had to eat right, have an annual physical exam, and get plenty of rest.

There's lots more known today about healthy lifestyles than what your mom or mine knew. I'll share some of the information with you here in Part 4. It isn't just what you eat, but also how you eat that matters. In addition to exercise, your attitude about your body is also important. Being in bed eight hours doesn't necessarily mean that you're getting a good night's rest. Your day affects your mind and your body while you're sleeping (or trying to).

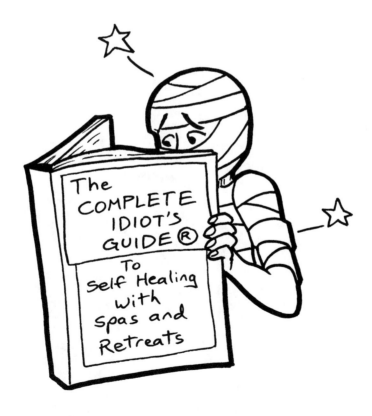

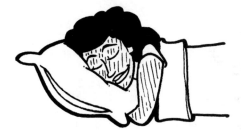

Chapter 10

Lullaby and Good Night

In This Chapter

➤ Understanding the importance of sleep

➤ Recognizing how sleep and stress are related

➤ Deciding how much sleep you need

➤ Getting a good night's rest

I recall taking my then-infant son to a kid's pizza place that featured a stage show of animatronic animals, loud music, and a roomful of rides and games. I became hoarse trying to talk over the noise. He slept through it all. If only we could continue "sleeping like a baby" as we grow up!

Why is it that babies sleep so well? "No worries," as the song goes, has to be one reason. Adults take their troubles to bed with them, consciously and unconsciously. Babies also get their measure of warm milk before sleep. What are you ingesting? If you can stay awake through this chapter, then maybe you'll have a better night's rest at the end of it.

Sleep Is Nature's Medicine

Sleep helps us. We need it

➤ To renew our bodies.

➤ To give our minds a rest.

➤ To interrupt and cut off whatever is creating stress for us now.

➤ To get ready to meet the new challenges of the next day.

One study showed that for healthy adults an average of eight hours of sleep a night is best. Less than six hours is not sufficient for most people's bodies to renew themselves.

Sleeping more than nine hours nightly may indicate illness or avoidance of something or someone who makes you anxious.

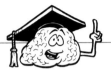

Mindful Moment

"Business affairs fly about like thick dust to belabor our lives; only sleep affords a little reprieve. As for seeing novel things in our sleep—traveling abroad and being able to walk without legs and fly without wings—it provides us also with a little fairyland."
—from *The Quotable Spirit,* compiled and edited by Peter Lorie and Manuela Dunn Mascetti (Macmillan, 1996)

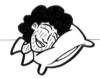

Take 5

Koalas sleep an average of 22 hours a day, longer than any other animal.

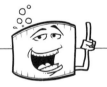

Jacuzzi Jive

REM sleep is the stage of **Rapid Eye Movement,** so named because during this time the eyes move rapidly beneath closed lids. REM phases occur at regular intervals and are associated with dreaming. The rest of one's sleep is spent in **non-REM** sleep. When you are sleeping but not dreaming, you are in the non-REM phase.

How much sleep do you need? Be conscious of your sleep cycle. When do you feel good? A good night's sleep can lower your anxiety and stress levels. When you awake refreshed, you are better prepared to cope with the worrisome situations in your life.

There are other reasons to get a good night's rest. Your brain needs to sleep and dream to remain healthy. Sleeping difficulties lead to fatigue, irritability, loss of concentration, and forgetfulness.

To Sleep, Perchance to Dream

Even when you're sleeping, your body experiences a cycle of waking, sleeping, dreaming, and waking again. Both light sleepers and heavy sleepers go into *REM* and *non-REM* sleep; you need both kinds of sleep to awake refreshed.

Your brain is awake while you are sleeping. When you are in REM sleep, your brain is as active as when your body is in the wide-awake, alert state. Scientists learned this by examining brain wave patterns of sleeping people and people who were awake. The brain wave patterns were the same, as shown in the following figure.

What is your brain working on at night while it is active? It's working on the substance of your life and the content of your dreams. This is why your mental state at bedtime is so important.

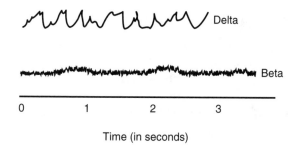

Brain wave patterns are different, depending upon the body's activity. Delta waves occur during restful sleep, but beta waves occur during both dreaming and waking.

Dream Along with Me

You hear people say, "I never dream." Everyone dreams, but people seldom remember what they've dreamt.

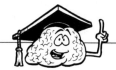

Mindful Moment

If you want to remember your dreams, attitude and preparation help. Show yourself you want to remember: Put paper and pen or a dream journal next to your bed so you are able to reach it easily at night. As you drift off to sleep, tell yourself you want to remember your dreams. If you wake during the night, write down the dream. In the morning, write down whatever you remember as soon as you remember it. To interpret your dreams, check out *The Complete Idiot's Guide to Interpreting Your Dreams* (Alpha Books, 1999) or other books on the subject. Some retreats offer lectures on dreams.

The content of your dreams contributes to a good or bad night's sleep. Scary movies or anxiety can lead to nightmares, disrupting your sleep and leaving you feeling fatigued in the morning. On the other hand, a calming soak and peaceful music (at your home or a day spa) can result in a wonderfully relaxed physical state and trouble-free mental state, and thus a super sleep.

When you're awake, you're not always conscious of how you act or why. You operate on auto-pilot or act to avoid your fears or other worrisome issues. Sleep, however, is a time when anything may come into your unconscious; you cannot censor what you don't want to face. Dreams are an opportunity to reconcile your conscious and unconscious states. Understanding your dreams may lead you to awareness and growth, healing and health.

Take 5

REM sleep has been found not only in mammals, but also in birds, reptiles, and fish. I wonder what a snake dreams about?

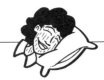

Take 5

Before purchasing a big-ticket specialty bed, consider contacting a medical supply facility (sometimes associated with drug stores) and first rent the item. Use it and see whether it helps. Check whether your health insurance carrier will cover the cost of purchasing one, especially if it's similar to a hospital bed.

Chill Out

When purchasing a futon, consider a thicker pad to allow for flattening over time. You may also stack several pads on top of each other. Also consider whether the style you are buying is convertible to another use (like a sofa) should you tire of sleeping on the futon later.

Sleep Like a Baby

The best sleep is one uninterrupted by internal or external distractions. What's bothering you? Before you can sleep, you need to remedy it.

Bed and Mattress

You know how important your bed is when you have to sleep somewhere else. You remember Goldilocks and the Three Bears, don't you? Mama's and Papa's beds were too soft and too hard. But yours doesn't have to be.

You have lots of choices these days for mattresses. There are orthopedic mattresses, air mattresses, waterbeds, and futons. There are mattresses with dual controls, so you and your partner can dial up different settings of firmness.

Pillows

Pillows come in many sizes, shapes, and styles: down, fiberfill, and even buckwheat hull pillows. There are specially shaped pillows (more like large headrests) that fit on either side of your neck and under your head.

Although it isn't usual to try out pillows in a store, they are wrapped in plastic to keep them dirt- and germ-free. If you feel comfortable, take a pillow and put it on a display bed and try it out. If you buy something that isn't right, take it back or buy another one. Pillows aren't that expensive to deny yourself many good nights' rest.

Bedroom

Do you enjoy your bedroom? "Why is that important?" you ask. Whether you recognize it or not, if you don't feel good about your bedroom, it just might be more difficult, unconsciously if not consciously, to snuggle in and get a good night's rest. Take a look around your bedroom. What don't you like? What would you change? What is wonderful and cozy and restful?

I'm not talking about hiring an expensive decorator, although if money is no object, I suppose that's solution. Rather, consider some inexpensive enhancements such as changing the lighting, wall color, or window treatments—anything that will make the room more inviting and relaxing for you.

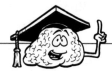

Mindful Moment

When rearranging the furniture in your bedroom, you may want to consult *The Complete Idiot's Guide to Feng Shui* (Alpha Books, 1999). Feng Shui is the art of Chinese placement, which considers the movement of energy in a living space. Meaning, literally, wind and water, Feng Shui seeks to achieve harmony and balance in the home, workplace, and garden by looking at the way the energies of these places and the people who inhabit them interact. When planning furniture placement within a home, for example, a Feng Shui practitioner will also consider the person's birth time, the influence of near and distant galaxies, and the rhythms of the sun, moon, and stars.

Room Temperature

You know how important room temperature is, especially if you sleep with someone who prefers a different temperature. If you are too cold or too warm, you will wake up.

Noise

If noise is keeping you awake, determine what is causing the noise and whether it's something you can control. If you live too near the highway or airport, or your furnace lets you know whenever it kicks on, the best you can do is cover up the noise.

One way to cover disturbing noise is to create your own soothing noise to counteract it. For example, I have a setting on my clock radio that allows me to listen to a variety of water sounds—waves, rain, or waterfalls—with a range of speeds. Such items are advertised in catalogues and department stores. They are inexpensive and work. (Of course, you *could* take off for a watery spa or retreat instead!)

Chill Out

If you're concerned about the possible health effects of electro-magnetic fields from electrical wires and appliances in your home, take Debra Lynn Dadd's advice in *Home Safe Home* (Putnam, 1997): Make electric blankets safer by using them just to preheat the bed; unplug and remove them before retiring for the night.

Another possibility is to buy or make a fountain for your room. These are available in many department, discount, and garden stores, as well as through catalogues. They come in a range of prices from very affordable ($40 to $60) to off the charts. You can also make one yourself, as you will discover in Chapter 15, "Nature Calls!"

Pollution

Sleeping is breathing. If you have difficulty breathing, you have difficulty sleeping. Clean up your bedroom air (if not your entire living space) and you just might sleep better. You might try:

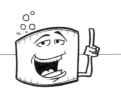

Jacuzzi Jive

A **HEPA air filter** means a high-efficiency particulate air filter. These filters remove potentially harmful particles from the air, but they don't remove gases that pollute the air.

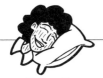

Take 5

You may be able to reduce the negative effects of breathing polluted air by taking antioxidants, drinking pure water, and using saunas and steam baths to eliminate the toxins from your body.

➤ Taking a self-healing break at a desert, mountaintop, or ocean retreat or spa: I'll show you in later chapters how to "import" them for your home.

➤ A *HEPA air filter,* either a free-standing model to clean an area like a bedroom or built into your heating and cooling system for your entire living space.

➤ An activated charcoal air filter system for gaseous pollution.

➤ A humidifier to bring warm, moist air into the room.

➤ Green plants: Dr. Andrew Weil in his *8 Weeks to Optimum Health* (Fawcett Books, 1998) recommends the spider plant, Boston fern, English ivy, and striped dracaena for removing gaseous air pollution.

➤ Removing any materials or items you know that affect your breathing, from animals and cleaning agents to composite construction materials (such as particleboard used in some furniture) and synthetic wall-to-wall carpeting.

➤ Dusting and vacuuming regularly (don't forget under the bed).

Bodily Aches or Pains

Do you know the cause of your aches and pains? If you smashed your fingers in a door, it's obvious, but if something else is causing you regular discomfort, it may be interfering with your sleep.

Check out

- ➤ Your mattress: Poor support stresses the body.

- ➤ Your pillow: It's the proverbial pain in the neck.

- ➤ Massage: Maybe a good rub at a day spa will help.

- ➤ A skilled practitioner who will manipulate your limbs, crack some bones, and re-align your body.

- ➤ Acupuncture: Find out what's needling you.

- ➤ Yoga: Gently stretch yourself into shape.

- ➤ Your mind: What you think manifests itself in how you feel.

Mental and Emotional State

It's up to you to check your worries at the door and not bring them to bed. A mind plagued by thoughts of the next day's test or presentation, a relationship, health concerns, or a difficult child is not at rest or ready for rest. An overactive mind defeats the quietest bedroom and the most comfortable bed. When you finally drift off to sleep, your anxieties may wake you in the middle of the night or haunt your dreams.

You need to find ways that calm you so you are able to invite a peaceful, deep sleep. You might try

- ➤ Changing your attitude: Your mind controls your body. If you approach bed with an "Oh no, not another awful night" attitude or, like my daughter, an "I won't be able to sleep anyway" attitude, you probably *will* have trouble sleeping. Of course, putting pressure on yourself like, "I have to go to sleep," or "Something must be wrong with me if I can't go to sleep" isn't what you're looking for here, either. Instead, every night calmly expect a restful, peaceful sleep. Soon, that positive thought alone will trigger your body's relaxation and sleep mode.

- ➤ Prayer.

- ➤ Taking a walk to "clear your head."

- ➤ Reading, but watch the content.

- ➤ Soothing sounds, such as music or water.

- ➤ Stretching to focus on your body rather than your mind.

- ➤ Breathing exercises designed for relaxation.

- ➤ Journaling: Write down your concerns so you are able to get them out of your head and onto paper.

- ➤ Visualization (using your mind or imagination to see yourself sleeping peacefully).

- ➤ Daily exercise.

Chill Out

Debra Dadd in her book *Home Safe Home* warns of plastics and their potential health hazards. Sheets, bedding, pillows, and mattresses may be made of polyurethane foam, polyester, or acrylic and treated with chemical fire retardants or a formaldehyde-based permanent press finish. These plastics are known to cause health problems in some people. Are they contributing factors to your sleeplessness?

Personal Comforts

What do *you* need to sleep?

➤ Do you need natural fibers such as flannel, wool, silk, or cotton? What touch do you prefer next to your skin?

➤ Do you need a teddy or animal (stuffed or real) with you each evening or when a sleeping partner is away?

➤ Do you need body oil or lotions that provide relaxing stimulation and scent?

Even if you generally sleep well, you may have difficulty when your routine is disrupted due to travel or absence of a sleeping partner. What gives you comfort at home and away? A better night's sleep may depend upon your answer.

Food or Drink

Notice when you drink. Doing so close to bedtime may be uncomfortable and keep you awake. Consuming too much liquid may require trips to the bathroom and interrupt your sleep. Consider not drinking two to three hours before bedtime. What you eat is also important. Stimulants, food additives, or pesticides on food may create sleeping difficulties.

Caffeine

Caffeine is a stimulant and is responsible for many cases of insomnia. Some individuals are so sensitive that a cup or two of a caffeine drink in the morning affects their sleep cycle that evening. Caffeine lurks in

➤ Coffee and tea.

➤ Chocolate.

➤ Colas.

➤ Prescription or over-the-counter medication such as decongestants and cold remedies (check labels or ask).

➤ Diet and energy booster products (check labels).

Pay attention to how much caffeine you consume and how close to bedtime you consume it. Many spas and retreats watch your consumption for you, serving only freshly prepared or vegetarian meals and forbidding all caffeine sources.

Pesticides

Pesticides are sprayed on some fruits and vegetables throughout the growing season to keep them blemish-free. However, pesticides, even regulated ones, are poison, and some of that poison may be left on your food, causing your sleep problems. If you have a problem with pesticides, try organically grown food (or grow your own). Health food stores and even supermarkets these days carry some pesticide-free foodstuffs.

Artificial Colors and Food Additives

Although processed foods are convenient, they often contain artificial additives, coloring, artificial flavors, nitrates, and sulfites, and they also may be packaged in plastic. If you know you eat lots of foods that contain these substances, you may want to eliminate some and see whether your health, state of mind, and sleep cycle benefit.

Drugs

Using drugs to sleep seems like a quick fix, but you're ignoring the dangers of possible addiction, alteration of moods, interference with memory and intellectual function, and the suppression of REM sleep, necessary for good mental health. Besides, when you wake up, you'll have to admit you've only covered up and not dealt with the underlying cause of your restlessness (assuming it's more than a bad mattress or pillow).

I bet there are more factors involved in not sleeping well than you imagined. Clearly, you cannot change everything at once—and you don't need to. Take a few moments to review the list and notice the factors that might apply to you. Then make one change at a time. Remember to expect the best: a wonderful, restful, rejuvenating, deep sleep.

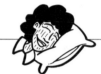

Take 5

Some health practitioners recommend the herb valerian, a mild sleeping aid, because it's not addictive. Valerian is available in capsule and tea form in health food stores.

The Least You Need to Know

➤ Sleep is absolutely essential for your physical and mental health.

➤ The best sleep is uninterrupted and peaceful, of about eight hours duration, with anxiety-free dreaming.

➤ All kinds of factors, from bedding and bodily aches and pains to emotional distress and pollution, can affect the quality and quantity of sleep.

➤ The most important factor in sleeping like a baby might just be a positive mental attitude.

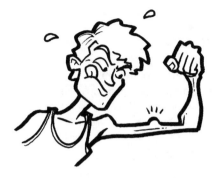

Chapter 11

Let's Get Physical

In This Chapter

➤ Getting in touch with your body

➤ Managing negative self-talk and using positive affirmations

➤ Treating yourself well with massage and mindful movement

➤ Understanding the benefits of exercise

➤ Choosing fitness options that are best for you

In this chapter I'll talk about taking care of your body, but don't expect details on the latest workout trends. I'll show you how to heal your body by changing the way you look at, talk about, and treat yourself. I'll also explain how you can enjoy a marvelous massage.

Next is movement. Whether you need a jump start or want to enhance your current workout, I'll introduce you to a variety of exercise forms. There are the slow, mindful movements of yoga and tai chi. Even if you have a difficult time getting motivated for physical activity, these might be just what you're waiting for. (To help your motivation, visit a spa and try a new workout or activity.) The chapter ends with a rundown of the exercise benefits to mind, body, and spirit, and help in sorting through both vigorous and not-so-active fitness options to find the ones that are right for you.

Mirror, Mirror on the Wall

What do you see when you look in a mirror? Do you see your inner beauty? Do you see your outer beauty? You don't see any beauty? Then I say it's time to start thinking differently about yourself.

Self-Talk

Self-talk can be destructive. If you're telling yourself you're stupid, make too many mistakes, don't know how to handle your job, are a terrible parent, or look ugly, you'll begin believing that. Your actions will reflect these negative beliefs. Your mood, outlook, and health will take a nose dive. You may hide in your room. At the worst, you may believe yourself an unworthy individual who doesn't deserve to enjoy life.

To change self-talk, you need to

➤ Recognize when you're doing it.

➤ Examine the thoughts in your mind.

➤ Determine whether your thoughts are facts or just your low opinion of yourself.

➤ Chase away the bad talk and substitute positive ideas.

Self-talk applies to all aspects of your life. In this chapter, however, I'll focus on how you feel about the way you look and move, your health, and anything else related to your body.

If on occasion, you see some merit to any adverse thoughts, address the issue. For example, if you notice your body is stiffer than it used to be, it doesn't necessarily mean you're becoming old or developing arthritis. It might be that you exercised too long or too intensely, or that you haven't exercised enough lately. Deal with those issues. Your conclusion that you are old or arthritic is a symptom; it's not the real issue.

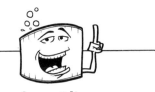

Jacuzzi Jive

Your **self-talk** is your internal thinking process. It's what you say out loud in your head. How much positive or negative self-talk you do affects your moods, your outlook, and your health. **Affirmations** are positive statements, or positive self-talk, that you repeat throughout the day and over many days until the content of the words becomes established habits and beliefs. The words send the message to your mind, telling yourself what you want to accomplish.

Affirmations

Emotional behavior is like physical behavior. Everyone has good emotional habits and bad emotional habits. With practice, you can change your bad habits. Act as if you believe your new thinking, and ignore the old feelings. There is a mind-body connection after all. (Read Chapter 13, "Heal Thyself," for a further discussion.)

To develop better emotional habits and better self-talk, try using *affirmations*. They reinforce changes you want to make and goals you want to achieve. Post your affirmations on your mirror, door, refrigerator, or wherever you will see and be reminded of them during the day. Say them upon waking and before drifting off to sleep. They'll take hold in your subconscious mind.

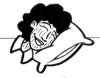

Take 5

If you think of, or write down, all your blessings or good moments, you'll spend all your time on wonderful thoughts, and there won't be any room for self-degrading talk. Maybe you could begin a joyful journal!

One example is this general affirmation created by French hypnotherapist Emil Coue. He said, "Every day, in every way, I'm getting better and better." Others might be:

➤ My mind and body are joyful, relaxed, and at peace.

➤ I release the negative energy from my body and embrace the positive.

➤ I let go of past hurtful emotions and create a bright future.

➤ I have all that I need to shape a satisfying body.

To create your own affirmation or series of affirmations, think of an affirmation as a fill-in-the-blank exercise. Try these beginnings to get you started:

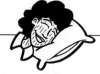

Take 5

An affirmation alarm clock, called the Affirmation Station, records your affirmation and then plays it back, in decreasing volume, for 10 minutes before you drift off to sleep. In the morning, the clock wakes you up by playing your affirmation in increasing volume for 10 minutes. For more information, call 800-779-6383 or go online at www.now-zen.com.

I love _____.

I forgive _____.

I can do _____.

I am a wonderful person because _____
_____.

In creating your own affirmations, follow these guidelines:

1. State them positively. ("I eat healthy foods to nourish my body," not "I am on a diet.")

2. Make them in the present tense. ("I move with grace," not "I want to move with grace.") The present tense tells you you already have what you want.

3. Make the statement short and simple. One sentence is best.

4. Aim for some drama and excitement in your statement. Give your body and mind something to hold on to.

5. This is your statement. Make it about you alone. ("I accept help when needed," not "I want others to help me.")

6. Be sure your affirmation is realistic.

7. Your affirmation states your goal, not a list of all your objectives in reaching that goal.

Now that you have a clear affirmation, believe in it, and trust that it will happen. Be aware of people or occurrences around you that may lead you to your goal. Don't worry about how it will occur; just know that it will.

A Temple Within

Don't get nervous. You don't have to do anything differently. In fact, you don't have to do anything at all. You *are* a temple.

In ancient times, people built monuments of stone to honor or house the object of their worship. These sacred places allowed people to feel closer to their holy ones. For example, Solomon built the great temple in Jerusalem that housed the Ark of the Covenant.

But Solomon knew that God was with the people wherever they were, not just in the temple. Fortunately so, because the temple was destroyed, rebuilt, and destroyed for good, except for the western wall. Later, followers of Jesus wrote about how God not only dwells in the place of worship, but in different ways also dwells in each one of us.

What's More Important?

Which do you believe?

➤ You are a body who happens to have a spirit.

➤ You are spirit who happens to dwell for a time in a body.

If you believe the first statement, you want to care for yourself so that you live as long as possible, don't you? If you agree with the second statement, then surely you need to respect your body so that it can provide for your higher spirit's purpose.

Reflections on Your Body

You can use a variety of sources as the basis for reflections about your body. If you're tempted to read through them all now, go ahead. But then come back later and reflect on each one individually. Notice that they come from different traditions, and some are not particularly spiritual. Use them to connect with your body and accept it for what it is—and perhaps even grow to honor and revere it.

Some Writings for Inspiration

Readings, workshops, and the comments of others may offer nuggets of wisdom worth considering for a longer period of time. I offer you a few thoughts which have given me pause:

> The body has to be looked after: one has to be very caring about the body and very loving to the body. And then, its very spontaneity purifies it, makes it holy.
> —Osho (1931–1990)

Sow an act, and you reap a habit.
Sow a habit, and you reap a character.
Sow a character, and you reap a destiny.
—Charles Reade (1814–1884)

You never identify yourself with the shadow cast by your body, or with its reflection, or with the body you see in a dream or in your imagination. Therefore you should not identify yourself with this living body, either.
—Shankara (788–820)

Do you not know that your body is a temple of the Holy Spirit within you, whom you have from God, and that you are not your own? For you have been purchased at a price. Therefore glorify God in your body.
—1 Corinthians 6:19–20

These bodies are perishable; but the dwellers in these bodies are eternal, indestructible, and impenetrable.
—The *Bhagavad Gita* (500 B.C.E.)

Meditation on the Body

This meditation is adapted from one used in a series of classes I attended. Because it is long, you would do well to tape record it so that you can play it back for yourself when you meditate. When you do, be sure to leave pauses after each step.

1. Begin by sitting tall, feet on the floor, hands comfortably in your lap.

2. Take a few deep breaths. Quiet yourself.

3. See how you feel.

4. Do a scan of your body, starting with your feet and going all the way up, just to notice how you're feeling.

5. Say hello to your body, to your feet, your legs, and your other body parts up to your neck and ears.

6. Take some time to appreciate, validate, and be grateful to your body for all it does for you. It pumps your blood, carries you around, works your kidneys, regulates your breathing, and does all those things you don't have to think about.

7. Try to get into a spirit of deep appreciation and gratitude for your body.

8. Listen to what your body has to say to you. Is there tension, pain, soreness, or discomfort?

9. What is your body trying to tell you that you need to pay attention to?

10. Focus in on one area of your body that really wants to communicate with you.

11. In your mind, finish this statement, "If this part of my body could speak to me, what it wants to tell me is ..."

131

12. Try to think of some things you could do to take care of the problem your body is telling you about. For example, if your heart is feeling constricted and lonely, you could decide to reach out to some people. If your head is hurting, maybe you are overworking your left brain.

13. Think of a plan to address the problem in your body.

14. Commit to that plan.

15. Put your body on release mode. See your body releasing built-up tension, pain, and discomfort. You could visualize a vacuum sucking up all the debris, see a garbage chute carrying all the negative stuff away, or see your blood clearing all the junk out of your body, down through your legs, and into the earth.

16. Release; release; release.

17. Anything you felt bad about in the past, release it. Release; release.

18. Release fear. Fear blocks your body. Release; release; release.

19. Think of somebody you're holding a grudge against. Where are you holding that unforgiveness in your body? Release it; release; release.

20. What is your most negative thought about yourself, whether it's from you or others? That negative thought is in every cell of your body. Release it; release; release. Let it flow out of you.

21. Now that you've released all these negative things, your cells are empty. They're like billions and billions of little chalices waiting to be filled. You will fill them with holy light.

22. Allow yourself to see a golden, radiant sun, and let the rays come down and fill up those cells.

23. Within yourself, look up at the central sun. See that place in the central sun where that ray comes from. Let a little miniature of the central sun float down on top of your head and begin to shoot the most intense bright light into your body.

24. Feel that holy light spread throughout your entire being.

25. Put your palms up, and allow that light to fill your mind, your heart, your legs, your arms, and every cell in your body.

26. Feel the brightness as it increases in intensity. It becomes brighter, brighter, and even brighter.

27. Approach the most brilliance you can imagine.

28. Let that brilliance fill your entire body and shoot out of your hands, so you are receiving and giving.

29. Let that brilliant light continue to cleanse you and burn away negative thoughts. In particular, let that sun enlighten you, shine away your fears, and allow you to really trust.

30. As the sun continues to shine on and through you, let yourself understand that your being and your skills originate in this sun, your God-given abilities.

31. Now let the sun set into the center of your body, where it continues to radiate light.

32. Allow yourself to feel the magnificence of your own divinity.

33. As you are in this light, feel its peace, its wisdom, its joy, its knowledge, its courage, its compassion, and its love.

34. Maintain your awareness of your peace, wisdom, joy, knowledge, courage, compassion, and love as you slowly open your eyes.

35. Come back into the room, bringing your focus to where you are seated. Notice how you feel.

36. Allow yourself to enjoy another undisturbed moment. When you are ready, rise or sleep.

37. Bring this center of love with you into the rest of your day, and radiate your peace, wisdom, joy, knowledge, courage, compassion, and love to others you meet.

Reflecting on Your Reflections

After a long meditation like that one, hold on to your feelings and thoughts. Use your experiences to do the following:

➤ Learn a better frame of mind and how to stay in it even when you're not meditating.

➤ Understand your body better and recognize when you need healing.

➤ Forge the connection between your body and your emotional, mental, and spiritual state.

➤ Join in the cosmic dance, giving and receiving every day.

➤ Record your feelings in a journal and compare them over time.

Your body will reward you for taking care of it. As you become at ease with the process, you'll be able to do quick body scans even while you're walking from your desk to a meeting or as your children are running up to you after school.

Now that you're more in touch with your body, you may want to consider some types of slow movement that combine your awareness of body, mind, and spirit.

Yoga for Everyone

Don't be frightened off from yoga by pictures of advanced yoga practitioners twisting themselves into pretzels. My husband has limited movement in his joints, but he participates in and benefits from a short, daily yoga routine of gentle stretching. Yoga grows with you in two ways: The more yoga you do, the better you are at it and the more benefit you get from it. You can do yoga, no matter what your age or fitness level.

At a weekend retreat, I led a morning wake-up routine using yoga and dance poses for women mostly over age 60. They hadn't done this kind of stretching before, but no one complained. Those slow and controlled poses offered a good stretch even for those who were more physically fit.

There are many types of yoga, and there are many good books, including *The Complete Idiot's Guide to Yoga* and *The Complete Idiot's Guide to Power Yoga,* so I'll mention only a few points here. (You can find a brief description of some simple yoga poses in Chapter 9, "The Children's Corner.")

Great Yoga at Spas and Retreats

You can have some wonderful yoga experiences at a spa or retreat that will get you off to a great start in yoga or enrich the yoga you may already do. I speak from experience here: I participated in a week-long retreat one year in California that included a daily yoga session. My husband and I also attended an intensive (30 hours) weekend yoga retreat in Hawaii.

Activities like yoga make you aware of your body and how it feels and how it is moving. In the process, your mind must let go of other thoughts, including those that may be causing you anxiety or distress. You may be able to do two things at once, like talk and walk, but you cannot think about two things at once!

Benefits Aplenty

The advantages of yoga are many:

➤ You don't need equipment to do yoga.

➤ You don't need special clothing (anything loose works) to do yoga.

➤ You can do yoga almost anywhere: at home, in the office, or while traveling on business.

➤ Yoga improves your physical condition.

➤ Yoga improves your mental outlook.

➤ Yoga can address specific problems such as a sore back or daily headaches.

Just remember, though, simply getting your body into some poses won't make you relax or tune into an inner space. You need some discipline, concentration, and the right attitude.

Yoga Basics

Yoga improves and conditions every part of the body. Yoga is a system of self-development which involves discovering truth, the truth of your purpose, of your being, of life, and of your relationship to and identification with the Supreme Being. In order to do this, yoga believes that your body and your mind, which tends to wander toward external objects, must be harnessed and directed.

Yoga as a philosophy is more than just bodily positions. The controlled breathing and slow, disciplined movements help you transcend your mind and body and achieve truth wherein the individual soul identifies itself with the supreme soul or God. The philosophy of yoga is that man, animals, birds, fish, trees, earth, rocks, and elements are one. Yoga as a philosophy also includes

➤ Diet.

➤ Moral values.

➤ Reincarnation.

➤ A relationship to a higher force.

However, even if you practice your own spiritual principles and use only the poses of yoga, you still will gain awareness and peace.

Tai Chi

Tai chi chuan, often called tai chi, is a Chinese form of moving meditation. Tai chi offers a calm awareness of the spirit, an alert mind, and a flexible, strong body. It helps you slow down and grow in patience. When you practice tai chi, you move the body's energy to promote good feelings.

As a practice in patience, try this tai chi walking exercise. How long can you wait until you take the next step? It's not a matter of thinking; the right time will show itself.

1. Stand with your feet comfortably apart, back straight and tall, and your head aligned over your neck and spine.

2. Hold your arms out in front of you as though you were holding a large ball.

3. Begin to walk forward.

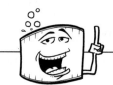

Jacuzzi Jive

Yoga is a practice developed in the East, using postures and controlled breathing to stretch and tone the body, improve circulation, calm the central nervous system, and experience a meditative and whole state of being.

Tai chi is a Chinese martial art form with a constant flow of energy, combining mental concentration, slow breathing, and graceful dance-like movements.

Take 5

The key to relaxation in tai chi is the idea of sinking your weight. Feel so bound to the ground that you are as one; feel that your feet have roots that go down as your body reaches up.

4. Hold your arms in front of you as you walk.

5. Place all your weight on the forward foot. Only then lift your back foot.

6. As the back foot is now the forward foot, wait until all your weight is shifted onto this forward foot before you lift your back foot.

7. As you move side to side, collapse into your hip and feel all tension moving down through your leg, through your foot, and into the earth.

As you move, keep your head level and try not to bounce. Practice patience, waiting until the time is right to take the next step. (This is a good motto for life, too.)

Feldenkrais

The Feldenkrais method of movement combines awareness, attention, and imagination. There is no goal to achieve, except to discover what makes your body comfortable and uncomfortable.

In each session, you isolate one body part, for example, your arm. You lie on the floor, see how far you can stretch your arm, and notice whether it is a complete or restricted movement or whether there is any pain. You can use Feldenkrais therapy to discover

➤ Where you are holding tension.

➤ How you can relieve tension.

➤ How to open up and let go.

➤ How to be comfortable in your body.

Chill Out

Be extremely cautious when operating a moving vehicle after a massage session. One time I was so relaxed that when a police officer stopped me for going through a stop sign, I replied, "What stop sign?" I know of someone else who had a car accident on the way home from a massage. Oops.

You can take a quick course in Feldenkrais or make it a lifelong pursuit like yoga or tai chi.

Maybe You "Knead" Massage

Massage relieves muscle contractions, stimulates circulation, and relaxes your mind and body. There are a variety of methods, and you can get lots more information from many good books, including *The Complete Idiot's Guide to Massage,* and, of course, at spas and retreats.

Touch is an incredibly important part of life. Animals and infants who grow up without touch (hugging, playing, sitting, kissing, holding hands) are emotionally stunted. Touch opens up pathways to emotion. When you are holding onto destructive feelings, touch can help you relax and allow those emotions to surface so that they can be dealt with and cleared away.

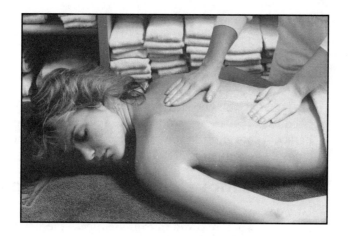

Show your body you love it by giving it a massage. Your body will welcome the healing touch, relief for aching muscles, and movement to release toxins.
(Image © H. Armstrong Roberts)

Your massage therapist is not a counselor, so you may not want to voice your stress or unhappiness. However, it is a good idea to let him or her know whether you're experiencing tension or pain. It may take only a light stroke for your body to release the pain, sadness, or tension in a river of tears. I know from retreats I've been on that men may experience a tearful release from massage just as often as women.

More Movement: Exercise

Exercise is good for you, body, mind, and spirit. A simple walk around the block lifts your spirits. Yoga and similar disciplines are great as calm, effective movement. Some days you may want a change of pace, or perhaps you prefer a more invigorating workout all the time. If you want company, inspiration, or great ideas from new teachers, enjoy a new or familiar fitness program at a spa. It can be like a shot in the arm (and the legs!).

It's Natural

Remember the fight-or-flight response from Chapter 2, "Simon Says Sit Down"? When your body thinks it is in danger, it goes into a stress response and produces hormones that put you in a state of height-ened physical arousal. You are now ready to fight or flee. However, because stressors today are more often psychological than physical, many people don't have

Take 5

In many cultures, abundant tears are expected to commemorate deaths, births, weddings, and tribal ceremonies. People who do not or cannot cry are considered hard-hearted and not very evolved individuals.

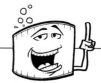

Jacuzzi Jive

I'm using **exercise** in a broader context here. I'm not concerned with exercise for weight loss, although that may happen. Neither am I focusing on strenuous physical activity. Rather, I'm talking about activities that offer mental or physical release of tension and thereby promote relaxation, stress reduction, and a sense of peace.

a proper outlet for release of this stress. You may want to punch out your boss, but it's frowned upon. You may be tempted to run away from another overtime assignment, but then you might also be "running away" from your job!

Chill Out

Exercise can be overdone. Randall Cottrell, author of *Stress Management* (Dushkin Publishing, 1992), cites a report showing that runners who trained more than 45 miles a week had stress hormones in their bloodstream. In fact, the levels were as high as those in patients suffering from depression or anorexia.

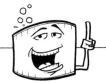

Jacuzzi Jive

Aerobic exercise, such as running or mountain biking, conditions your heart and lungs because you are taking in more oxygen to help your body cope with high levels of exertion. **Nonaerobic** exercise, such as yoga or slow walking, does not raise your heart rate, is more serene, and does not require greater amounts of oxygen to fuel your body's active needs.

Besides, you're moving anyway when you're stressed out. When you're feeling stressed, do you tap your feet, tap a pencil, rub your fingertips together, or suddenly need to get up and go somewhere, anywhere? These behaviors are all little ways to get rid of extra nervous energy.

A Little Movement Won't Kill You

One positive way to deal with stress is daily *exercise*. The muscular work involved in exercise breaks the stress response in your body. Studies show that exercise eases tension, regardless of how fit you are. A series of studies in the 1960s at the University of Southern California called it the "tranquilizer effect." And exercise addiction has none of the deadly health risks associated with the pill variety.

Other benefits of physical exercise include: improved breathing (deeper, fuller breaths), increased stamina, better digestion, increased energy and less overall fatigue, decreased appetite, a better frame of mind, improved ability to think, and easier and better sleeping. With a clear head, satisfied body, and positive attitude, you can approach any event with confidence.

Range of Motion

So what kinds of activities do I recommend? You can choose from

➤ Competitive sports.

➤ Individual activities.

➤ Controlled movements (such as tai chi or yoga).

➤ Mind sports (such as puzzles, crossword puzzles, or chess).

➤ Creative outlets (such as painting or woodworking).

Whether you choose *aerobic* or *nonaerobic* exercise, you may experience

➤ A sense of control or achievement.

➤ A break from daily worries.

➤ An opportunity to socialize.

Just be sure you find the activity pleasant. If you're using the activity to calm yourself, you don't want to choose something that upsets you. Therefore, you need to know yourself. If you can't stand losing, don't go in for competitive sports because you can't win all the time!

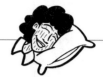

Take 5

Energize your brain with exercise. Studies show that aerobic exercise increases thinking ability.

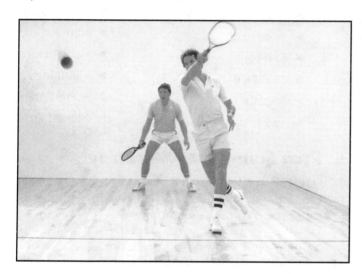

Engaging in activity is one way to relieve stress. If you are concerned about your performance, however, watch that you don't increase your stress level by playing competitive sports.
(Image © Artemis Picture Research)

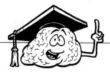

Mindful Moment

After a hearty laugh, your heart rate, blood pressure, and muscular tension drop below their normal levels. As Norman Cousins said in his book, *Anatomy of an Illness* (Norton, 1979), just 20 minutes of hearty laughing gave him two hours of painless sleep. He called laughing "internal jogging," a kind of sedentary aerobic exercise. (That's jogging anyone can get into!)

Chill Out

Pressuring yourself to add a major exercise routine to a life already in a state of high stress isn't a great idea. Begin gradually. Even a five-minute walk at lunch, for example, is great. Increase the time you exercise over a period of weeks. Don't use time pressures as an excuse! It's precisely because you have such pressures that you need physical activity.

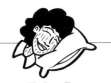

Take 5

Make a daily appointment with yourself, even if for only 15 minutes. Schedule it. Put it on your calendar and do not cancel!

Surely you can find an exercise you enjoy in this list:

➤ Laughter (sounds great to me)
➤ Bicycling
➤ Walking
➤ Golf
➤ Swimming
➤ Fencing
➤ Bowling
➤ Gardening
➤ Jogging
➤ Tennis
➤ Basketball
➤ Baseball
➤ Handball
➤ Squash
➤ Paddleball
➤ Table tennis
➤ Pool
➤ Badminton
➤ Volleyball
➤ Dancing
➤ Playing an instrument
➤ Singing
➤ Photography
➤ Horseback riding
➤ Jumping rope
➤ Calisthenics
➤ Climbing stairs
➤ Weight training
➤ Martial arts

Pick Something, Already

Don't get stuck trying to choose an activity. Surely you can find something that you like. If you don't like one thing you try, choose something else. It's okay to switch. Some people switch regularly; it's called cross-training, which encourages you to include different activities each week so that you use different sets of muscles.

Next, decide if you'll go it alone, or get a friend or group for company. Then, see if you'll exercise

➤ At home, with or without a video or TV show.
➤ In the neighborhood, streets, or park.
➤ At a local health club or gym.
➤ At a spa, wellness center, or retreat.

If you're interested in doing something different or need some extra motivation, consider kicking off your exercise routine at a spa or retreat. These places have staff who are friendly, knowledgeable, and available to meet your needs.

The Least You Need to Know

➤ Your health—physical, mental, and spiritual—is more than exercise and healthy living; it's a matter of your body image.

➤ Monitor your self-talk, and use affirmations and reflections to achieve your goals and connect with your spiritual self.

➤ Take care of the temple that you are with massage and mindful movements such as yoga, tai chi, or Feldenkrais.

➤ Physical exercise releases stress and tension, elevates your mood, and adds to overall health.

➤ Spas and wellness centers are excellent for enhancing your body awareness and introducing you to new forms of movement and exercise.

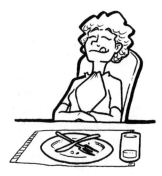

Chapter 12

Restful Repasts

In This Chapter

➤ Avoiding stress–filled foods

➤ Making healthy food choices

➤ Feeding your spirit as well as your stomach

➤ Making mealtimes more special

Just about every supermarket tabloid and woman's magazine has headlines promoting weight loss, delectable desserts, and quick recipes for the person on the go. These are hot-selling topics to be sure, but isn't there more to food? Yes, much more.

There's the connection between your emotional state, your physical state, your nutritional needs and habits, and a spiritual consciousness, for example. This chapter explores some aspects of food far removed from speedy meals, calorie counting, and fat grams.

Food and Feelings

If you're trying to get your life under control and become more relaxed and at peace, take time to examine your eating habits, not just your diet. Change your thinking, your feelings, and your behavior regarding food. Time away at a spa or wellness center with healthy food and nutritional information can get you on the right track.

Emotional stress affects your eating habits. Some people are "emotional eaters." When the going gets tough, they go into the kitchen, the cabinets, or the fridge and eat. People eat for comfort, as a pick-me-up when they're blue, as a distraction or a break, and for a special treat when all else fails. The problem is, people often eat the wrong foods during such times, and these foods can add to their stress.

Caffeine Culprits

Certain foods can cause your body to go into a stress response, just as though you were reacting to a stressful event, especially if you're not used to having that food. The most common kind of food that causes this response is caffeine, which may be found in coffee, tea, chocolate, colas and some other carbonated beverages, and certain over-the-counter medicines, such as products for weight control, colds and allergies, pain relief, and menstrual aids. If you're already under stress and reach for one of these foods, you may unknowingly increase your stress response rather than help soothe it. Too much caffeine can cause anxiety, an inability to concentrate, irritability, and intestinal upset.

To calm you (not pump you up even more), soothe stomach upsets, and make you feel better overall, try the following instead of caffeinated foods:

➤ Licorice or a licorice extract (called DGL), available in health food stores

➤ Herbal teas, such as chamomile or peppermint

➤ Japanese green tea, which contains about a third of the caffeine found in black tea

➤ Dim lights and soothing music

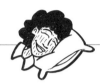

Take 5

Studies show that green tea appears to offer anticancer effects, as well as helping to prevent strokes.

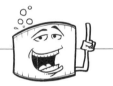

Jacuzzi Jive

The **B complex** is a group of 10 vitamins that primarily works with enzymes. Together, these vitamins change the food you eat into nutrients your body can use.

Sneaky Sweets

Ah dessert! It's associated with good times: birthdays, anniversaries, and other celebrations. It's no wonder then that when you're a little down, you might reach for a sugary sweet, hoping it'll cheer you up.

The B Vitamin Robber

But high levels of sugar aggravate the stress you're already feeling. When your marvelous mechanism (your body) has incoming sugar, *B complex* vitamins have a role in breaking down that sugar. Those vitamins are not in most sweets, so your body goes looking elsewhere for them. Problem is, your body also uses B complex vitamins to control stress. When you take in too much sugar, you use up some of your B vitamins to break it down and may not have enough B vitamins left over to meet other bodily needs. In other words, your quick sugar fix is a bad idea!

Sugar Highs Lead to Sugar Lows

There's another reason why too much sugar means trouble. When sugar is ingested, the body produces insulin to break down the sugar and distribute it (diabetics can't produce enough insulin, so they need to take it as a medication). If you take in lots of sugar, your body produces lots of insulin, which can send your blood sugar to below normal. This unhealthy state is called *hypoglyce-mia*. Symptoms include anxiety, irritability, fatigue, trembling, and/or increased heart activity.

Bottom line: When you're feeling stressed, don't reach for sugary food. If you need a sweet, try fruit, which contains natural sugars, for example. Then go out, get some fresh air, and take a short walk.

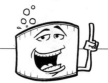

Jacuzzi Jive

Hypoglycemia is a level of blood sugar (glucose) too low for normal function. Not itself a disease, hypoglycemia is a symptom of a problem and must be treated. Brain function, for example, is especially dependent on adequate levels of glucose in the blood.

Calming Catastrophes

There are other foods people use to calm themselves. Let's look at some of them. These items may not increase your stress response as caffeine and sugar do, but lots of them in your diet can lead to other health problems.

Forget the Fat—Mostly

A slice of pizza here and a handful of buttered microwave popcorn there adds up. When you reach for the snack food, check the labels. Although your body needs some fat, too much fat—especially saturated fat—is not good and is associated with heart disease, cancer, obesity, and diabetes. Healthier eating trims the fat and relies more on monounsaturated fats, the kind found mostly in olive and canola oils. These fats also may have beneficial effects on your cardiovascular system.

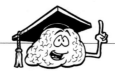

Mindful Moment

Herbs may be more than just pleasant taste sensations; they are gaining popularity and credibility as agents of healing and health. For more information on the possible benefits of herbs, check out this Web site: www.herbsthatheal.com.

Shun the Salt

Snacks and prepackaged and processed foods contain large amounts of salt (look for sodium on the label). Too much salt can cause swelling, fluid retention, and weight gain. Most authorities also agree that salt should be limited in persons suffering from hypertension (high blood pressure).

Do you need even more salt on those fries? If you can't resist that favorite yummy that helps you feel good, see whether it is available in a low-sodium variety. When you are doing the cooking, try substituting spices, seasonings, and herbs in place of salt.

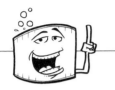

Jacuzzi Jive

Simple carbohydrates are called sugars and include honey, jams, syrup, table sugar, candies, soft drinks, and fruit juices. **Complex carbohydrates** are starch and are found in whole grains, vegetables, seeds, legumes, and beans.

Curb the Carbs

It's okay, even healthy, to eat carbohydrates. When you're stressed, carbohydrates can help your body produce serotonin, which calms your nerves. But not all carbohydrates are the same. You need to know which ones to enjoy and which to avoid.

There are two major types of carbohydrates: simple and complex. Simple carbs are broken down quickly into sugar in your body. Examples of simple carbs are corn syrup, fruit juice, white sugar, white rice, and white flour. Eating too many simple carbs puts too much sugar into your body too quickly and may cause the high insulin/low blood sugar reaction described earlier.

On the other hand, complex carbs break down more slowly and are higher in vitamins, minerals, and fiber. Find them in whole fruit, whole grains, legumes like peas, beans, and lentils, and whole-grain breads and cereals.

Take 5

A professor of mine was fond of saying, "The whiter the bread, the sooner you're dead." The adage describes the better choice of complex carbs found in whole grains.

Ax the Alcohol

If you're not ready to become a teetotaler, at least monitor how much you drink to calm down after a hard day. The Dietary Guidelines for Americans recommend that men drink no more than two drinks daily. Women are limited to one drink. A drink is defined as $1^{1}/_{2}$ ounces of whiskey, 5 ounces of wine, or 12 ounces of beer.

Excessive alcohol can stress your liver. It also depletes B vitamins (needed to control stress, remember?) and many trace minerals, not to mention the extra calories in it. Consider trying some new teas or juices to add variety to your beverage options instead.

A Matter of Taste

We all don't eat alike. Yet all of us are interested in lowering our stress levels. We're also searching for nutritious foods that can keep us healthy and maybe even slow the aging process. Which one of today's popular dietary approaches suits your taste?

The Vegetarian Diet

A vegetarian is someone who avoids eating all animal products or someone who refrains from eating a few select animal foods. Types of vegetarian-style eaters include:

➤ **Vegans:** Eat no animal products, meat, dairy, or eggs.

➤ **Lacto vegetarians:** Eat no meat and eggs but eat dairy.

➤ **Ovo lacto vegetarians:** Eat no meat but eat dairy and eggs.

➤ **Semi-vegetarians:** Eat no red meat but may eat chicken, turkey, and fish, as well as dairy and eggs.

Vegetarian diets are usually healthier because they are low in animal fat, high in fiber, and naturally high in vitamins, minerals, and other nutrients. Vegetarians generally have a lower incidence of high blood pressure, cancer, diabetes, arthritis, and obesity.

Not everyone can adjust to a vegetarian diet, however. Some people report fatigue, an inability to eat the amount and variety of food needed to get enough of all the important nutrients, or not having enough enzymes in their body to break down all that roughage. Sometimes digestive problems are a result of changing to a vegetarian diet too suddenly. If you can't stomach this diet, you might want to put the emphasis on grains, legumes, vegetables, and fruits and gradually cut out meat.

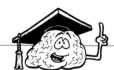

Mindful Moment

I bought into the social consciousness aspect of the vegetarian diet in the early 1970s after the publication of Frances Moore Lappé's book, *Diet for a Small Planet*. The book includes recipes and a message of how you can reduce world hunger by adopting a meatless diet.

The Macrobiotic Diet

The macrobiotic diet classifies each food as either yin or yang, the forces of energy controlling the world, and works to balance them. A follower of the macrobiotic approach eats a diet that is up to 85 percent whole grains and vegetables. All meat, eggs, dairy products, caffeine, sugar, alcohol, and processed foods are absent from the grocery list.

The macrobiotic diet classifies each food as either yin or yang, the opposite yet complementary forces of energy controlling the world. In addition, the methods of cooking are classified as more yin or more yang. The aim of macrobiotic cooking is to create harmony in each meal by balancing yin and yang.

In general, the animal kingdom is more yang. The vegetable kingdom is more yin. Hence, salt, minerals, eggs, meat, poultry, and fish are more yang. Vegetables, nuts, fruits, spices, and sugar are more yin. The food near the middle, especially cereal grains, have a more equal balance of yin and yang.

A macrobiotic diet is popular among people looking for holistic approaches to diseases such as cancer, diabetes, and heart disease. In addition, followers of this diet, as described in *Macrobiotic Cooking for Everyone,* by Edward and Wendy Esko (Japan Publications, 1980), believe the diet is an important part of an alternative lifestyle, which could transform the world into a more harmonious and more peaceful place.

If you're intrigued by macrobiotics, I suggest you do your research before you plunge in, because this diet demands a good understanding of nutrition and a strong personal commitment. Take a weekend or night class or go to a workshop on macrobiotics at a spa.

A to Z Diets

New and old approaches to nutrition collide and become re-invented. The Atkins Diet, for example, promotes the consumption of high amounts of fat and protein, restricting most carbohydrates. The Carbohydrate Lover's Diet does just about the opposite. The Zone Diet is similar to the Atkins Diet, but the Zone Diet allows you to eat more carbohydrates.

The Pritikin Diet supports a low-fat vegetarian cuisine and excludes all meat, poultry, nuts, and whole eggs. Touted as being beneficial in lowering cholesterol and blood pressure, as well as in controlling diabetes, this approach also includes regular exercise and stress reduction. The Stillman Diet is referred to as the water diet. One of these dietary regimes may appeal to you, or you may want to take what makes sense to you healthwise from each of them and incorporate that into your own eating style.

Chill Out

If you change your eating habits, consult a dietician or naturopath in order to ensure that you are receiving a correct balance of vitamins and minerals.

Take 5

Have you ever compared the tastes of a fresh vegetable, a frozen vegetable, and a canned vegetable? Try it some time.

To Your Health

Don't think that you have to follow one so-called healthy diet or, if you do follow one, that you have to eat that way your entire life. No one healthy diet is right for everyone. However you choose to eat, consider these ingredients of your own recipe for healthy eating.

Freshness First

I know what it's like to cook for six people, each of whom has his own food likes and dislikes. I can be lured by the quick and easy solution of prepackaged foods, take-out, and delivery. However, I remember the first time I tasted a fresh pea that I had grown. I was sitting on the ground, stripping the peas from their pods, and depositing them in a bowl. Somewhat apprehensively, I put one beautifully round, green pea into my mouth. It was so unlike the salty, mushy canned stuff I was raised on. Those fresh peas were bursting with flavor and texture.

Another time, I visited a peach orchard in Colorado at the height of the season and sampled a fresh peach from the orchard. I have never, before or since, tasted such a heavenly, juicy peach. My entire being rejoiced at the treat I was giving it.

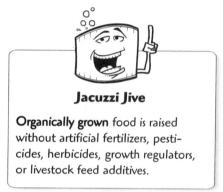

Jacuzzi Jive

Organically grown food is raised without artificial fertilizers, pesticides, herbicides, growth regulators, or livestock feed additives.

Both alternative and conventional medicine agree that fewer processed foods and more complex carbohydrates make a healthier diet. Consider *organically grown* food to minimize your intake of potentially harmful chemicals such as pesticides and growth hormones. Eating a diet high in complex carbohydrates will fill you up and lessen your desire for processed sugars.

Positive Protein

Your body needs protein for cell growth and repair, for your immune system, and to help keep your blood sugar level stable. Proteins are a part of your hair, nails, skin, muscles, bones, and DNA. Whether you get your protein from plant, animal, or dairy sources is up to you, although most health experts recommend that you eat animal protein in moderation.

It wasn't until I began using the recommendations in *Diet for a Small Planet* that I realized plants could be a source of protein. You need to learn how to combine plants, however, to eat the right amount of nutrients from them. Find a cookbook that guides you and enjoy some new recipes while you're at it. Try to have meatless meals several times each week.

Vote for Variety

Eating a greater variety of foods is more interesting and inviting, not to mention healthy. The colors on your plate are more than aesthetically pleasing; they represent various minerals, vitamins, and other nutrients important for your health.

Get out of a food rut. If it's the same old bagel and coffee for breakfast (that's a problem right there), experiment with something new. Eat a different fruit each day. Try a new vegetable or a new recipe each week.

Add variety to your herbs and spices to season your food. Visit your library (I still prefer the touch of a book to the glare of the screen) or the Internet and compile lists of new-to-you herbs. Then use them.

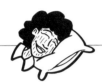

Take 5

Enjoy laughter and good company. As Proverbs 17:22 says, "A merry heart doeth good like a medicine. But a broken spirit drieth the bones."

Eliminate the Negative

If you're not prepared to cut off your supply of caffeine, alcohol, salt, refined sugar, or saturated fats, then limit them.

Savvy Supplements

The Complete Idiot's Guide to Living Longer and Healthier notes a recent survey that found that only 1 percent of the respondents were getting all the recommended vitamins and minerals from their food. That means all of us could benefit from nutritional supplements.

The saying, "You are what you eat," has merit. Food fills emotional needs, has a strong impact on your physical makeup, and affects your psyche. If you want to examine your eating patterns, get advice, or try a different cuisine, go to a spa, wellness center, or retreat that features healthy eating workshops and menus.

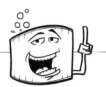

Jacuzzi Jive

To **fast**, as used here, means to completely or partially abstain from nourishment.

To Eat or Not to Eat

Around the world, and in both Eastern and Western cultures, people *fast*. People use fasting for a mix of spiritual and secular reasons, including the following:

➤ Inducing visions and dreams

➤ Gaining discipline over the body

➤ Initiating or maintaining contact with a divine power

➤ Repenting or purifying oneself

➤ Expressing devotion and worship

➤ Preparing for an important event

One more reason for fasting is to connect with all the world's people. When you approach a smaller plate or none at all, you consider those who do not have enough to eat and take time to examine your values and how they are expressed in your eating. Organizations such as Bread for the World and Oxfam, which sponsors an annual fast the Thursday before Thanksgiving Day, help people see alternatives.

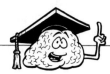

Mindful Moment

Many religious traditions include fasting during some time of their year. Buddhists list fasting as one of the 13 practices that can serve as an aid to leading a happy life. In the Islamic tradition, Muslims observe the ninth month, Ramadan, by not taking liquid or food in the hours between dawn and sunset. Fasting is one of the "good works"—one of the recognized duties of the devout Muslim. For the Jews, fasting is an outward expression of inner penitence; on Yom Kippur, the Day of Atonement, Jews fast and pray for forgiveness of their sins. For Roman Catholics, fasting is still required on certain days of the year.

Whatever your motivation, you might try a simple fast. You may choose to

➤ Go without food and liquid all day.

➤ Eat only one normal-size meal.

➤ Cut back on your portions.

➤ Eat no meat for the day.

➤ Eliminate sugar, salt, alcohol, and caffeine for the day.

➤ Consume only liquids, such as vegetable juices, broths, herbal teas, or water, during the day.

If you try a fast, your attitude is more important than your degree of fasting. Don't look at it as depriving yourself. Rather, reflect on how it

➤ Is healthy.

➤ Helps you appreciate what you have.

➤ Gives you a small understanding of hunger.

➤ Might move you to volunteer or help others.

➤ Frees up eating time to use in other ways.

➤ Might be a sign of an inner conversion to something beyond the everyday.

Finally, don't advertise your practice. This is an inner exercise. You're not fasting to gain sympathy or applause.

If your experience is positive, or at least not a total disaster, try a fast again. Some people fast once a week to give their digestive and intestinal tracts a rest. You may try a monthly fast. If you introduce a fast on a regular schedule, whatever that schedule, your body will welcome it as part of its natural rhythms. Your mind also will be relieved knowing it won't have to plan as many meals.

Detox Now and Again

Your body has its own built-in *detoxification* system. Toxins that dissolve in water are flushed out in your urine; fiber scrubs the colon. As blood circulates through the body, toxins it has picked up are carried to the liver, which is the body's primary filtering organ. Even your skin gets in the act: It releases toxins by sweating.

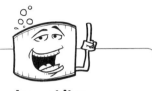

Jacuzzi Jive

Similar to a fast, a **detoxification,** or **detox,** plan helps the body rid itself of toxins that may accumulate from food preservatives, caffeine, alcohol, environmental pollution, secondary smoke, and pesticides and other chemicals in food.

The Body's Response to Detox

Regardless of whether it's called a detox plan, the diet you get at a spa or retreat might just be one. For instance, one retreat I went on served only vegetarian meals: no meat, no dairy, and no eggs; only water and herbal tea to drink; no sugar, salt, caffeine, or alcohol; and limited calories. Yet the group kept up an exercise and yoga regimen and hiked 10 to 15 miles daily. On the fifth and sixth days, the group was offered small amounts of protein.

I experienced what might be a typical reaction to such a diet:

➤ Increased urination

➤ Lightheadedness

➤ A slight headache

➤ Mild nausea

The staff said they knew when the group was detoxing, because by the third or fourth day, they could smell it! (Remember, the skin also releases toxins.)

I did have an unexpected reaction to alcohol as a result of my week, however. I am, at best, a mild drinker. I avoid alcohol, but I drink a glass of wine on occasion and a glass of beer even less frequently. I had no intention of eliminating alcohol, wine, and beer from my life. I just went on retreat. When I returned home, I tried a glass of wine and found I had lost all taste for it; it was awful. For two and a half years, I lived happily without drinking any alcohol.

Some Detox Guidelines

Setting up a simple detox program for yourself doesn't have to be complicated. You might, for example, eat meat, fish, vegetables, and fruit but eliminate the following foods from your diet:

➤ Sugar and artificial sweeteners

➤ Grains, breads, and cereals

➤ Soda (or pop, depending on your part of the country)

➤ High-starch foods such as corn, peas, potatoes, bananas, and peanuts

➤ Butter, margarine, and oils

➤ Sweetened fruit juices

➤ Coffee, black tea, and alcohol

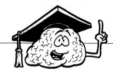

Mindful Moment

When you drink a glass of juice, every part of that juice nourishes and touches every part of your being. Indeed, that juice becomes magnificently transformed; it becomes one with you and is you. How you treat and view your food is how you treat and view yourself and, by extension, others.

Conscious Cooking

How do you eat? When? How often? How are you feeling when you eat? What else are you doing while you eat? Are you hurried or deliberate? Are you upset or at peace?

Do you think at all about the food itself? Where does it come from? How did it come to your table? Who was involved in its production? Consider the existence of life-giving plants and animals that in their dying sustain human life. How is it that one seed produces a tomato and another produces a stalk of wheat? This thinking is being conscious of creation, the creation that also created you.

The mysteries of life are all around you, if you but have the eyes to see. What a gift you give yourself when you approach your meals in gratitude and in awareness of all the forces that come together in that moment. A change in attitude, awareness, and insight promotes harmony within your body and soul.

A number of years ago I watched a simplified version of a traditional Japanese tea ceremony. It added another dimension to my appreciation of what is put before me. Although I am used to giving thanks, I now also notice the colors and variety. I also started using serving dishes rather than placing the pots on the table, as I was raised. Finally, I am more deliberate about remembering all the people, from sower to harvester to grocer, whose lives and care went into the food before me. Eating can be a spiritual exercise, if you let it.

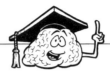

Mindful Moment

The Japanese tea ceremony is based on Zen Buddhist philosophy, and has its roots in the twelfth century, when Zen was reintroduced from China. Its name in Japanese, *cha-no-yu*, means "the way of tea." In the sixteenth century, Sen-no Rikyu, the greatest of the tea masters, applied the four fundamental principles of Zen to "the way of tea." These principles are harmony, respect, purity, and tranquility. The surroundings are an important part of the ceremony, which is conducted in a tea house, or as practiced today, in a special tea room within the home. The most formal ceremony takes four hours, and two types of green tea are served.

In the book (and film) *Like Water for Chocolate* by Laura Esquivel, Tita infuses her emotions in the food she prepares. You, too, can share your sense of gratitude, love, and joy through your food by how you approach the table:

➤ Take a moment to express or just silently feel the gratitude for what is before you.

➤ Chew slowly to savor the flavors and textures and appreciate the natural taste of the food.

➤ Appreciate the table setting, the company, and the cook.

➤ Eat only when you are hungry.

➤ Eat with people you enjoy and only if you are not upset.

Food is a necessary part of life, and being thankful for its abundance is appropriate. In your moments of deeper reflection, if your thankfulness becomes wonder or reverence, that, too, is appropriate.

Do You Have Atmosphere?

Your home is your castle. Do you treat yourself like royalty? What kind of atmosphere do you create for yourself?

Atmosphere is important. Don't you feel happier and more joyful when you put a tablecloth on the table, set out fancy china, and add candles and flowers? I do. If how you set the table lifts your spirits, why not celebrate all the time, not just on special occasions.

To set a happy and relaxed table, pay attention to

➤ The tablecloth or placemats, napkins, dishes, serving dishes, and glassware you use.

➤ Flowers, centerpiece, or candles.

➤ Soothing music.

➤ Time: Don't hurry or answer the telephone during mealtime.

➤ Talk: Encourage pleasant conversation and don't argue!

➤ Sitting a bit after the meal instead of jumping up to clear the table as soon as you've finished.

Look over your table and acknowledge your dining companions. Taken together, you have created a living, beautiful tableau. Appreciate your efforts and your life. Be grateful and content.

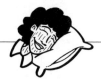

Take 5

When you rate a restaurant, don't you include its atmosphere: decorations, lighting, seating? If atmosphere is so important when eating out, shouldn't it be important when you're eating at home?

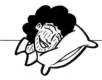

Take 5

For children, serve milk in wine glasses. Change tablecloths or table runners with the seasons or for holidays. Let children create their own special placemat (have them draw or paint a picture and then laminate the picture).

The Least You Need to Know

➤ Monitor your intake of stress- and anxiety-causing foods, especially caffeine and sugar.

➤ Food is an essential aspect of life. Develop a different relationship—even a spiritual one—with food by following a fast or a detox program on occasion and by being aware of and grateful for the hands that produced that which you enjoy.

➤ Find a healthy diet for you by eating a variety of the freshest foods, taking nutritional supplements, and avoiding pesticides and contaminants.

➤ Take time to create a joyful, relaxed atmosphere for your meals.

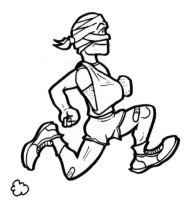

Chapter 13

Heal Thyself

In This Chapter

➤ Understanding wellness

➤ Preventing physical illness

➤ Introducing spiritual healing

➤ Wellness centers you can visit

If only we could drop a few coins into the wishing well, wish good health for ourselves, and it were so. The good news is that simple lifestyle changes can make a big difference in your health. You can't change your genes, but many important health factors are under your control: your diet, activity level, stress level, alcohol or drug use, living environment, and your values and spiritual practices.

This chapter explains how the concepts of wellness and holistic health are connected to traditional and alternative medicines and to spiritual healing. You'll explore the trend toward wellness centers and find out how they offer you opportunities for self-healing. Finally, you'll be introduced to a selection of wellness centers across the country.

In Search of Wellness

Remember the old saying, "An apple a day keeps the doctor away"? I'm not convinced that that's all it takes, but I do think it's true that I can influence my health. Indeed, this belief is at the core of *wellness*.

Drinking from Your Own Well

Wellness is more than the absence of disease. It is a positive state of being that also includes emotional, mental, and spiritual health. These dimensions are all interrelated.

Wellness, then, incorporates a range of behaviors, including

- Fitness.
- Proper nutrition.
- Stress management.
- Social support.
- Self-worth and purpose.
- Spirituality.
- Prevention of illness.
- Health education.

Self-healing and wellness are within your grasp. You influence your health with every lifestyle choice you make.

An Ounce of Prevention

You've probably heard the adage, "An ounce of prevention is worth a pound of cure." Whether you use only conventional medicine or complement it with alternative practices, health care professionals today agree that the patient has an important role in his well-being. Your actions can help prevent many of the conditions that caused death and disease in the past. This is why there is more interest in good nutrition and regular exercise and in reducing or eliminating smoking and drinking than ever before.

Prevention is important for another reason. Most infectious diseases are under control in this country, thanks to advances in immunization. The stress-related conditions, however, need more attention. In Chapter 2, "Simon Says Sit Down," you read about how stress can suppress your immune system and contribute to a host of ailments. Physicians can treat the symptoms, but the patient must prevent or control the stress causing the reaction.

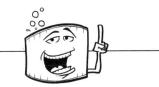

Jacuzzi Jive

Wellness is the intentional and consistent effort to stay healthy and to achieve your highest potential for well-being. When you practice **self-healing,** you accept the responsibility for and make the lifestyle changes necessary for emotional, mental, physical, and spiritual health. Another aspect of self-healing for many is belief in and use of mind-body techniques such as biofeedback and meditation.

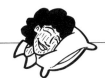

Take 5

Talk with your parents and relatives to get details about your family's medical history. It's good information to have, and it can alert you to lifestyle changes that may help prevent disease for you.

Finding Wellness

New musicians re-record old music. Fashions that went out of style are popular again. So, too, many ancient methods and beliefs about healing are being rediscovered. What this rediscovery means is that more choices are open to us than ever before. More medical choices are available, and spiritual practices can be included as an important part of our physical well-being.

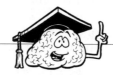

Mindful Moment

Physicians today continue to take the Hippocratic oath, named after the fifth-century B.C.E. Greek physician Hippocrates who emphasized environmental causes and treatment of illness as well as the importance of emotional factors and nutrition in health and disease.

Healing Temples

The ancients journeyed to one of the many temples of the Greek healing god Aesculapius when they were physically or emotionally ill or troubled. For 800 years throughout Europe, the Near East, and the Mediterranean, temple medicine was the primary source of healing.

Healing was a sacred process, a communion between the individual and the gods. To prepare for it, a person would purify himself through cleansing and fasting. He would withdraw from the unhealthy habits of daily life, listen to the stories of miracle cures, ask for advice regarding diet or herbs, and pray for a healing dream. The individual was viewed as a whole person, and mind and body were treated together.

Eastern Philosophy

Old Chinese and Indian texts show how important harmony is to wellness. The familiar yin-yang symbol of balance and harmony illustrates this concept. It was important to have harmony between the individual and the social and natural worlds—between diet, exercise, meditation, and relationships.

Eastern practices rested on the belief that

➤ Positive thoughts can increase our capacity to heal.

➤ Negative thoughts can impede healing.

➤ Medicine and spirituality, when used together, are more effective in helping people heal, as well as maintain health, than when either is used alone.

Holistic Medicine

Each part of you taken together creates the being you are. All parts influence and affect each other. Rather than treating a person piecemeal, *holistic health* offers a perspective different from traditional medicine by ministering to a person's whole being. Holism states that mind, body, and spirit are inseparable. As a result, holistic healing examines an individual's attitudes, beliefs, values, support system, and environment.

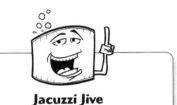

Jacuzzi Jive

Holistic health emphasizes wellness, prevention, and patient education. It focuses on the whole individual and his environment and emotions, his capacity to heal himself, and his role as an active partner in his health.

It also embraces the spiritual aspects of health and illness. For example, you might reflect on the meaning of or learn a lesson from an illness. Continuing a spiritual practice during illness can help you

➤ Endure the illness.

➤ Increase inner strength.

➤ Increase insight and understanding.

➤ Prepare yourself for healing or releasing life.

When this transformation occurs, you heal yourself, spiritually if not physically, and become an inspiration to others. Other people are able to look at how you handled your crisis and may gain some insight about how to deal with their own.

The actor Christopher Reeve is one contemporary example. After a horse-riding accident left him a quadriplegic, he decided to maintain a hopeful and helpful profile for himself, his family, and others, even resuming his professional career. This life of hope is a testament to the unleashed power of the spirit.

The holistic approach to healing is alive and well in 12-step groups. For example, in Alcoholics Anonymous (AA), a disciplined process of recovery occurs when members commit to look within themselves and to make attitudinal and lifestyle changes.

Minding Your Body

The National Institutes of Health reports that "mind and body are so integrally related that it makes little sense to refer to therapies as having impact just on the mind or the body" (from the *Alternative Medicine: Expanding Medical Horizons* report, 1992). So when someone tells you to quit complaining because "it's all in your head," that person may have a point. What can you do that doctors cannot? You can monitor your thoughts, mend your mind, and mind your body. This valuable prescription is free and without side effects.

Mind-Body Conversations

Science has confirmed what ancient healers knew: The mind talks with the body and in that talk, directs the body's behavior. The brain uses the central nervous system and the body's chemical messenger system to convert the content of the mind into nerve impulses and bodily responses.

Biofeedback offers an example of how the mind-body connection aids healing. Initially, an individual is connected by painless electrodes to a machine that monitors the body's response. While meditating, or using additional relaxation exercises, the machine feeds back or signals a patient when his body is showing a relaxation response. After training, the individual is able to use mind exercises to calm the body without the need for the machine.

For additional information on biofeedback training, contact the Association for Applied Psychophysiology and Biofeedback in Wheatridge, Colorado, at 303-422-8436.

Chill Out

Not everyone who uses mind–body techniques to treat an illness succeeds. For a discussion of why, read Dr. Caroline Myss's book, *Why People Don't Heal and How They Can.* For a religious discussion of pain and suffering, refer to the book of Job from the Hebrew scriptures, or Harold Kushner's *Why Bad Things Happen to Good People.*

Emotions Count

Emotions affect bodily responses. Science has shown that the chemicals in the brain can be turned on and off by certain mental states. Your feelings of stress, helplessness, and anger, for example, affect these chemicals. The same is true of the opposite emotions of peace, confidence, and joy. So what does this mean? It means you have the capacity, through your attitudes and actions, to regulate your body's responses.

Belief Counts

Belief in the outcome is essential to healing. Healings recorded in sacred writings describe the seeker's belief in the outcome. *Who Gets Sick: How Beliefs, Moods and Thoughts Affect Your Health* by Blair Justice, Ph.D. (Jeremy P. Tarcher, 1988) collects the scientific evidence and reports that beliefs can actually change the cells of the brain and affect the neurotransmitters that help determine health. One example from the medical journals (Klopfer, Bruno, "Psychological Variables in Human Cancer," 1957) illustrates how belief and outcome are connected. A patient dying from cancer was no longer responding to medications. The patient heard of a new miracle drug and participated in an experimental study. After only one dose of the medicine, the patient responded, to the surprise of the physicians. The tumor shrank rapidly, and the patient's vitality returned.

The patient later read a report concluding the drug was ineffective. He quickly relapsed. When doctors offered him a double dose, the patient again improved. After a second article labeled the drug worthless, the patient relapsed, and he died several days later.

The placebo response (that a person becomes well even when given a sugar pill, for example, because he believes it is an effective medication) is one of the most widely known examples of mind-body interactions in contemporary scientific medicine. Studies have also documented the opposite, or nocebo, effect. In one example mentioned in *Quantum Healing: Exploring the Frontiers of Mind/Body Medicine* (Bantam, 1989), surgeons assumed that an anesthetized patient could not hear and was not influenced by what was said during the operation. It was discovered, however, that the unconscious mind heard every word. When the surgeons said aloud that the condition was more serious than they had thought, patients tended to not recover. Today, standard operating procedure is to refrain from negative comments during surgery. In addition, the more positive the opinions prior to surgery, the more positive the outcome for the patient.

Additional medical cases provide fascinating reading. One describes a woman who breaks out in an allergic reaction when she flies through the air space of the state she connects with her allergy. Dr. Bennett Braun, research psychiatrist and specialist in the field of multiple personalities, has studied and verified different physical characteristics from warts, scars, and rashes to colorblindness and epilepsy in the same person, depending upon which personality is dominant. Researchers are looking for ways to explain these occurrences. Some believe that the mind-body connection is the answer.

Take 5

Meditation is so effective in reducing tension and stress that the National Institutes of Health in 1984 recommended meditation instead of medication as the primary treatment for mild hypertension.

Mind-Body in Practice

The National Institutes of Health lists and recognizes these mind-body therapies as having scientifically established beneficial effects: psychotherapy, support groups, meditation, imagery, hypnosis, biofeedback, yoga, dance therapy, music therapy, art therapy, and prayer and mental healing.

Mind-body techniques such as relaxation methods, visualization or guided imagery, *biofeedback,* and meditation are easy to learn. All are based on the ability of the mind to control the body and many of its functions. What an easy way to get the stress out!

Alternative Paths to Wellness

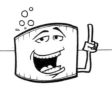

Jacuzzi Jive

During a **biofeedback** session, a special machine gives the individual continuous information about her biological responses. She uses the information to learn to control her body's responses.

Both traditional and holistic physicians may complement conventional treatments with alternative therapies. For example, medication may be used in a serious episode for an individual with asthma, but the physician may suggest lifestyle changes to reduce the number and severity of such episodes. The physician might examine psychological influences, or teach the individual relaxation techniques, or make changes in the individual's exercise and diet to eliminate foods that stress the system.

Holistic practitioners use additional methods. These methods include

➤ Massage and chiropractic massage.

➤ *Osteopathy*.

➤ Acupuncture.

➤ Herbs.

➤ Homeopathy.

Spiritual Well-Being

Spiritual health provides a unifying power that integrates the other dimensions of wellness. Therefore, the relationship between spirituality and wellness is meaningful in your quest for a better quality of life.

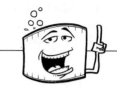

Jacuzzi Jive

Osteopathy is a system of medical treatments based on the belief that physical manipulation of bones and/or muscles can alleviate problems by realigning body parts into their proper positions. **Homeopathy** is based on the idea that "like cures like." Consequently, a patient is given a very diluted solution of a substance that causes symptoms of his disease.

Boosting Your Spiritual Well-Being

How might you increase your spiritual health? Try these suggestions:

1. Be aware of your thoughts. Monitor them, especially negative ones. Learn how to understand and influence your belief systems. Use the personality review in Chapter 3, "Let's Get Personal," to identify concepts you inherited from others.

2. Increase your consciousness by tuning into your body and life and energy. Be aware of your energy, aura, and chakras.

3. Make moments of silence a part of each day.

4. Recognize that an inner force guides you to become more conscious and that a divine force is part of your every thought and action.

5. Get to know better the nature of the God within you.

6. Understand how you participate in the creation of whatever you experience in your life, including your health.

7. Adopt a daily spiritual practice such as prayer or meditation.

You don't enhance your spiritual life through a business-as-usual approach. You need to spend some time each day on your spirit. You need to give it your attention on retreat and at home on a regular basis. Practices such as prayer and meditation nourish your energy system and help unite your mind, heart, and spirit.

You need a healthy spiritual life and a healthy physical life. This is not an either/or situation. You can benefit both by visiting a spa or a retreat. Another option is visiting a wellness center.

Chill Out

Watch out for noise pollution. Guests at a new $900-per-night resort deep in the desert of northern Africa report that the most important luxury of their stay is the silence. Only when you give yourself the gift of a few moments of silence do you realize what you are missing and how intrusive and upsetting all that daily noise can be to body and soul.

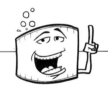

Jacuzzi Jive

Wellness centers are places where people come to learn about wellness and how to change their attitudes and their behavior so they can be as healthy as possible. Neighborhood wellness centers offer drop-in classes and programs; others welcome guests for days or even weeks at a time.

Seeking the Cure

As people search for self-healing, their paths will differ. In former times, people took the cure in mineral baths. Modern times offer more variety. Spas offer beauty and body treatments. Resorts have added fitness and recreational activities. Spiritual retreats may offer workshops in addition to silence. *Wellness centers* provide guidance in staying healthy.

Wellness is a concept first popularized by John Travis, M.D., who established the first wellness center in California in the mid l970s. Such centers emphasize the promotion of health rather than the treatment of disease and educate people in self-healing and self-care.

Wellness centers offer lots of educational programs, with classes and workshops and activities for mind, body, and spirit. The holy is not neglected in holistic work. All wellness centers help you find your healthy lifestyle, but they do it in different ways. The following sections provide a few examples.

Wainwright House

Advertised as the oldest, nonprofit, nonsectarian, holistic education center in the United States, Wainwright House is located on five acres of lawns and gardens overlooking Milton Harbor on Long Island Sound. It has weekend and weeklong programs for groups of 16 or fewer participants. Topics of past sessions included meditation, use of time, intuition, life challenges, and Celtic spirit. It hosts nationally known speakers such as Matthew Fox and Shakti Gawain.

Wainwright House
260 Stuyvesant Avenue
Rye, NY 10580
914-967-6080
www.wainwright.org

Kripalu Center for Yoga and Health

Kripalu Center, another nonprofit organization, uses yoga as the center of its wellness program. Yoga instruction, including how to make it a part of daily life, and related education on topics of wellness and bodywork, self and spirit, and outdoor fitness are described in its 74-page catalog of offerings. Located in the Berkshire Mountains of western Massachusetts, Kripalu also offers a popular weekend or weeklong retreat and renewal program that you design by choosing those activities of interest to you. Workshop topics include those appropriate for individuals, couples, families, lesbians, and gay men.

Kripalu Center
Box 793
Lenox, MA 01240-0793
Phone: 800-741-7353
Fax: 413-448-3333
www.kripalu.org

Omega Institute for Holistic Studies

From well-known speakers such as Ram Dass and Andrew Weil to holistic medical doctors, Chinese herbalists and acupuncturists, and massage, movement, and fitness instructors, Omega offers a five-day "wellness week." In the evening, guests join together for a dance, film, or other gathering. Guests have a choice of accommodations from cabins, dormitories, or campsites while staying on the 80-acre site of rolling hills, trails, and a lake in upstate New York.

Omega Institute for Holistic Studies
260 Lake Drive
Rhinebeck, NY 12572
800-944-1001
www.omega-inst.org

The Raj

You may be surprised to find an Indian-oriented (as in India) facility in Iowa, but that's what The Raj is. Guests receive evaluations from both a Western doctor and an Ayurvedic physician, who prescribes a personal detoxifying program that balances exercise, nutrition, herbal treatments, and bodywork. Located on 100 acres of meadows and woods, The Raj also offers aromatherapy, skin treatments with ingredients imported from India, and vegetarian cuisine with, you guessed it, Indian flavors. Special programs for weight loss, diabetes, asthma, and hypertension are available.

The Raj
1734 Jasmine Avenue
Fairfield, IA 52556
800-248-9050
www.theraj.com

Harmony Hill Wellness Retreat Center

This wellness facility offers general programs for women in transition (menopause) and stress reduction and renewal, but it especially targets persons who are living with cancer and their family support and other caregivers. Three- and five-day retreats are available on this 12-acre property at the Hood Canal overlooking the Olympic Mountains. Three labyrinths, two outdoors and one indoors, help guests connect spirit and body.

Harmony Hill
7362 E. Hwy 106
Union, WA 98592
Phone: 360-898-2363
Fax: 360-898-2364
E-mail: harmony@halcyon.com
Web site: www.harmonyhill.org

Hollyhock Farm

If islands are your thing, try Hollyhock Farm on Cortes Island, 100 miles north of Vancouver in British Columbia, Canada. Courses vary from two to five days, but the central theme is improving life through involvement in the arts, enhanced relationships, spirituality, and healing mind, body, and soul. There are also weekend retreats for couples. The interactive approach is the key here, with exercises, games, discussion, psychodrama, plays, storytelling, and music. Unstructured retreats are also available. Hollyhock Farm is 48 acres of forest, gardens, orchards, and beachfront. Cortes Island is known for its rich marine life.

Hollyhock Farm
Box 127
Manson's Landing, Cortes Island
BC Canada VOP lKO
604-935-6465

The Inner Voyage

If you want to ship out entirely, try The Inner Voyage, a holistic experience at sea. It's a fantastic way to find self-healing (unless you get seasick). A family member went on a weeklong cruise and raved about it. There were well-known speakers, workshops, mind-body exercises, gourmet and vegetarian cuisine, and an array of holistic services. Leave your cares and cell phone behind. The Inner Voyage is sponsored in conjunction with *New Age* magazine; call 800-546-7871 for schedules and information.

Sah Naji Kwe Wilderness Spa

If you don't want to get lost at sea, but do want to get lost, perhaps this facility, which made *New Age* magazine's top 10 holistic retreats list in their 1999 Special Issue, will work for you. It's more rustic and rugged than the others and approaches healing by learning from native practices. It's located in the Northwest Territories in Canada on the arctic shoreline of Great Slave Lake, and guests stay in platform tents heated by a wood stove. You may choose to dine on local delicacies such as caribou and moose or opt for vegetarian or Oriental fare. Bodywork, meditation, clay baths, pipe and sweat lodge ceremonies, and canoeing and hiking round out the program.

Sah Naji Kwe Wilderness Spa
Box 98, Rae-Edzo
Northwest Territories
Canada
867-371-3144
www.wilderness-spa.com

The Least You Need to Know

➤ Wellness is your intentional effort to achieve and maintain not only physical health, but also mental, emotional, and spiritual health.

➤ Wellness is found not on an either/or path, but on a both-and-one path. You need spas and retreats to foster spiritual and physical health.

➤ Self-healing is within your grasp if you use a variety of mind-body healing techniques and disease-prevention strategies and attend to your spiritual health.

➤ Wellness centers and holistic, educational facilities use the lessons of Western and alternative therapies to help you achieve optimal well-being.

Part 5
Getaways for Homebodies

Sometimes you just want to stay home. You go to work. You go to meetings. You go to the store and run errands. You attend countless school events. It would be nice to go to a spa or retreat, but who has the time to plan such a trip? Can't you linger in your robe, forget about shaving, and not worry whether it's a bad hair day? Certainly!

When you prefer staying home, for any number of reasons, you don't need to miss out on the comfort and benefits of a spa or retreat experience. I'll share some ways to turn your ordinary bathroom into a spa (no renovations necessary). You'll discover how to take a small space in your home or use your backyard or the woods nearby to create a sanctuary. Besides, in between your spa and retreat visits, you'll need some relaxation to keep you going in your normal, everyday environment.

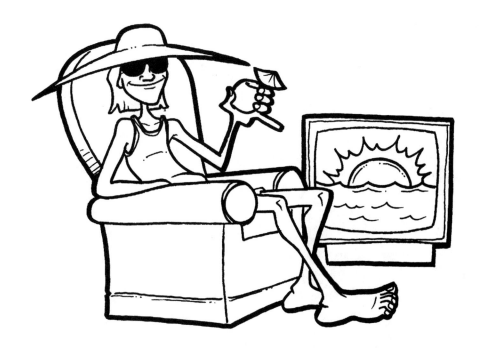

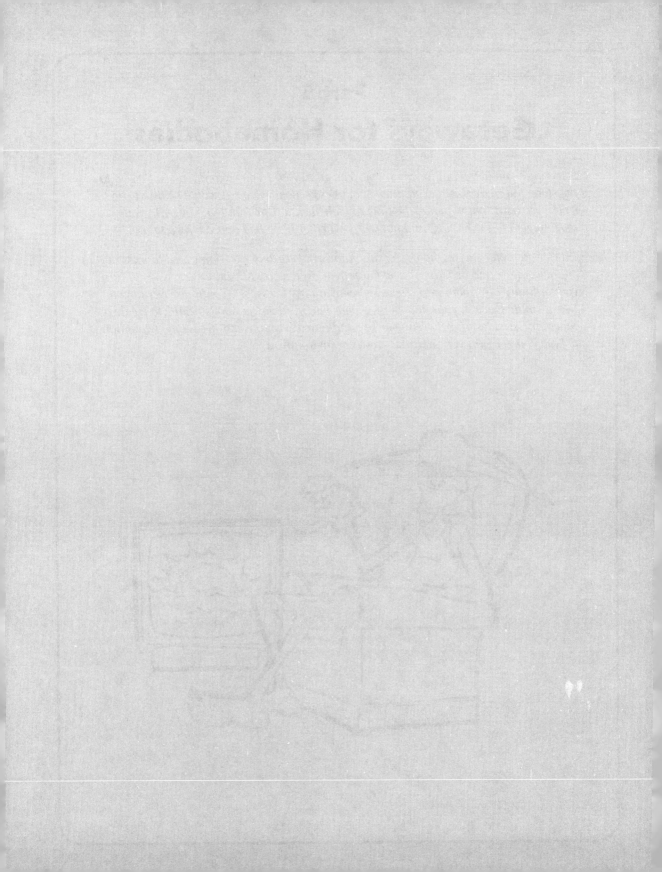

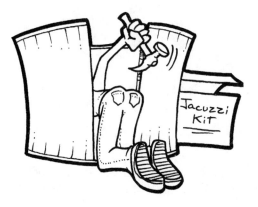

Chapter 14

Creating Your Home Spa and Personal Retreat

In This Chapter

➤ Basic supplies for your at-home spa

➤ Lifting your scents-es with aromatherapy

➤ Self-massage and facials

➤ Finding quiet retreat spaces

➤ Shrines and home altars

There's something about leaning back and having someone else do the rubbing, scrubbing, kneading, and polishing. I'm not talking about housework—I'm talking about rubbing and scrubbing the skin until it glows, kneading tired or achy muscles, and polishing fingers and forgotten toes. Then you collapse in a heap of glorious bliss before a meal someone else prepared and will later clean up.

You can read about these experiences in Part 6, "Take Me Away from Here!" and dream about them any time you want. But because it's highly unlikely you'll be spending your entire life at the spa or on retreat, let me show you how to bring the flavor of a spa or retreat experience into your home anytime you want. Get ready to create fabulous moments at home!

Doing It at Home

So what is it that you'll be imitating at home? Spas generally offer

➤ Scrubs and rubs.

➤ Aromatherapy.

➤ Soothing baths.

➤ Healthy meals.

➤ Fitness.

Retreats also offer

➤ Quiet.

➤ A spiritual dimension.

A bathroom with a bathtub and a shower is an ideal setting for your home spa. Stock your shelves with spa supplies so you are ready to indulge yourself at the hint of a free moment or two. Your basic supply list includes

➤ Soft towels (splurge on them).

➤ Candles: scented and unscented.

➤ Scrubbers: body brushes, loofahs, *pumice*, sea sponges, scrubbing mitts.

➤ Cosmetic scrubs.

➤ Facial mud.

➤ Moisturizers: foot and hand cream, body lotion, face lotion.

➤ A few essential oils, perhaps lavender, peppermint, and chamomile.

For manicures and pedicures, find a basket or other pleasing container, and use it to hold

➤ Nail scrub brush.

➤ Nail files.

➤ Emery boards.

➤ Buffers.

➤ Polish, if you use it.

Whether you do your nails on the balcony or in front of the stereo, everything is together. Have basket, will travel.

Now that you're stocked up, let's see how to use what you have.

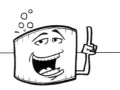

Jacuzzi Jive

Pumice is a light volcanic rock used in solid or powdered form for smoothing, scouring, and polishing skin. It may be a hand-size stone, in granular form in creams, or on a handle, similar to a hairbrush. **Cosmetic scrubs** are creams or lotions containing small particles used to cleanse your skin. An **exfoliant** is a substance that sloughs off dead skin cells.

The Ins and Outs

When you avail yourself of your home spa or retreat, create a ritual as you enter or leave this block of special time. It's a symbolic way of shutting the door on the world and your worries. Identify your entrance into your sanctuary, a place of inner peace, relaxation, vitality, and wellness.

Simple yet potent ways to signify your entrance are to

➤ Light candles or incense.

➤ Ring a bell.

➤ Play special music.

Once you have entered your space, ignore all outside distractions.

When you finish, resist the temptation to rush back into the stream of life. If you're groggy from a soak, it may be difficult to rush anyway. Create a ritual for this in-between time. Perhaps you will

➤ Write in your journal.

➤ Read from an inspirational book.

➤ Ring the bell a second time.

➤ Turn off the music.

➤ Extinguish the candles.

Create a graceful transition from your sanctuary into the world. You will return to the people in your life with greater energy, peace of mind, and serenity.

Treat Your Tastebuds, Too

Gourmet, vegetarian, low-fat, or other special meals are part of the spa experience, but you won't find recipes in this chapter. There are so many cookbooks available for you to try! I suggest that to add to the luxury of your day, you don't cook at all. Order a fabulous meal and have it delivered. When you leave your sanctuary, it will be waiting for you on a table you earlier set with candles, flowers, china, and crystal. Enjoy.

Scrubs for Glowing Skin

Your outer skin layer is dead. The dead cells, which look like tiny white flakes, are rubbed away and replaced constantly. Gently rubbing away these skin cells can improve the appearance of your skin. For lots of hints and good advice, check out *The Complete Idiot's Guide to Beautiful Skin* (Alpha Books, 1998) and many other good books.

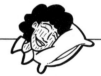

Take 5

Spa Discoveries, The International Spa of the Month Club, brings the spa experience to your home. The club offers a newsletter profiling a featured spa, health tips, wellness, stress management, fitness, spa recipes, and monthly shipments of two full-size spa products from destination spas around the world. Members receive discounts on products and spa accommodations. Call toll-free 800-823-7727 or check its Web site at www.spadiscoveries.com for more information.

Rinse the Gray Away: Full Body

Think of your skin as looking like the shower door after too many showers. A film builds up, and the shine vanishes. Here's one way to rinse away the film:

1. Before you bathe or shower, run a dry body brush from your toes to your neck in long sweeps. Watch the dry flakes as they fly off. (If you have sensitive skin, you may wish to skip this step because the brush may be irritating.)

2. For areas that need additional attention, dampen and use a skin scrub or pumice to smooth extra dry or rough places. Or scrub while the skin is still damp following your bath. Work in the scrub with circular movements, slow and firm. Scrubs are available fragrance-free or scented, with pumice or other natural abrasives to slough off dry skin. Rinse.

3. Finish with a moisturizer after every bath or shower for soft, healthy skin. Choose the richest, gloppiest moisturizer and use just a little too much.

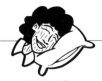

Take 5

Skin that's been exfoliated and moisturized until it's soft and smooth takes fake tanning lotions beautifully; there's no streaking or excess color around ankles, knees, and elbows.

Salt Scrub for the Body

My local day spa uses salt scrubs to exfoliate skin cells, and you can, too:

1. Use a base oil of jojoba, macadamia, or hazelnut; even vegetable oil will do. Add $1/2$ cup of table or Kosher salt.

2. Wet yourself thoroughly in the shower.

3. Rub the salt mixture over your body (not face) using your hands, a loofah, or a washcloth. Rub gently in circles moving from your extremities toward your torso.

4. Rinse salt off thoroughly.

5. Pat yourself dry with a clean towel and apply a rich moisturizer.

Chill Out

Don't use a salt rub right after shaving—ouch!

Don't Forget Your Feet

This is a rescue package for dog-tired, rough feet:

1. Fill a bowl with warm water and add bath foam or foot soak.

2. Rub some body oil into your feet, and put them in the water. Relax. Soak for at least 15 minutes.

3. Pat your feet dry. Use a granular foot scrub or a pumice to remove dry or rough skin.

4. Smooth on rich lotion. (You don't need special foot lotion.)

5. If you wish, cool your feet with a quick foot spray before putting on shoes or slippers. With such gorgeous feet, go ahead and wear sandals.

Face It

This easy face routine doesn't take much time:

1. Cleanse your face thoroughly with lots of inexpensive cleanser. Wipe away most, but not all, of the cleanser with damp cotton or a damp washcloth.

2. Use a glob of exfoliating cream or gel and work it over your face in small, circular movements. Rinse.

3. Cover your face with too much moisturizer, and leave on for 20 minutes. Then wipe off the excess with tissue.

4. Once a week, skip step 2 and instead use a beauty mask to brighten and restore skin tone. After you rinse, do step 3.

Sensual Smells

Smells are all around us. Certain smells even affect our moods. Fragrance can be used in the bath (or shower) and on the body for *aromatherapy*.

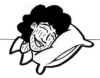

Take 5

While your feet are soaking, close your eyes and cover them with a cucumber slice or two, write in your journal, read your mail, or return calls from friends.

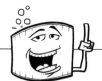

Jacuzzi Jive

Create a **beauty mask** by covering your face (not the eyes) with a product such as mud or facial cleanser that dries on the skin. Masks penetrate pores, absorb dirt, exfoliate dead skin cells, and tone skin tissue. When dry, wash off with warm water. For a **mud bath,** immerse your unclothed body into mud, or spread on mud and let dry for benefits similar to a mask.

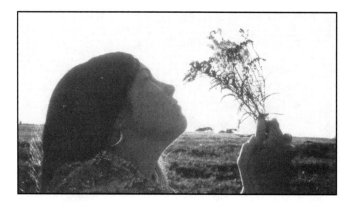

Fragrance is used in the bath (or shower), on the body, as aromatherapy, and in cooking. For self-healing, choose scents that relax and renew you.
(Image © H. Armstrong Roberts)

175

How Your Nose Knows

When you take a deep breath, the scent, the essence, is picked up by the hairs that line the nose. Through the olfactory system, the essence travels on nerve impulses directly to the brain. At the same time, the molecules of the scent mix with oxygen in your lungs.

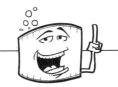

Jacuzzi Jive

Aromatherapy uses pure essential oils, either absorbed through the skin or inhaled through the nose. The term also describes scent-oriented therapies that use plant oils. **Essential oils** are fragrant oils made from plant sources, such as flowers, leaves, and bark. Only oils made by steam distillation are technically pure essential oils. Different essential oils are thought to have different, potent effects on body, mind, and spirit.

Chill Out

Some people have allergic reactions to essential oils. Test an oil first by mixing it with a carrier oil. Place a small amount not on your face but on the underside of your wrist, leaving it on for 24 hours. If any reaction occurs, wash it off immediately. Avoid oils on your face if you have acne-prone skin.

The part of the brain that identifies scents is the same area that controls the emotions and influences endocrine and immune system activity in the body. It is also located next to the area of the brain that's responsible for memory. It's no wonder then that you may recall scents from some long-ago time, even if you have no specific memory of them. Indeed, real estate agents suggest putting a drop of vanilla in the oven or on light bulbs when showing your home because the smell reminds folks of cookies baking or Grandma's house, both delightful remembrances of "home."

Putting You in the Mood with Oils

Oils have a variety of properties, including:

➤ Calming

➤ Stimulating

➤ Creating an optimistic mood

➤ Acting as an aphrodisiac

➤ Anti-inflammatory

➤ Antibiotic

By inhaling specific *essential oils,* you can change your mood and perhaps even heal a variety of stress-related physical symptoms.

Essential oils may be placed in the following:

➤ Diffuser

➤ Potpourri burner

➤ Bathtub

➤ Cotton ball in a plastic bag for keeping in your purse or briefcase so you can sniff it throughout the day

When mixed with a unscented carrier oil, essential oils can be used in massage, which brings both smell and touch to heal mind and body. Suggested carrier oils are ones with a vegetable base or avocado, jojoba, and sesame oils.

Judith Sachs' book, *Nature's Prozac* (Prentice Hall, 1997), suggests using these oils for these conditions:

➤ Bergamot or geranium for depression and anxiety

➤ Chamomile or mandarin to calm agitation

➤ Jasmine or mandarin if you feel hopeless

➤ Orange or peppermint for fatigue or lack of energy

➤ Sandalwood or tea tree for relaxation

➤ Lavender for insomnia, tension, anxiety, and rashes

➤ Gentian if you're easily discouraged

➤ Heather if you're obsessed with your own troubles

➤ Rose if you're depressed (a new take on "stop and smell the roses!")

Chill Out

Don't ingest essential oils or place them directly on your skin unless they are first mixed with a carrier oil.

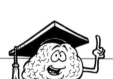

Mindful Moment

Ayurveda (Sanskrit for "science of living") is the oldest (over 5,000 years old) system of scientifically based health care. Ayurveda combines diet, exercise, meditation, herbal therapy, aromatherapy, and music therapy into a philosophical system of energy balancing to enhance health and avoid disease. Essential oils are used to harmonize an out-of-balance personality. Best-selling author Deepak Chopra has popularized Ayurveda in the Western world. His books include *Creating Health, Quantum Healing,* and *Unconditional Life.*

Herbs Work, Too

The use of herbs for medical conditions is the most ancient form of health care known to humankind. Common herbs growing on your windowsill or in your garden also can be used for aromatherapy, teas, baths, facials, and wraps.

For teas, purchase herbal teas in ready-made packets or buy a teaball and make your own. I like to use a mixture of mullein leaf, lemon balm, chamomile, peppermint, rosehips, and stevia. If you grow herbs, use

➤ Peppermint or chamomile for stomach upset or to improve digestion (my Grandmom always kept these two herbs on hand).

➤ Chamomile or hops as a sleep aid.

Make an Herbal Sachet

Make a no-sew sachet for under your pillow, in your car, even in your shoes. Take a piece of fabric, about six inches square. Fold it in half, right sides together, and seal two sides with fabric glue. When the glue is dry, turn the sachet inside out. Then fill it with potpourri, fresh pine needles, or fresh herbs and close the remaining side with a bit of glue.

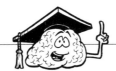

Mindful Moment

Extensive scientific documentation now exists regarding the use of herbs for treating conditions including those of the female and male reproductive systems, indigestion, insomnia, heart disease, cancer, peptic ulcers, rheumatic and arthritic conditions, chronic skin problems such as eczema and psoriasis, anxiety and tension-related stress, hypertension, and allergies.

It's a Wrap!

This herbal wrap is a bit messy (it's easier in the summer when you can go outdoors), but it's manageable. You will need a lounge chair on a water-tolerant floor. Cover the chair with a blanket and then a plastic sheet (a clean shower curtain or drop cloth works well).

To cook the herbal mixture, combine two gallons of boiling water and four cups of dried herbs and let it steep for 20 minutes. Any herbal combination you like may be used. *The Complete Idiot's Guide to Beautiful Skin* suggests a mixture of rose petals, chamomile, elder flowers, peppermint, yarrow, and lavender. After 20 minutes, strain out the herbs, close your sink or bathtub drain, and pour in the scented water.

Soak a flat twin-size bedsheet, folded so it fits into the liquid. Wring it out until it's wet and warm but not dripping. Get a partner and have him or her unfold and

Take 5

Pretend you are away at a day spa. Turn off the phone, turn on the answering machine, ignore the doorbell, cancel appointments, and enjoy the peace and quiet.

wrap the sheet around you, loose enough so you can remove your arms if needed. Then wrap the plastic over the sheet and finally cover yourself with the blanket. Lie on the lounge chair for 15 minutes (or longer, but don't get chilled as the wrap cools).

Candles Create a Scents-ual Atmosphere

Walk into any department or discount store today and you will find scented candles, mood candles, or healing candles. Use candles when you eat, bathe, exercise, meditate, pray, or even work.

To soak in a tub surrounded by a collection of candles of differing sizes and heights is wonderfully decadent. Candles provide pleasing fragrances and spiritual connections even when the lights are on. (I used scented candles while writing this book.)

Take 5

Could it get easier? Pre-packaged herbal and aromatherapy mixtures are available in stores for your bath. Just tear open the package and add to the water.

Soaking Away Stress and Strain

Make time to soak. Let the water melt away your cares. Professional spas offer aromatherapy, herbal, mud, and whirlpool baths. Each method has its own relaxing and cleansing properties.

A special bath requires a little preparation:

1. Take a pre-bath scrub. It gets rid of all the gunk and prepares the skin to absorb the benefits of the substances you add to your bath water.

2. Enhance the bath water with any of these:

   ➤ Add a few drops of essential oil to your bath water.

   ➤ Add herbs or other self-healing material to your bath in a cloth container made of cheesecloth or muslin. Try pine needles, lavender, rose petals, or citrus peel in your bag.

   ➤ Add sea salt or powdered seaweed.

   ➤ Try two cups of vinegar (apple cider, rice, or wine) to tone and cleanse the skin.

   ➤ Use oatmeal or cornstarch for itchy skin. (It's a time-honored chicken pox remedy.)

   ➤ If you have a Jacuzzi, use it.

Chill Out

If you have children and are applying a facial mask, warn them. I really scared my son one time!

3. Multiply your benefits by wearing a mud mask in the bath. Or try whipped egg whites, cucumber slices, or warm cooked oatmeal and honey on your face to draw out the impurities.

4. Take advantage of your just-soaked and softened hands and feet and give them a manicure or pedicure.

For Hands and Feet

When you can't take a full bath, give your extremities a mini bath. Soak your fingertips or feet for 5 to 10 minutes in a bowl of warm water. Treat this soak as you would any bath: Add herbs, essential oils, or flower petals. Then do the following:

1. Scrub your hands or feet and nails with a nail brush.

2. Rinse well and apply lotion or oil.

3. Gently push back cuticles with a cotton swab.

4. Trim and shape nails.

5. Buff your nails.

6. Polish your nails if you wish.

Your skin will glow, and your energy will show!

Soaking Wet with Steam

Steam makes you sweat. When you do, the toxins that have been building up inside you come out through your pores. *The Complete Idiot's Guide to Massage* offers this suggestion for making a steam tent at home to replicate a sauna or steam bath: Pour a gallon of simmering, steaming water into a large bowl or pot that's sitting on a thick towel. Add scents if you wish and have a chair and a large woolen blanket handy.

Take off your clothes, unless it's okay to get them sweaty. Put the bowl on the floor, the chair near it, and sit with the blanket over you, the chair, and the bowl. Relax and breathe deeply for 10 to 20 minutes. If you're really adventurous, get out of the heat and right into a cool shower.

If this sounds like too much trouble, do what I did as a kid: Pour the hot water and scents into a well-stoppered sink, and put a towel over your head and sink. Or if you want to sit, put the water in a bowl, place the bowl on a low table (with towels underneath the bowl to protect the table's finish), and throw a towel over your head and the bowl on the table.

You Knead a Rub

Massage dissolves tension and helps alleviate pain. When you need some quick massage relief, help yourself. Here are a few quick rubs for headache, jaw, and foot pain.

My Head Aches!

Often, headaches around the forehead originate where muscles at the base of the skull meet the neck. Move your fingers all around your scalp as though you were giving yourself a good shampoo. In fact, do this self-massage whenever you wash your hair.

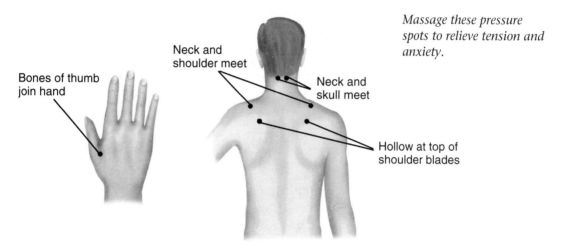

Massage these pressure spots to relieve tension and anxiety.

Neck and shoulder meet

Bones of thumb join hand

Neck and skull meet

Hollow at top of shoulder blades

Quit Your Jaw-ing

You may carry tension in your jaw. When you are angry or stubborn you may "set your jaw." You may clench it or grind your teeth, putting big stress on the jaw. To bring immediate relief to a stiff and painful jaw, open and close your mouth to feel your jaw joint. Then press on this joint or rub it gently in a circular motion.

Energetic, Tension-Free Feet

Long ago I learned a trick for energizing myself by massaging one spot on the bottom of each foot. I gladly pass it along. Until you learn where this magic energy spot is, remove your socks as well as your shoes. Gently bend your toes and notice a crease across the ball of your foot. Now draw an imaginary line down from the space between your big and next toes. Where the lines intersect, you will feel a hollowed-out place on the sole of your foot. Gently massage that spot with the thumb of your opposite hand. Switch feet and thumbs and repeat.

If your feet need relief, pull and spread your toes like the massage pros. Sit so you can grab your foot by interlacing your fingers between your toes. At first, it may be difficult to find enough room between your toes for your finger; your toes may be literally too cramped. As you repeat this exercise, your toes will become more flexible and less intent on holding together. (Don't forget to switch and get hold of your other foot's toes. You will, of course, need to use your other hand.)

Your feet work so hard for you. Here's one last instant stress remedy for your feet:

➤ Add two drops of lavender essential oil to some body lotion.

➤ Massage the lotion into your feet with small, circular movements.

➤ Gently pull each toe.

Retreat to Your Sanctuary

Your sanctuary is your special place, which your body and soul will learn to know well. When you enter it, your energy begins to run. Look at your home with new eyes to find an area of retreat.

Sacred Space

You don't need a great deal of space to create a nook or area that has a quiet and hidden feel to it.

1. Convert your junk, storage, or infrequently used guest room into a haven. Fill it with large comfy floor pillows or a squishy chair or couch. Include dim lighting or candles. Add a home altar if you wish (see the following "Shrines and Altars" section) or a fountain. Teach the family that this room is a quiet-only place.

2. A closet may be large enough (indeed, my children have on occasion slept in them). Use candles or battery-powered lights or even strings of white holiday lights. Mount a small wall shelf or hang a tapestry, picture, object, or momentos for use as a meditation focus.

3. Create an area off a hall or larger room. Find space by thinking differently about your furniture placement. You can create barriers or dividers with tall plants or trees, movable screens, large vases with tall flowers or feathers, or bookcases, breakfronts, hutches, or armoires.

4. Use covered outdoor space, such as a porch, patio, balcony, or deck. Use the same techniques of arrangement and furnishings as you would indoors.

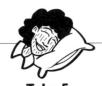

Take 5

Meet regularly with like-minded seekers to support your spiritual practice. Form your own spiritual group. Size is unimportant: One or two others is enough.

Furnish with Care

You want an atmosphere of repose and refreshment. Typical furnishings include candles and/or incense, flowers or plants, and beautiful photographs, objects, or artwork. If you choose to use even a corner of a room, mark it and gather together symbols of your intentions in that space. Find a basket or trunk and gather your reading, journals, or prayer books.

Shrines and Altars

Shrines and home altars recall home worship spaces of earlier times and reinforce the intimacy of and connection with an unseen world. They may also be places to gather a collection of sentimental souvenirs acquired over the course of a lifetime. Such a space causes you to slow down and pause, think, and see a picture of your life. Locate your shrine or altar anywhere you feel it lives, wherever it feels right.

Shrines may be placed just so or rearranged as you add or subtract items. Wherever and however it is displayed, such an area is a continuous reminder of your life and the source of all life.

The Least You Need to Know

➤ You can create your own home spa in your bathroom with your tub, shower, and some basic supplies.

➤ Enjoy soaks, mud masks, facials, body scrubs, manicures, pedicures, and self-massage in the privacy and comfort of your home.

➤ Use herbs or essential oils for fragrance, relaxation, and healing in teas, baths, facials, and wraps. Light a scented candle, too.

➤ Arrange your furniture, plants, and favorite objects to define a quiet, hidden retreat space at home.

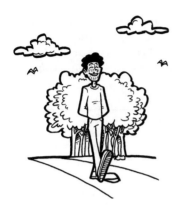

Chapter 15

Nature Calls!

In This Chapter

➤ Walking as meditation

➤ Soothing, stress-relieving water

➤ Fountains and pools as peaceful places

➤ Bring nature indoors, close to you, for health and renewal

When you step into a wood, field, or glen, it's as though you step across an invisible boundary into a sanctuary of safety and peace. The quiet is noticeable in its pervasiveness. In all this quiet, the sound of a waterfall or a gurgling stream somewhere out of sight immediately captures your attention.

Nature beckons you wherever you are. Can't you feel the energy? The holiness of the unspoiled earth is in your bones: Play in the mud, splash in puddles, and build tree houses! Hail the first buds in springtime, marvel at the bending and stretching of plants as they reach out for the life-giving light, and delight at the ever-changing colors of the landscape. In this chapter, you'll find ways to use the healing energy of nature. You'll learn how to meditate while you walk, create peaceful sounds with fountains and water gardens, bring nature indoors to release tension and worry, and have some plain old fun.

Your Own Nature

We are all part of nature. The same energy that flows through us flows through the entire universe. Like nature, we have rhythms. We have daily cycles of wakefulness, productivity, and rest. We have seasons, as Anita Spencer calls them in her book

Seasons (Paulist Press, 1982), which are larger chunks of our lives through which we move. At mid-life, as we saw in Chapter 3, "Let's Get Personal," we may go through a metamorphosis, just as a caterpillar becomes a butterfly. We have periods of intense work and times, as in winter, when we need to lie fallow and gather our strength for the next blooming. Honor your rhythms.

Holy Ground

I am holy ground,
for within me resides the Holy One
who is both Mother and Father to each of us.

I am holy ground,
for I seek to avoid the evil ones and evil ways,
and live so as to give glory to our Creator.

I am holy ground,
for I am filled with the love of the One who created me,
unconditional love which is, forever and ever.

I am holy ground,
for I, too, am love.

I am holy ground,
for I seek to forgive others
whether or not they forgive me.

I am holy ground,
for the Spirit works in and through me
to heal my sisters and brothers.

I am holy ground,
for my spirit, too, was before, and is after,
and does not end, but is, forever and ever.

I am holy ground,
and you are, too.

(© Linda Short, The GLAD Collection, 1994)

Recently, I attended a presentation by a Lakota Indian. He reminded us that the Indian (his term, so don't get on me about political correctness) walks in harmony with all of the earth, because every rock, tree, and plant is also a living spirit. Indeed, he began this talk, as he does every talk, by taking out a stone, setting it before him, and keeping it in view as a focal point. He explained that the stone teaches him that it is an ancient spirit that has lived long before he was born, lives today, and will live long after he leaves the earth.

I found his explanation humbling. Here we sit, convinced that our idea, job, or relationship is the most important aspect of our lives. Is it really? Doesn't the stone put things in a different perspective? We are more like the flower, which fades, withers, and soon dies. It's urgent, then, that we bloom while we can.

Walking Meditation

Slow down your spirit, and let it drink in the heady wine of creation. Thoreau had his pond. Frost had his woods on a snowy evening. Religious figures across traditions had desert and mountain retreats for solitude and renewal.

Go to your favorite outdoor spot and reclaim the art of moseying for yourself. If you mosey down a path and pass a turtle sitting on a log, stay and see who moves first, the turtle or you. If you see a butterfly, watch its darting moves and landings until it leaves your sight. If you pass flowers, stop and smell them.

Even when you need to complete something or be somewhere quickly, step slowly. Stepping slowly can be a moving meditation. Not all of us can sit for a long time, and even in traditional monastic settings, sitting meditation is mixed with walking meditation. Both are valid. What is important is what is in your mind.

You can practice informal walking meditation anywhere. Just walk normally on a sidewalk, down your office hall, in the woods, with your children, or with your dog. While you walk, remember that you are here, now, in your body. Remind yourself to note this moment, allow distractions to pass, and observe each step you take. If you find yourself starting to rush, slow your pace. Appreciate where you are now.

When you walk, you make an impression on the earth, literally. Think of the footprints you leave behind on the beach: They're different when you walk, when you run, when you walk backward, and when they are erased partially or completely by the waves. As you walk through life, what kind of footprints are you leaving behind?

Chill Out

Smell flowers. Pick them only if they are your own. Wildflowers don't last, anyway. They are meant to live free, untamed lives wherever you find them.

Take 5

Many conditioning experts now believe that it's possible to achieve maximum fitness without entering a gym or buying fancy equipment by using walking as your regular exercise. The National Institutes of Health recommends 30 minutes of moderate exercise on most, preferably all, days of the week.

Life-Giving Waters

I love water. I can stare endlessly at a stream, a lake, or the waves of the ocean. Water has always been a source of serenity. It is also essential to all life.

In religious traditions, water symbolizes a life-giving quality. The floods washed the earth clean, bringing forgiveness and permitting renewal. The Israelites moved to freedom through the parted waters of the Red Sea. Water is used in baptism, a sacrament that cleanses a Christian of original sin and brings him into the church. In Islam, wadu is a ritual washing before prayer. Hindus from all over the world travel to India to drink from and bathe in the Ganges river, and pray, "May your water … Soothe our troubled souls."

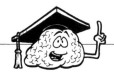

Mindful Moment

"He learned from [the river] continually. Above all, he learned from it how to listen with a still heart, with a waiting, open soul, without passion, without desire, without judgment, without opinions."
—from *Siddartha* by Hermann Hesse (1877–1962)

The sight, scent, and sound of water refreshes and calms while giving pleasure, whether in the excitement of a fountain, the gentle movement of a river, or the reflections of a still pool. My friend's son made her a lily pond in her backyard in the city. She eats breakfast out there, drinks tea there, and congregates with visitors there. Perhaps you might try to create a watery environment that soothes your soul and refreshes your spirit.

Water gardens and fountains are quite popular today. Books, articles, television segments, and your local gardening center offer advice and supplies on how to create a wet world suitable for your home or apartment (and your thirsty animals). If you want the presence of water (more than in your sink or shower) without the work, go out and buy a ready-made fountain. Then you can listen and enjoy while you skip ahead to the next chapter. If you want to create a watery space yourself, read on.

Container Water Gardens

Water gardens need not be grand affairs; small ones are just as delightful and involve less maintenance, especially if you choose containers. There are many books and magazine articles on building ponds and pools, indoor and out, and you can buy such things ready-made.

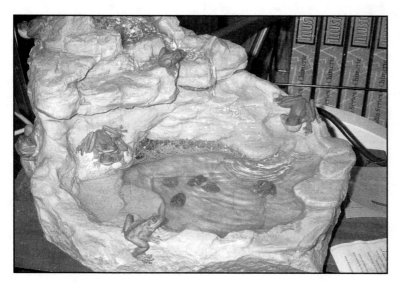

Purchase one of the many fanciful or simply elegant water fountains or make your own to bring the sound, sight, and scent of soothing water into your home.
(Photo courtesy of Wondrous Things, Croton-on-Hudson, NY)

To create a container water garden, you need a waterproof container. The larger the container is, the heavier the garden will be. (Carry any buckets of water lately?) Try using a metal basin, terra cotta or ceramic pot, or wooden barrel. If your pot of choice has a drainage hole, just plug it up. Use fine concrete in the hole and cover it with a waterproof sealant. Wooden barrels may be waterproofed by lining them with a piece of pond liner secured just above the water line. Just about any container that is clean and holds water can be used for a water garden.

Next, carefully choose the location of your garden. You won't be moving it anytime soon. Consider whether it is in a convenient spot (are you able to enjoy it, hear it, see it) or near an electrical outlet if you want to create bubbles or a fountain, whether there is sufficient sunlight for the kinds of plants you want, and whether the floor can withstand water spills.

Before you start pouring in the water, decide what else you want in your water garden. Water lilies may be the most desirable, decorative, and coveted of all water plants. No wonder, their brilliant blooms are hypnotizing. For an outdoor container garden, look for the smaller sizes of lilies that tolerate shallower planting depths. For example, miniature lilies require only nine inches of water; the largest ones need water at least three feet deep.

When you add the lilies to your container, you can leave them in their boxes if the boxes are the open-sided, aquatic ones. Ask about these boxes where you buy the flowers. So the boxes don't sit on the bottom of the container, put a brick or a second box in the bottom of the pond container as a stand.

If you want fish, figure out the surface area of your garden. The number of fish depends on the area of the water. Each square foot supports one two-inch fish. The same area will hold greater numbers of smaller fish. A small goldfish in an outdoor water garden controls mosquito larvae. Otherwise, maintenance is minimal. Plants in a small tub block much of the sun and thus control algae growth.

You will need to top off the water occasionally as it evaporates (or as pets drink it). Your indoor container garden will add humidity to your home, which is particularly important in the winter when heating dries out your home and your nasal passages.

Chill Out

If you have young children, be sure all water containers are childproof or out of reach. If you use terra cotta pots in or around an outdoor pond, take them inside during the winter so they don't crack from the cold.

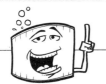

Jacuzzi Jive

A **bubbler** is a small submersible pump. It may be adjusted to create a quiet or a vigorous bubbling action in the water. Other types of pumps have a jet head that is adjustable to create a shorter or taller fountain of water. Look for pumps in stores carrying garden or aquarium supplies.

Fountains for Tabletop, Floor, or Outdoors

You can make a fountain as easily as a water garden by adding a surface or submersible pump, or you can purchase a self-contained fountain to hang on a wall or sit on any indoor or outdoor surface: shelves, stands, or floors. Use a *bubbler* if you wish your water to remind you of a babbling brook. If you choose a jet head, you can direct the water flow through a simple spout or straight up as in a traditional fountain.

Depending upon the size of your water fountain, you'll need to deal with the problem of weight. Small tabletop fountains can be made from containers like small flowerpots or even salad bowls. Arrange your stones (or perhaps shells collected from some long ago trip and gathering dust in a display basket) and add your bubbler according to its instructions. That may be all you need.

The construction of a fountain in a basket was demonstrated on Christopher Lowell's *Interior Motives* television show. It followed these steps:

➤ Select a waterproof bowl.

➤ Add a pump and rocks to bowl.

➤ Put the bowl inside a basket.

➤ Place moss around the bowl.

➤ Add spider plants, ivy, or other plants that will root in water.

Whenever you use a pump, arrange your materials to hide the pump's wiring. Other details you might include are a candle, a little waterproof kerosene lamp, a bell, or a religious artifact. Look through some magazines, displays, or books, or just use your imagination.

In-Ground Ponds

If you are ready to try an outdoor, in-ground pond, there are two ways to begin: Dig your own hole and shape it, or dig your hole and plant a pre-formed mold. Molded ponds are available in weather-resistant plastic or fiberglass. You could even recycle a child's small rigid swimming pool.

Location

Before you begin digging, ask some questions about the location of your pond. Do you want it

➤ Near a sitting area?

➤ Visible from the house?

➤ Accessible to a hose?

➤ In the sun or mainly in shade?

When you have a place in mind, take a string, rope, or garden hose, and lay it out on the ground in the shape you want. Play with the shape by changing the outline until you find the perfect shape.

Take 5

Have a water party and let each guest create his own tabletop water haven.

Take 5

If you have an old carpet, line the hole with it before you add sand. It acts as a great protective mat. A dark-colored liner looks more natural than a light or bright one.

Digging

Take a deep breath. Now it's time to dig. (Remember, you can always fill your hole, re-seed, and keep your lawn.) Work around the outside of your shape. Dig from the outside edge toward the center. Your deepest area will be in the center.

For a simple pond, just dig a hole. Remove any sticks or stones likely to puncture or damage the liner. Remember, water is heavy, so there will be a lot of pressure down onto the ground. Cover the dirt with at least one inch of sand.

If you're using a preformed mold, dig a rectangular hole large enough to accommodate the mold. You still need sand on the bottom. You may also need wedges to keep your mold level if it is an irregular shape. Make the hole deep enough so that the mold sits at least one inch below ground level. Add water to the mold to add weight and keep it at its original depth while you backfill. Keep checking the mold with a level while backfilling around the mold. Lucky you: Skip ahead to the "Finishing" section.

Lining Your Hole

If you've dug a hole, the next step is to line it. A liner is made of heavy-gauge PVC or rubber that molds itself to the shape of your pond. Think of flipping dough into a pie pan. The dough is flat and large enough to more than cover the pan. When the rolled dough is put into the pan, it sinks and settles in to match the shape of the pan. Instead of cutting off the excess dough hanging over the edge, however, you will hold your excess liner in place with rocks, paving, or sod.

After placing the liner in the hole, stretch it across. Help shape it by tucking and folding. Anchor it with bricks or rocks at the edges. As you gradually add water to the pond, the liner will tighten. Slowly release the anchoring weights.

As you fill the pond with water, smooth out wrinkles and pull out major creases in the liner. Helping hands are desirable at this stage (actually they're helpful throughout the whole process!). Once the pond is full, you'll know how much surplus edging material you have. Cut away some of the excess, leaving about a foot around, which you will hide under edging slabs, rocks, or whatever you choose.

Finishing

Decide what else you may wish to add to your pond besides water. Pond liners are nontoxic, so you needn't wait to add plants, fish, or a bubbler or fountain. Finish the pond with a rock edging or a border of crushed stone, if you wish. Put plants around the border, and then pull up a chair, put up your feet, and enjoy— maybe even splash your feet in your new pond.

In-Ground Ponds with an Edge

The basic pond is great, but if you want to add a variety of plants in the pond itself, you may need some shallower water. You can create shallow areas by digging a hole with ledges. In effect, you will dig a hole with steps down into it.

Shallower water depths allow for plantings such as reeds, rushes, cattails, iris, and pickerel weed. These marginal plants love the water, as long as it's not too deep. Sit these plants right in their containers on the ledge for "planting" in the pond.

Chill Out

Be sure the liner is large enough for the depth, width, and length of your hole, *plus* a margin of an extra foot or two around the edges.

Take 5

Avoid putting the fish directly into your pond. Instead, let the bag they are in float on the surface until the temperature of the water inside is the same as the pond's. Release the fish and sprinkle the water with fish food. Don't be concerned if the fish hide instead of feeding right away. Eventually, they'll get used to their new surroundings. To survive over the winter, goldfish need a water depth of at least 1 to $1^1/2$ feet somewhere in the pond.

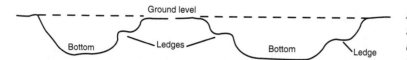

Add a ledge to one or both sides of your pond to accommodate plants that thrive in shallow water.

Rocks, Shells, Sand, Feathers, and Nests

Encourage serenity and contemplation by bringing the outdoors inside. Natural objects will remind you of your connection to all of life and will serve to calm your mind in the midst of endless distractions. These natural forms can help focus your mind for meditation or prayer as well.

Towering Stones

A couple summers ago my family took a vacation on an island off the Maine coast. Other than the one telephone in the hotel lobby where we stayed, there were no electronics. We spent our stay absorbed in the water, forest, and trails that circled the island.

An interesting find was an area of stone towers made by unseen hands and left at the water's edge. Our children added their own. A stone tower is a unique way to bring the ancient wisdom and power of stone into your dwelling or yard. It's like a free-form totem, one that you can change at a whim, like a child's building blocks.

Use stones as well to rid yourself of worries or troubles. First, collect a few stones from a trip or walk. Choose one of these stones and give it one of your worries. Then throw away the stone, and your worry with it.

Soothing Sand

Isn't sand delightful? Sand art, sand paintings, and sand tables are all fun ways to use sand. You can play with sand, too. Add a drop of food coloring to make your own pigmented sand. Allow yourself play time. Recapture your sense of wonder, daydream, and remember your innocence. Forget about making something. Forget schedules. Let your tension and worries slip through your hand and leave you, just as the grains of sand fall gently through your fingers.

Fragrant Pine

There's something about standing in a pine forest or a redwood forest and being dwarfed by the trees, and then looking up and being greeted by fingers of light stretching down to welcome you. If you enjoy the fragrance of pine, bring in clusters of branches and use the needles to make a scented bath oil. Here's how: Purchase baby oil and clean a pleasing glass jar. Then transfer the oil to the jar and add a handful of fresh pine needles. Seal it with a stopper or cork, and let the mixture sit for four weeks before you use it in your bath. Replace the old needles with new ones from time to time.

Have Nature Come to You

If you don't live near a grand expanse of nature, appreciate what you do have. Gather up a leaf or two in the fall and make leaf prints. Grow small gardens on the window sill. Bring flowers into your home. Receive the gifts of the wonderful fragrances and vibrant colors as they cheer and refresh you, and be reminded of that unseen something that nourishes all of creation.

The Least You Need to Know

➤ When you experience the gifts of the natural world, you are drawn closer to your spiritual nature.

➤ Walking, whether in the woods or down the street, is a way to meditate while moving.

➤ Water—its sight, scent, and sound—relaxes, refreshes, and renews you; use it in or around your home for serenity and contemplation.

➤ When you can't go to nature, have it come to you by bringing stones, shells, leaves, flowers, and sand art into your home.

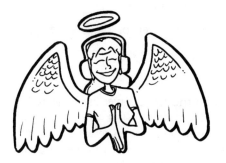

Soulful Sounds

Music and dance are the two best-kept secrets for health and healing. The body receives the good vibrations from the music, and all the chakras, the body's energy centers, are invigorated, from the first up through the seventh. By opening and strengthening your flow of energy, you can push out blockages of stress, negative attitudes, ill health, and detrimental habits. Then, pure, cleansing energy is able to flow unobstructed.

This chapter looks at the role of music and dance in various cultures and across time for prayer, for healing, and for health. Because "music is the soul's own speech," I'll listen in as you discover your voice and your soul's own melody.

In the Beginning

No one can say when music began, for it was in the world hundreds of years before anyone invented writing. That fact itself testifies to a fundamental connection between music and the human spirit. Silence is golden, but I can't imagine a world without sound!

The first sound you heard was your mother's heartbeat; it was music to your ears. Then you heard other sounds, which were the voices of those outside the womb. One of those voices belonged to your mother. It's amazing how a child can pick out his mother's voice from among a crowd (and how well he can ignore it).

What music is in your life today? Do you create any? Whether for healing or for enjoyment, music can lift your spirit.

The Wave

You hear sound when vibrations that move through the air as waves are collected by your outer ear. The shape of the ear is like a funnel, and that's what it does: It funnels the sound from the outside to the middle ear. The middle ear then sends the sound waves to the inner ear, which passes the messages to the brain. The brain interprets the messages as sound. When the sound is a rhythmic sequence of pleasing sounds, it's music.

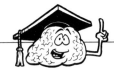

Mindful Moment

Tuva, a former Soviet state between Siberia and Mongolia, maintains a folk music tradition called xoomei, or the Tuvan art of "throat singing." The singer produces two or more tones simultaneously, a sound which is said to possess a unique and otherworldly beauty. Although the style of singing is not unique to Tuva (Tibetan and Inuit singers also practice throat singing), Tuvan singers have become unusually adept, occasionally producing a third rhythm sound in between the deep, guttural drone and the shifting series of high harmonics that is the melody line.

The Voice

It's believed that the first music was vocal. Think about it: You don't need anything but yourself to create this music. You yell to your mate, your offspring, the mastodon.

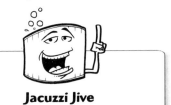

Jacuzzi Jive

Pitch refers to the highness or lowness of a tone.

One day you're surprised when your yell echoes back to you. Perhaps early man did what I did as a kid—kept yelling but changed his *pitch*. Repeat that exercise in different ways and you have the first bars of the first crude song.

Early tribes practiced their sounds, shouting and chanting during hunts, even as accompaniment to dance. Just watch how a two-year-old creates steps to sound; perhaps that's what prehistoric humans did.

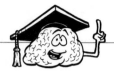

Mindful Moment

Gourd rattles, scrapers, and bull-roarers, which are early instruments, have been found in Europe in deposits that were made 30,000 years ago. A bone flute-like object, found in 1995 in Slovenia, is thought to be 43,000 to 82,000 years old.

The Instrument

After you start using your voice, then you involve other parts of the body. Clap your hands. Stomp your feet. Slap your thighs. Now you are in a state of ecstasy, moving all around and not paying attention, just moving, and you hit a stick, or a stone, or two stones together. Now you're using instruments.

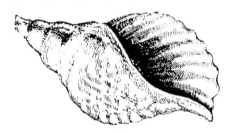

The ancient conch shell trumpet is still used in ceremonies from Mexico to Polynesia.

Music of the Spheres

Music offers a door to the sacred realms without getting involved in complicated belief systems. Soothing background music

➤ Aids meditation.

➤ Offers a respite from the daily pace.

➤ Can be a shortcut to the solace and stability provided by religious traditions.

In purely musical terms, no difference exists between sacred and secular music. They both arrange notes, harmonies, and tempos. Sacred music, however, generally has three purposes:

➤ It praises a deity, requests mercy, or offers thanks.

➤ It raises listeners and performers to emotional and spiritual heights.

➤ It celebrates.

The music is not an end in itself; it's a vehicle for worship.

Raise Your Voices

St. Augustine said, "When we sing, we pray twice." It isn't enough to hear the instruments; we must join in as witnesses connecting heaven and Earth.

Throughout most of human history, the sacred words of religions have been sung, not written. They were taught to the next generation in song. Navajo priests are called "singers." *Shamans* use music as their primary means of contacting the spirit world. Priests and monks sing during Christian masses, the Buddhist *pujas*, Islamic calls to prayer, Hindu sacrifices, and other ceremonies that form the basis of the world's religions.

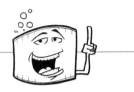

Jacuzzi Jive

Shamans are priests or medicine men who contact and influence the good and bad spirits of their traditions. **Puja** is the name given to certain Buddhist prayer rituals.

The Taize Experience

Taize is a sung prayer named after the town in France where it originated. The community of monks in Taize live a life of prayer and contemplation, and they share time, thoughts, and routine tasks with thousands of visitors each year. In some parts of the United States, you can find special Taize liturgies. I have danced to some Taize music.

The hallmark of Taize is its musical style: simple songs whose words are sung over and over and over again. The repetition frees up and focuses the mind, much like repeating a mantra does. In this way, the songs aid prayer and nourish the inner journey.

Chill Out

Some people, way back when, thought music could be the sound of evil spirits as well as good ones. As religion and worship developed, these thoughts were incorporated into some belief systems. Even today, some faiths believe music leads to depravity, so they shun it.

Your Own Song

The singing group The Mamas and the Papas reminded its listeners to "make your own kind of music and/sing your own special song/make your own kind of music/even if nobody else sings along." Your song and your voice is deep within you, just as your connection to the divine is deep within you. You know where to look: inside yourself. No operations or fancy equipment are needed, just put on your meditation or prayer cap. Seek and ye shall find.

Each one of us is gifted with a unique voice that we bring to the world through our life, regardless of our current station, education, or culture. What we keep searching for outside ourselves is within our knowing; indeed, it is within. Taking quiet time just in your own free moments or on retreat or during your spa visit allows you to go within.

In her book, *Women Who Run with the Wolves* (Ballantine Books, 1992), Clarissa Pinkola Estés talks about searching for the lost pieces of ourselves. She calls them bones, noteworthy, I think, because bones are an integral and necessary part of our bodies. We search to find the missing bones so we may, indeed, become whole.

Are you looking, or have you found your song?

Playing the Score

Finding your melody and your voice is only the first step. Your next decision is whether to play it or shelve it in the section marked unsung hopes and dreams. The finding and the playing of "our song" give us joy, peace, and health. We rejoice, but perhaps we also wait in hope of discovering more pieces of ourselves, more bones.

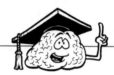

Mindful Moment

Members of many religious traditions hold that there are heavenly connections to religious music. Some believe that it is divinely inspired, for example, as in the nada-brahman "God-as-sound" of Hinduism. Music may be used during creation, as in the drum playing and cosmic dance of the Hindu god Siva Nataraja or in other tales of gods who "sing" their creations and creatures into existence. Sometimes music moves in the opposite direction, from Earth to the heavens, as in the case of the Tibetan composer Mi-la-ras-pa (1040–1123), whose songs are said to have been taken to fill the Tibetan Buddhist heavens with music. (Pretty good gig, huh?)

From Mozart to Rock 'n' Roll for Relaxation

If you didn't know it before you picked up this book, you know it now: Relaxation is beneficial to your health. Music can put you in a relaxed state if you choose the right style for you. Massage therapists play music while they knead you. Some people use music as an aid in prayer or meditation. Classical music and rock 'n' roll are very different styles, yet both can trigger the body's relaxation response—it just depends on how you use the music.

Mozart created beautiful music, but it seems that there's more to his music than beauty. In a 1993 preliminary study, researchers at the University of California discovered that musical training helped

➤ Improve scores on IQ tests.

➤ Organize the firing patterns of neurons in the brain, stimulating creative right-brain thinking.

➤ Increase focus and concentration.

➤ Reduce stress.

➤ Calm the nervous system.

Weekend Musicians

Across the music spectrum, rock 'n' roll is relieving stress and relaxing men and women by providing an invigorating and fun outlet for their pent-up emotions. The Weekend Warriors program, dreamed up by an ex-rocker from California, is franchised to more than 100 music stores throughout the United States.

Interested wannabe musicians (talent or auditions are not necessary) sign on for five weeks. They are settled in groups and given instruments, a place to practice, and a professional musician as coach. As a kind of graduation ceremony, the group gives a live concert at a local club.

Participants say it's a fun, social way of getting rid of stress. The experience also creates friendships that increase participants' sense of belonging and lessen their loneliness, thus improving both emotional and physical health.

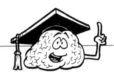

Mindful Moment

Although dancing during worship is not common in the United States, faith and frenzy abound in other corners of the globe. Each year, the Fez Festival of World Sacred Music attracts thousands to Fez, Morocco. Last year the series of concerts included whirling dervishes from Turkey, Greek Byzantine chants, Irish chants, Andalusian Jewish songs, American spirituals, Indian ragas, and Sufi songs from Azerbaijan and Uzbekistan.

Healing Sounds

One Earth Day I attended a presentation called "Spoken Flute" given by a member of the Cheyenne River Lakota Tribe of South Dakota. With chant and instrumental flute music, he offered healing to us and to the earth.

The Navajo believe that in their healing chants, the voice is wind, the greatest cosmic force. The singer calls upon the deities of the mountains, sky, Earth, and animal and plant kingdoms to bring harmony and restore health to a sick person.

Music aids healing in another way. I began this chapter by mentioning the mother's heartbeat as the first sound, or music, people hear. A musical beat is an outward parallel to a heartbeat. Just as colicky babies calm down when held to hear the heartbeat, so do we when we're out of sorts and hear the "heartbeat" of music. The National Institutes of Health (1992) and other sources report the beneficial effects of music. Indeed, some hospitals use music as therapy for their patients. When patients listen to music that mimics the heartbeat—when it has, for example, a repeating bass line—they experience decreased blood rate, decreased heart rate, decreased stress level, and lessening of pain.

Dance to the Music

I can't end this chapter without mentioning dance. It's almost impossible to feel down when you're dancing. You get an aerobic boost, beat the blues, and charge your battery when you're keeping time to a good beat. You don't need a partner or a dance floor, just a bit of cleared space. Add a wild, quick beat and improvise. You'll be jazzed.

Dance as Ritual

Dance has been part of religion for a long time. As it is natural to use your voice to sing to God, so in dance you use your entire body to praise and pray. In Psalm 150, God's people are told to "praise him with timbrel and dance." After the Israelites passed through the Red Sea, the Bible says that Miriam the prophetess "took a tambourine in her hand, while all the women went out after her dancing with tambourines …" Most famous perhaps is the dance of David before the Ark of the Covenant as it was carried in procession to Jerusalem.

The aims of sacred dance include

➤ Offering dance to God.

➤ Finding the festive nature of life and religion.

➤ Integrating body and soul.

➤ Affirming the body.

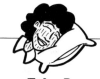

Take 5

Try danced prayer with young children. In classes I taught, I suggested a simple prayer. I took it line by line, asking the children how they felt their bodies wanted to move to express the line. The girls and boys were receptive and excited about this different prayer form.

A Wellness Dance

Dance is used as therapy and may be included in activities offered at a wellness center. Sometimes people don't dance because they have a body image that needs healing: They don't like their bodies or are ashamed of them. This exercise was used in a class I took that was designed to heal and teach body acceptance:

1. Begin by lighting candles and turning off lights. Light as many candles as you wish.

2. Choose a quiet, slow piece of music.

3. Begin standing, sitting, or kneeling, whichever is your preference.

4. Close your eyes.

5. Remain as you are for a few moments, just listening to the music.

6. Give your body permission to move. Try to avoid directing your bodily movements.

7. Allow yourself to flow freely and naturally with the tempo of the music.

Beginning in this way is to begin in a safe, nonjudgmental, private environment. As you allow yourself to move, your body and your mind react positively. When you become more comfortable, you may change the music, gradually increasing its tempo. The next stage may be to leave the lights on and finally, to open your eyes. At that point, Arthur Murray watch out!

Dancercise

If you don't know who Richard Simmons is, you must be from another planet. He's the king of dance music exercise. No wonder he's so popular—dance exercise works. Singing all the lyrics you still remember takes your mind off your aching body. Remember, your mind cannot think two thoughts simultaneously.

Dancing is fun and healthy. It relaxes you, drives away your stress (as long as you're not self-conscious about how you look on the dance floor), and tightens up your muscles. For these reasons, your wellness center or spa may offer dance classes or dance exercise. When you get back home, you'll have a great excuse to spend all night at the dance club.

The Least You Need to Know

➤ Music and dance activate all the chakras to energize, heal, and uplift.

➤ Each of us has a unique song to sing: the talents, gifts, and purpose that we offer to the world throughout our lives.

➤ Calming music lessens pain, decreases stress, and lowers heart and breathing rates.

➤ Dance is used for prayer, for therapy to heal our bodies, for exercise, and for just plain fun.

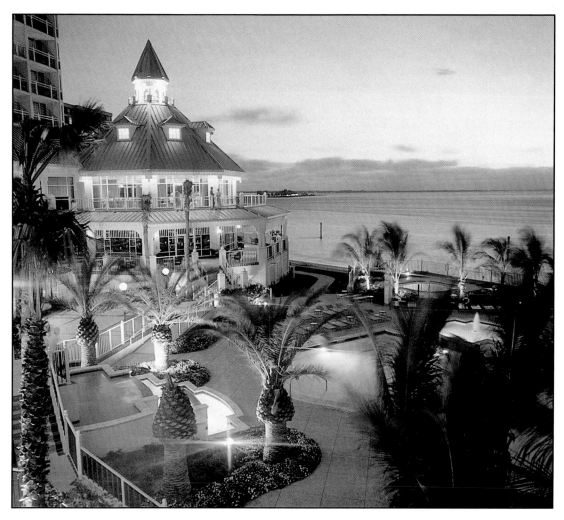

At the end of the day, appreciate the peaceful splendor of the sunset and allow a sense of gratitude to well up within you. A rejuvenating, restful sleep follows, as this feeling of peace, joy, and thanksgiving stays with you.

(Sanibel Harbour Resort and Spa, Florida; courtesy of Spa Finder)

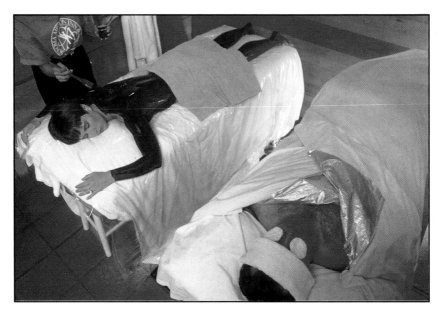

This is your special getaway to treat yourself well. Soak in the spa's beauty treatments and let someone else care for you.

(Sonoma Mission Inn and Spa, California; courtesy of Spa Finder)

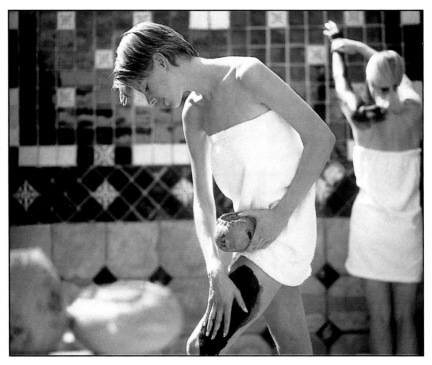

After a visit to a spa you'll be a pro at giving yourself a mud treatment. What a great way to bring the spa experience home with you!

(Ojai Valley Inn and Spa, California; courtesy of Spa Finder)

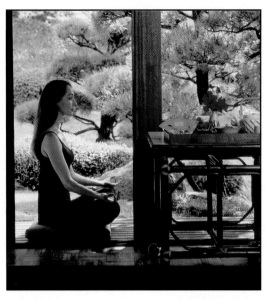

Breathe deeply and let the fresh-scented air calm and cleanse your body and spirit. Look closely. This scene could be outside your home, your hermitage, your retreat, or your spa.

(Golden Door, California; courtesy of Spa Finder)

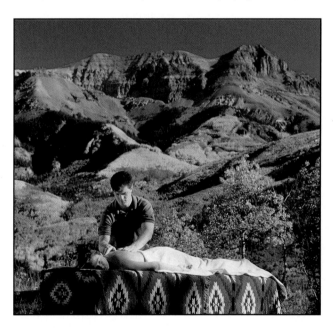

Become one with nature as your body is massaged and the gentle breezes caress your spirit and blow away every trace of stress and anxiety. Arise recharged by the same powerful, healing energy that flows through the universe.

(The Peaks Resort and Spa, Colorado; courtesy of Spa Finder)

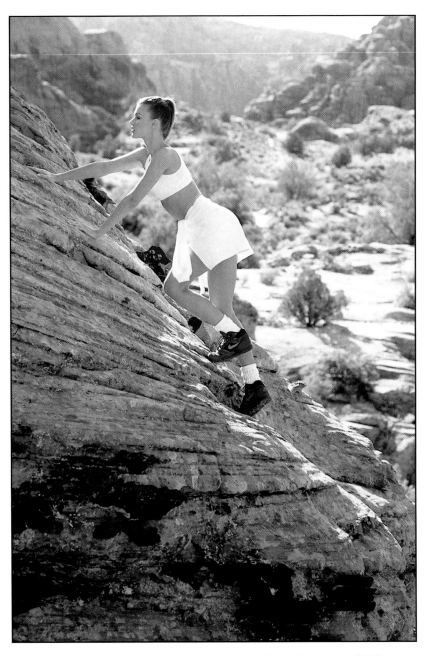

You don't need extravagant equipment to climb rocks, just a child's willingness to scramble on all fours. When you try this exhilarating exercise, get in touch with the strength deep within you and within the ancient stone.

(Green Valley Fitness Resort and Spa, Utah; courtesy of Spa Finder)

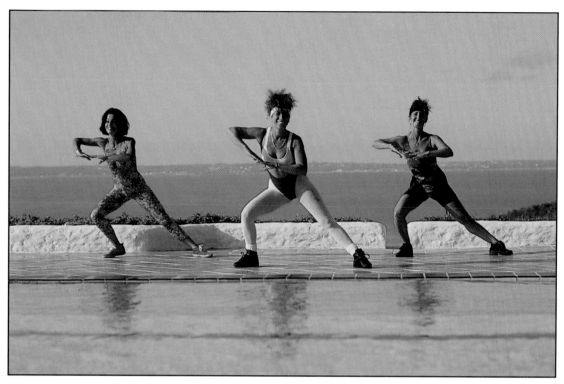

Water is a source of serenity and life. Even while your body is exercising, allow your mind to be aware of your surroundings and your spirit to drink it all in.
(Privilege Resort and Spa, St. Martin; courtesy of Spa Finder)

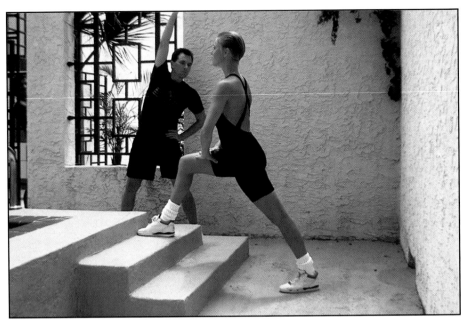

If you need encouragement or direction in shaping a fitness program that is right for you, find help at a spa or wellness center or at a class near your home. Sometimes it's just more fun to work out with someone else.

(Safety Harbor Resort, Florida; courtesy of Spa Finder)

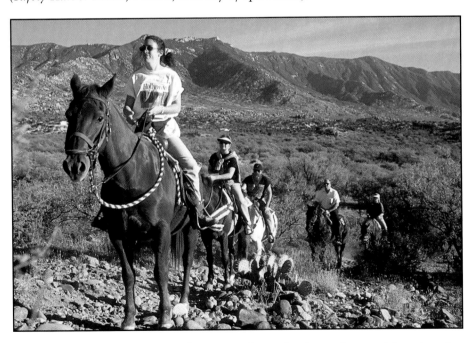

Horses are sensitive creatures who can teach us about ourselves and how to get along in life. And if your back can take it, riding is one wonderful way to get your daily quotient of fun and pleasure.

(Miraval, Life in Balance, Arizona; courtesy of Spa Finder)

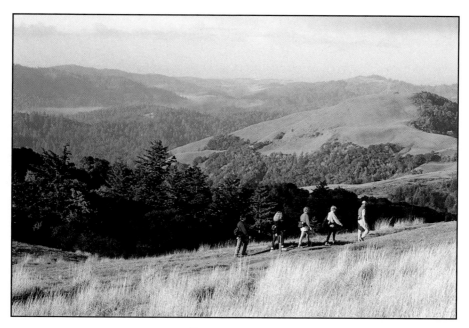

You can practice informal walking meditation anywhere (and get effective exercise besides), whether it's on a mountainside with spectacular views, or along the byways near your home. While walking, consider the kind of footprints you are leaving behind; if you wish a world of peace, joy, and hope, walk in the same way.

(The Lodge at Skylonda, California; courtesy of Spa Finder)

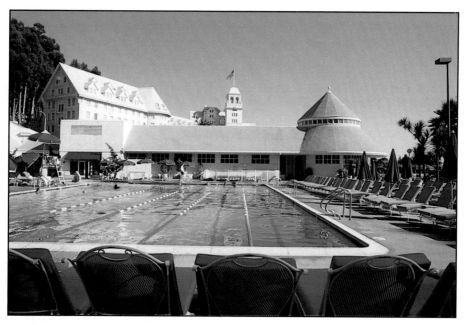

Water: cool, sparkling, soothing, and renewing. Splash like a child or swim hard and then let the world go by as you catnap poolside.

(The Claremont Resort and Spa, California; courtesy of Spa Finder)

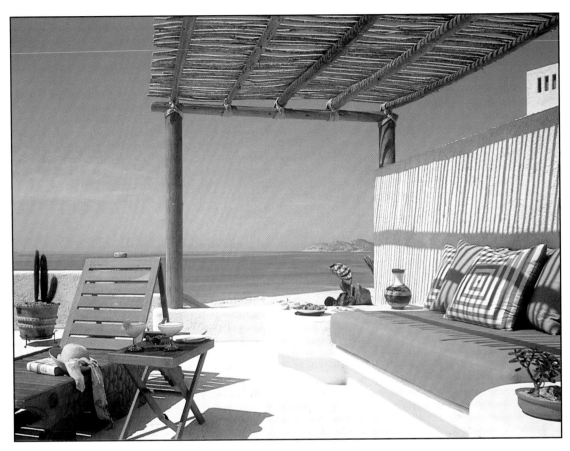

Look closely. There's the book you always wanted to read, an inviting chair, a refreshing drink, and heavenly solitude. There's only one thing missing—you! Plan your spa or retreat getaway today.
(Las Ventanas al Paraiso, Mexico; courtesy of Spa Finder)

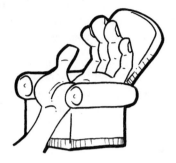

Chapter 17

Hand-y Ways to Relax

In This Chapter

➤ Using your hands for self-healing

➤ How energy flows can reduce stress

➤ Releasing tension through words

➤ Getting a grip on life

Hands enable you to reach out and touch all of life. You

➤ Handle it.

➤ Get a grip on yourself.

➤ Lend a hand.

Not only in language, but also in tangible ways hands are used to heal, comfort, anoint, and bond.

In this chapter, we'll look at how your hands are conduits for the energy flowing through your body. I end with a list of suggested activities that help release unwanted and negative energy and help keep your energy flowing freely for maximum health. Not surprisingly, all the activities use your hands.

Handling Energy

Hands are the conduits of tremendous amounts of energy. That's why energy practitioners, including massage therapists, can heal through the power of touch. We are all able to provide comfort or reassurance with only a gentle pat or the wordless brush of the hand.

It is possible to heal ourselves and others with our hands because this healing hand energy comes from the Source. It is called by different names, including cosmic energy. Because it is divine energy, it is appropriate that it enters the body through the seventh or crown chakra, which is the link to the higher self and the Higher Power.

The greater portion of energy in your upper body, your higher center, is this divine energy. When you draw it in, this pure energy, some say white light, enters through the crown chakra. It flows down the neck and splits at the shoulders, flowing out through each arm and hand. Another portion of it continues through your middle body.

Divine energy enters the body through the crown chakra and exits primarily through the hands.

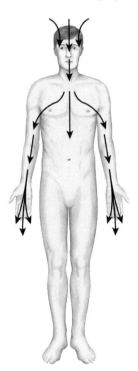

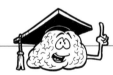

Mindful Moment

When people pray, "Make me a hollow reed," they are making an analogy with the flute, which takes wind and creates sounds of praise and healing. They ask that God's love flow freely through them, like wind through a flute, to others and carry away self-centered desires, grudges, and jealousies.

Depending upon your body's position, you give this exiting energy back to yourself in a shower of healing. When you pray or meditate, for example, the increased energy you transmit as you unite with the divine flows through you and back to you through your hands.

Letting Your Energy Flow

It's time for you to get a grip on your energy and your life. Many studies have shown that mental states are linked to physical conditions. Practitioners in the East have worked with energy and used its flow to eliminate stress- and disease-causing blockages for centuries.

Most often we notice our flow of energy, or lack of it, by the sensations in our hands. Whenever I sit down to type, I feel the energy in my fingers. When you engage in a particular activity that uses your creative energy, you may notice your body beginning or increasing its energy flow as you start the activity. That energy plays an important role in calming you down and healing what ails you in body and soul.

There are more beneficial ways to deal with unwanted and negative energy buildup than by chewing fingernails or cracking knuckles. From magic to macramé, clay to cooking, there's an almost endless variety of hand activities to suit your taste, temperament, and time.

Please, don't start complaining that you don't have enough time. When something is important enough, you find a way to make it work. The suggestions I offer in this chapter are merely a sampling. All use your hands. This is where energy may be blocked and where it builds up when you are nervous or under stress. Using your hands helps make the energy flow.

Get Down, Get Dirty, Get Gardening

Gardening gets you into direct contact with the soothing, vitalizing aspects of the earth. You don't have to dress up, shave, or wear makeup, and you can raise fresh vegetables for dinner! A garden is also a time-honored place to use for meditation or prayer.

Gardens teach us that we need to revel not only in the results, but also in the process itself. I still marvel at and am excited by the first shoots of spring reaching for the life-sustaining light. Read *The Complete Idiot's Guide to Gardening* (Alpha Books, 1999) for more enlightenment.

Gardens

➤ Delight the senses.

➤ Change with the seasons.

➤ Are an oasis.

Whether you have lots of acreage, a small yard, patio, or windowsill, you can transform your space into a vision of serenity.

Gardening gets you into direct contact with the soothing, vitalizing aspects of the earth. (Photo courtesy Linda Short)

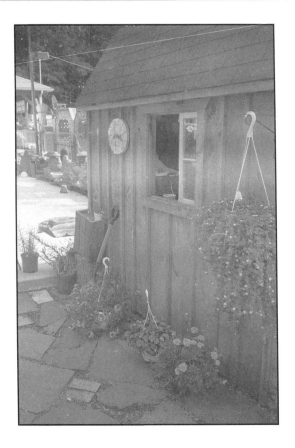

Make the Space Inviting

Define your area with edging materials, stone, or border plantings. Professionals create pathways, even through the smallest area. Yes, you want to be able to admire your garden and sit near it so that you can have quiet time for contemplation, but you need an inviting way to enter it and walk through it as well. Even a short path will do. Use paving stones in various shapes placed close enough so you're forced to shorten your steps and slow down.

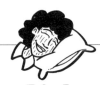

Take 5

Make paths curved, not straight. You see more of the garden, the walk is a bit longer, and curved paths are more aesthetically pleasing.

Add a chair or bench, perhaps a light source for nighttime visits, and a focal point such as a large rock, a piece of wood, a group of shells, or a garden sculpture. Together these things create a pleasing place where your body and soul want to spend time.

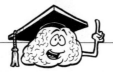

Mindful Moment

For over a thousand years, the cottage garden enriched the English countryside with its colors, fragrances, shapes, and textures. Traditionally almost everything these gardens grew was destined for the table. During the nineteenth century, these gardens became a haven for simple, hardy plants grown in profusion. Anyone was welcome to wander in and discover many surprises and delights in these gardens.

Add Water

A pond is tranquil and lovely to look at. The flowing water of a fountain helps absorb the noise of neighbors, traffic, and other unwanted distractions. (To learn how to build your own pond or fountain, read Chapter 15, "Nature Calls!") You might want to treat the birds (and you!) to a birdbath. Elevate it on a pedestal or place it right on the ground.

Add Sound

If you've added water to your garden, you may already be enjoying trickling, bubbling, or gurgling sounds. If not, or if you wish to add more sound, consider wind chimes or bells. Trees or tall grasses also make soothing sounds when the wind blows through them.

Use Rocks

I have a natural rock outcropping behind my house. Last fall I spent a few days removing moss and dirt from its facade so I can now enjoy its simple strength.

If you wish to follow the Zen tradition, make a garden entirely from gravel or sand raked around deliberately set stones. More practically speaking, this kind of garden is great for areas already covered with concrete, hard-to-cultivate areas, and people who suffer from soil-borne allergies. It's also very easy to maintain.

Take 5

To find a natural arrangement for a group of garden stones, Jeff Cox in *Landscaping with Nature: Using Nature's Designs to Plan Your Yard* (Rodale Press, 1991) recommends placing them according to the pattern of notes in a simple melody. The mood of the tune you pick should match the landscape. Select a few bars of music. Each note correlates to a rock: The higher the note's pitch, the taller the rock; the more emphasis on the note, the bigger the rock; the greater the space between notes, the more distance between the stones.

Ease of Maintenance

If you love gardening, make your garden as big as you can. If you want a more manageable garden that requires little attention, herbs are delightful low-maintenance plants. They do well in a garden, in pots, or in window boxes. They require little water (watch the pots and boxes, though, because they shouldn't dry out completely) and tolerate poor soil. Or grow perennials. I enjoy working outside in the garden, but I switched to perennials long ago. You might mix perennials and annuals, so you have the ease of plants that come up year after year with a few new delights each season.

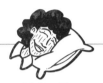

Take 5

Cut down on weeding and conserve water by using mulch, newspapers, or plastic around the plants.

Take 5

To create a flower arrangement of Oriental grace, choose three flowers of three lengths, symbolizing Earth (shortest), humans (middle), and heaven (tallest), and place them in a simple vase.

Chill Out

Place the bed of stone inside a relatively flat but interesting container to keep the stone from spilling or being kicked around.

Add Pleasant Scents

In the movie *The Mask of Zorro,* the elder Zorro's daughter, played by Catherine Zeta-Jones, remembers the smell of the flowers that her father, played by Anthony Hopkins, put into her crib when she was an infant. Scents evoke memories long after the event has passed out of our mind. (The calming, energizing, and healing power of scent is the basis for aromatherapy.) Add plants with a variety of pleasing scents, such as lavender, lemon balm, mint, and Lily of the Valley (sometimes called May Bells).

Splash Color Around

Emerson said, "Earth laughs in flowers." Fill the garden or balcony area with colors you love. Color by itself can be restorative, and it is the most immediately sensuous aspect of a garden.

Create an Evening Garden

Create a garden you can enjoy after the sun goes down, not only in fall and winter when there's less daylight, but year 'round, particularly if you're not often home before dark. For example, you might have a bed of white stone, with one large, interestingly shaped rock and a lantern beside it.

The lantern would protect the flame of a scented candle placed within. The stone is light-colored because it's more easily seen than a darker one at night. You might also use light-colored plants, such as bellflower and garden spires. The garden need not be big, so it can sit nicely in a backyard, on a balcony, on a porch, or even in a windowsill. End your day under the stars. Perhaps a shooting star or Peter Pan will visit one evening.

Writing: Going with the Flow

Writing is a useful tool for opening up one's creativity and problem-solving ability. Writing exercises may

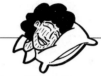

➤ Stimulate positive thinking.

➤ Help generate ideas.

➤ Enable you to take creative risks.

➤ Break through blocks.

➤ Give you confidence to implement creative ideas.

Take 5

Keep your desk or writing surface supplied with colorfully decorated or textured writing papers. Their beauty will invite you to use them more often, and you will enjoy writing more when you do so.

When you write about any stress you may be feeling, you release them from your mind. The negative energy flows out of your body through your hands and your general well-being improves. (Recall the discussion in Chapter 13, "Heal Thyself.") This kind of writing isn't journal writing—the kind you might do when you're recording reflections and occurrences. Rather, it's writing that draws attention to and focuses on your worries, tensions, and problems.

Ready, Set, Write!

The following writing exercises are for fun. No one will grade or even review what you write. Don't worry if you can't spell, and don't be concerned with how much you put on paper. Take out pen or pencil or turn on your computer, and let the writing begin. Use these ideas to get you started:

➤ List uses for an empty can or for a shoelace.

➤ Try writing with a group, working with others in pairs or threes. Take an ordinary object, for example, a key. Invent a new use for it. Give it a name. Write some promotional copy, explaining its benefits.

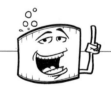

➤ Flow write by writing for 20 minutes. Set a timer or the beeper on your watch so your focus is on the writing and not on the time. Once you begin to write, you may not stop. Write whatever and everything that comes into your mind. Do not edit or censor. Write exactly what you think. The words flow from your mind, through your arm, hand, writing implement, and onto the paper. If you get

Jacuzzi Jive

Haiku is a Japanese verse form which, in English, consists of three unrhymed lines of five, seven, and five syllables respectively (totaling 17 syllables), often on some subject in nature.

stuck, continue to write what you last wrote until a new thought comes to mind. When you finish, notice where you began and where you ended. These are the important ideas that deserve attention.

➤ Often nature images creep into our flow writing. Choose one of them and write a *haiku*. After you've written it down, give it power by speaking it aloud to someone else.

➤ Write your unconscious. Your brain continues to function, apart from your dreaming, while you sleep. For this exercise, have paper and pen at your bedside. Immediately upon awaking, write whatever comes to mind. Do this for 10 to 15 minutes. These thoughts are the concerns that were last addressed by your unconscious. Continue this practice for a week (or longer) and notice any patterns in your writing.

➤ Write letters. I don't mean letters using typewriters or e-mail. I mean good, old-fashioned, pen-and-paper letters where you can feel the pen and the texture of the paper. A wonderful benefit is that you will receive letters in return, which will put a smile on your face and give a lift to your spirit. Use your Sabbath time (see Chapter 4, "Time Won't Let Me") or lunch break to take a real break and shift gears. Don't write about work!

Calming Clay

Whether you use play dough you make yourself, purchase clay at a department, craft, or art store, or go to a pottery studio, clay is another no-experience-necessary outlet for your frustrations. You need no special skill or ability to enjoy clay. It's like playing in the mud.

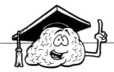

Mindful Moment

This play dough doesn't separate and get slimy like some other recipes. Mix 1 cup salt, 2 cups flour, and 4 teaspoons cream of tartar in a heavy pot. Add 2 tablespoons oil and 2 cups water. (Food coloring is optional.) Mix continuously as you cook on low to medium heat. As the mixture cooks, it will become rubbery and pull together in a large ball. Take it off the heat and spoon it out of the pot onto a sheet of foil to cool. Knead it slightly to smooth it out. Dough will last months if kept in an air-tight container. If left out in the air, it will crystallize and harden.

The clammy, cool nature of the clay balances the heat of your energy (something like dousing a flame) and calms you. The clay focuses on and releases the energy in your hands while you knead and pummel and pull and roll. Don't make anything; simply enjoy the mushy feeling of the clay as it squirts through and around your fingers. Spend most of your time working the dough. If you wish, mold something in the end.

Handbuilding

Fashioning clay by hand is called handbuilding. Traditionally you use coils (rolled pieces of clay like long snakes) and slabs (flat, rolled-out pieces of clay cut to size). Combine the forces of nature with your clay: Collect leaves, for example, and gently push them onto the surface of the clay. Enjoy their prints long after the leaves have dried and crumbled.

For Prayer or Meditation

Clay may be used with prayer or meditation. The clay becomes the object of attention, to focus the mind and set aside distractions. To begin, play slow, quiet instrumental music. Do not intend to work or fashion the clay, but rather allow the clay to fashion itself using your hands. When you conclude your prayer, notice how the clay looks and recall your thoughts during the process.

More Hand-y Ways to Relax

There are many more ways to encourage the flow of stress and negative energy from your body. Here are just a few:

➤ Painting

➤ Cooking and bread making

➤ Needle crafts and sewing

➤ Building and repairing

➤ Performing magic tricks

➤ Decoupage

➤ Playing an instrument

When you feel tired and stressed, notice how your hands feel and what you do with them. You may discover you could benefit from some simple hand-y ways to release and control your energy and your emotional state. You may even find a new passion!

The Least You Need to Know

➤ Your hands are a major block, preventing negative energy from flowing out of our bodies.

➤ Manipulation and use of your hands permits the release of stress and tension, enabling self-healing.

➤ Activities such as gardening, writing, and working with clay are excellent ways to focus on your hands and get them involved in creative activity.

➤ When the energy blockages in your hands are removed, the divine energy may flow freely throughout your being, bringing you peace and serenity.

Part 6
Take Me Away from Here!

How are you feeling? Do you look edgy, pale, out of sorts? Is work a crazy place; does home give you little relief? A spa or retreat may be just what you need to cure what ails you.

Whether you use sick leave or vacation time or just a weekend or a day, Part 6 will get you where you need to be. It takes you through the ins and outs of spas, retreats, and pilgrimages. There are questions to help you narrow the search for your ultimate getaway and sample destinations to entice you away from home (if you still need any further convincing!).

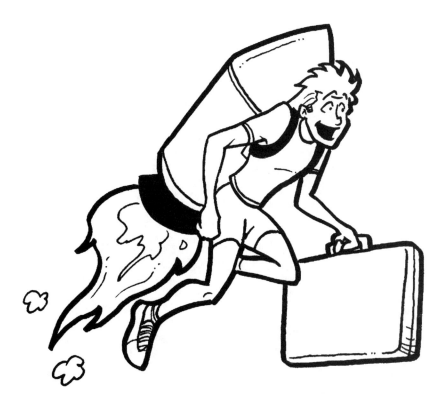

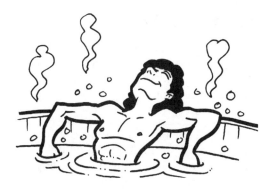

Chapter 18

Sparkling Spa-cial Spas

In This Chapter

➤ Not all spas are alike

➤ Get ready for luxury

➤ Spa programs and services

➤ A sample spa day

➤ For men as well

What is it about spas that either excites or repels people? Guests rave about the beauty treatments, services, and pampered attention shown them. But many who've never been to a spa say they wouldn't be caught dead at one. I have a theory about these strong reactions.

One of my theories has to do with the seemingly luxurious, expensive, wasteful side of spas. When spas began way back in the times of mineral baths, natural hot springs, and such, only the rich went and took the cure. The spa appeared to be a mere extension of their extravagant lifestyle.

Then along came various religious sects, including the Puritans, who made people feel pretty guilty, if not downright sinful, for spending time and money on themselves. "We need to do and accomplish and work," the people in these sects said, "We don't need to fritter away idle moments under creams or in saunas."

The thing is, as society heats up, each of us tries to keep pace with it, and it's taking its toll on us. Cars need maintenance to keep from overheating or falling apart, and so do we. We need tune-ups and sometimes major overhauls to be able to care for our families, our jobs, and our world.

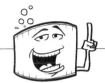

Jacuzzi Jive

As a philosophy, **hedonists** believe that the principal good and highest aim of society or the individual is to seek pleasure. **Hedonism** has come to be described as the self-indulgent pursuit of pleasure as a way of life.

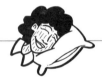

Take 5

If you believe you are good at mind and spirit care, but tend to neglect your body, be warned: You're a package deal and need to care for the whole package.

Chill Out

Not all day spas are created equal. Some are little more than hair or nail salons capitalizing on the spa boom. Visit first and ask for a tour. Give the place the once over, and you'll know if you want to go back.

How Puritan Are You?

Are you a Puritan, a *hedonist,* or, more likely, somewhere in between? The answer will help you understand how open you are to trying a spa and what you need to overcome to be comfortable about going to one (if indeed you're not quite sure yet).

Try this. When you have time on your hands, how do you feel? Can you relax or do you need to be doing something? If you always need to be busy or worrying about this or that, you're not alone. This tendency does mean, however, that you might not want to or be able to lie still for a massage, for example. You need to move, to accomplish something. The good news is that there's a spa for you, too. In fact, it's probably types like you that got the spa industry to include fitness and outdoor programs such as kayaking, mountain biking, and hiking in their agendas.

Spas also offer you a place and time to recover from an unhappy event or to celebrate a joyful one. This time is not self-indulgence, but good, old-fashioned taking care of yourself. It's what the medical establishment has been telling you: Take care of yourself, eat right, exercise, and calm down. Spa treatments touch your body, and in that touch, bring you energy and healing for a healthier and happier life. So go ahead and meet your own needs. It's doctor's orders!

A Spa by Any Name

Today, many types of facilities call themselves spas. Although most all of them have mud packs and herbal wraps, these things are often secondary now to, say, the nutrition program. You might attend a "resort spa" because it is a resort, and the fact that it has spa services is a bonus.

Major Categories

Spa Finder is a spa travel and reservation company that books spa vacation packages for the spas it represents. Its many spa listings can be found in Appendix A, "The Spa Finder Directory of Spa Retreats and Spa Resorts." Spa Finder uses these major divisions to classify the spas it represents:

➤ Spa retreats

➤ Resort spas

➤ Luxury spa retreats

➤ Luxury resort spas

➤ Weight management retreats

➤ New Age retreats

➤ Adventure spas

➤ Spas abroad

➤ Spas at sea

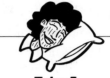

Take 5

Sample spa life at a day spa, which offers you many of the same services without the expense of an overnight stay. When you find it the grand affair that many do, I bet you'll want more and a longer spa stay.

Other spa reservation or information services use different categories.

These facilities may offer Japanese mud baths, holistic therapies, New Age philosophy, martial arts, yoga, massages, relationship or employment classes, workshops on coping with specific medical conditions, and more. Many spas offer weekend, as well as weeklong, programs.

Special-Interest Categories

If you are interested in a specific activity or service, ask for it. Some spas have a particular focus, for example:

➤ Stress management.

➤ Quitting smoking.

➤ Vegetarian cuisine.

➤ Fasting.

➤ Lots of pampering.

➤ Sports: Ask about your interest.

If you're thinking about combining a spa stay with your vacation, there are also listings for

➤ Honeymoons.

➤ Most tranquil spas.

➤ Most scenic locations.

➤ Popular tourist destinations.

➤ Gambling locales.

➤ Spas on the beach.

You will find a spa that meets your every desire.

Targeted Guests

Sometimes you may want to travel solo or with others who shares your situation. Different spas may be best for men, women, seniors, families, or mother/daughter stays. They are all spas, but they aren't all alike. The listings in Appendix A introduce you to the possibilities and allow you to narrow your choices.

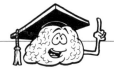

Mindful Moment

The International Spa Association reports that growing numbers of men are de-stressing in spas. Once the domain of women, spa clientele is now 25 percent men. "Men are discovering the health benefits of a facial or a body wrap," said spa consultant Michael Ternet in a recent issue of *USA Weekend Magazine*.

First-Day Jitters

When you enter a spa, you leave your daily life behind. You may need a day to become adjusted to your new surroundings, but then so will everyone else.

Queen—or King—for a Day

Years ago there was a television show called *Queen for a Day*. The winner received prizes that made her wishes come true. Folks who have hit the big jackpot sometimes aren't comfortable when they get their wish. You, too, may be a bit anxious when you realize you are where you wished to be!

Your anxiety is normal. After all, you probably traveled a distance and are tired, maybe even jet-lagged. Perhaps you're also a bit out of shape and feel a little self-conscious about it. Everyone else (except for perhaps the repeaters) is a little anxious, too.

To add to the confusion, fit young guys and good-looking women are treating you like a king or queen. You thought you were just a regular overworked guy or gal trying to pay the bills. If that isn't enough, the place is gorgeous. Now that you have them, use those servants, uh, staff, and ask questions to ease your way.

Leave Life Behind

Don't leave *all* of life behind; please continue breathing. You are here (wherever here is) for a change of pace:

➤ Put work out of your mind.

➤ Take a notebook to jot down any creative thoughts, business ideas, or personal insights that come into your head.

218

➤ Enjoy the people.

➤ Make the most of body treatments: Prepare for them and linger afterward.

➤ Try something you haven't done before.

➤ Focus on your goal, if you set one for yourself.

In other words, turn your mind away from home and give this experience your full attention.

Second Thoughts

As you're settling in, you may have some second thoughts about being here. Maybe you're afraid you haven't dressed right, won't be able to keep up with the workouts, will have to eat food you dislike, or will be showing more of your body than you'd like. Put the fears out of your mind.

Clothing

Some spas provide standard outfits. Otherwise, folks wear casual stuff like shorts, T-shirts, sweats, and robes. If you need to dress or change for dinner, you'll know ahead of time. At resorts, dress like you would on vacation; that's where you are, after all.

Workouts

I've attended a program considered to have one of the most challenging workouts, so, believe me, I know about performance anxiety! However, most spa goers are beginning an exercise regimen or are beginning again after taking some or lots of time off. Spas expect guests to be at different levels of fitness. If the workout is too difficult, speak up and find something more your speed.

Meals

Fortunately, spas realize that you need good food and instruction to help you eat healthier and maintain your desired weight level. You won't starve. Spa food is delicious, nutritious, and sufficient. Some spas offer all-you-can-eat buffets; others serve all guests the same menu. If you're hungry, ask for more.

Chill Out

Some spas offer "oxygen bars," where you eat up pure oxygen for body cleansing. But be careful if you have a lung condition: Dr. Marsha Gordon, author *of The Complete Idiot's Guide to Beautiful Skin*, writes that oxygen doesn't cleanse the body and could be dangerous.

Jacuzzi Jive

The term **bodywork** refers to therapies such as massage, deep-tissue manipulation, movement awareness, and energy balancing, which are used to improve the structure and functioning of the body.

Bodywork

Bodywork is a problem for many people. Often you're surrounded by great-looking staff and are embarrassed to bare your less-than-perfect body. Take a breath. Not all body treatments require disrobing. For example, some types of massage are done in light clothing. Then there are movement-awareness techniques like the Feldenkrais Method (see Chapter 11, "Let's Get Physical") or yoga done clothed.

If you plain aren't ready for touch-y treatments, try a visualization class to release tension from your body.

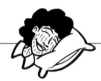

Take 5

A massage therapist doesn't know he's crossed over your comfort line unless you tell him or her, so if something's a problem, make your voice heard. Ask for someone else if a particular therapist isn't responding to your concerns.

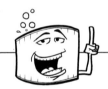

Jacuzzi Jive

Hydrotherapy uses the healing power of water along with massage or movement or simply soaking, steaming, or spraying. **Reflexology** uses massage on one part of the body (typically the feet, hands, or ears) to affect the health and function of other body areas. **Herbal wraps** involve sheets soaked in teas made from herbs that are wrapped around the body to induce you to sweat and release toxins.

If, however, you choose a body treatment that works best with no clothes on, rest assured that you undress in private. In addition, staff are trained to drape you discreetly so you won't feel exposed. (Besides, it gets chilly in your birthday suit!)

Services, Services, and More Services

Fortunately for me, this is an introductory book, so I can't cover every treatment you could possibly enjoy, considering all the spas worldwide. In any case, it seems like somebody's dreaming up new services daily, so if I did try to list them all I'd have a list with no end in sight. Then I couldn't get away for my massage and my facial, manicure, and pedicure package!

General Scheduling

When you make your spa reservation, ask about services and scheduling. Depending upon the facility and its promotions, some services may come as a prepaid package. Others may cost extra. Yet other spas ask you to pay individually for each service you choose, whether that's a class, a salon, or a spa service. (Read Chapter 21, "Finding Your Way at a Spa or Retreat," for the kinds of questions to ask about programs and services.)

If you stay at a resort or other facility with many guests, you will need to schedule appointments for various treatments. Don't assume you can walk in and be served; it's unlikely. Find out how far in advance appointments may be made and under what conditions they may be cancelled. Help with scheduling may be part of your orientation to the facility and its services. If it isn't, ask if you need guidance.

Thanks to *The Complete Idiot's Guide to Beautiful Skin*, I offer a few suggestions about when to schedule particular spa treatments for maximum benefit:

➤ **Massage.** Schedule massage after workouts, especially if your muscles aren't used to such workouts, or at day's end. You're not much good after a massage, and rest and sleep are best.

➤ **Other relaxers** (aromatherapy, hydrotherapy, reflexology, herbal wraps, facials). Schedule these for late afternoon when you're winding down anyway.

➤ **Beauty sessions** (hair, cosmetics, manicures, pedicures). Schedule them for the last day if you'll be swimming or sweating during your stay; you don't want to damage the results. You'll also look great for going home.

Chill Out

Be sure any facial you have is gentle and doesn't pull your skin. If you have sensitive or allergy-prone skin, say so. Some facials use fragranced lotions that can wreak havoc on sensitive faces. If you're acne-prone, ask for oil-free products.

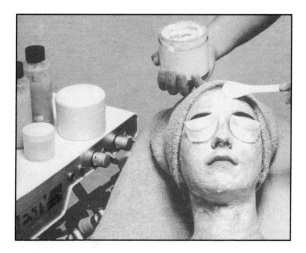

Let your entire body relax as you and your eyes experience the soothing effects of a cucumber beauty treatment in the spa's salon.
(Image © H. Armstrong Roberts)

Salon Services

Larger resorts, spas, and wellness centers usually divide their services between the salon and the spa area, and there are often separate reservation and appointment procedures.

Typical salon services are the visible beauty treatments, which include

➤ Hair services: shampoo, cut, set, style, conditioning, scalp treatment, coloring, frosting, braiding, and permanent/body wave.

➤ Facials.

➤ Neck massages.

➤ Manicure, nail wraps, and nail tips.

➤ Pedicures.

A foot reflexology treatment is a spa service, but it is sometimes given as an add-on to a pedicure in the salon.

Spa Services

If you follow the advice in this chapter, you won't be using the salon until the end of your stay. What will you be doing in the meantime? If you have fitness classes or educational workshops, you'll spend a fair amount of time there. Here's how your day might go:

➤ Rise between 8 and 9 A.M. and choose a morning swim, a meditation or yoga class, or a tennis lesson for the next hour or so.

➤ About 10:30 you may decide to lie around the pool, journal, or read. Or take another class—something new—if you feel ambitious.

➤ Take lunch outdoors around 1:00 P.M.

➤ How about a slow walk, meditation, or a nap after lunch?

➤ Feeling rested, you're ready for the gym or for pointers in healthier eating or stress relief.

➤ Now for a massage or a facial. Perhaps it's about 5 P.M.

➤ Enjoy a long, relaxing dinner.

➤ Dance, walk, read, journal, talk.

➤ By 9 P.M., retire for a long, deep sleep.

Indulge your curious and playful side and enjoy several new activities tomorrow.

When you're not eating, sleeping, resting, doing, or listening, there are the spa services. These services are often called by alien-sounding terms, such as the European Thalasso program. Sometimes the names sound exotic: "Ocean breeze facial," for instance, might only mean a facial outdoors. Let's see if I can't clear up some of your confusion.

Massage

Massage has been around forever, but maybe the no-clothes, touched-by-a-stranger bit is what gets to so many people, or maybe it's the massage parlors that are busted on cop shows where sex is being sold instead of a rubdown. But when you get over your anxiety and try massage, you will sigh with pleasure and tension-free relief and wonder why you ever waited so long.

➤ **Clothing optional.** Although a massage is best performed on bare skin (except for Shiatsu and Trager massage, which are performed with clothes on), if you can't disrobe completely, leave on your undergarments. If even that's too skimpy, you will be happy to know that almost any type of massage can be performed over light clothing, especially if your arms, legs, and neck are uncovered. If it's only a quick relaxation massage, you haven't the time for the dressing room scene anyway.

➤ **Session length.** Most massages last about one hour. Check with your spa; it may offer shorter or longer sessions.

➤ **Touch.** Massages range from a light, feathery touch to firm, deep-tissue massage. If it ever feels as though you're getting the hair rubbed off your legs, feel free to complain. If you can't relax, you can't enjoy the benefits.

➤ **Gender.** You don't need to explain to anyone why you'd prefer a massage therapist who is of your same sex or of the opposite sex. Personal preference demands respect.

➤ **Method.** With soothing music playing, your body is covered with a towel and sheet or sheet and blanket. When the therapist is ready to use massage oil on a part of your body such as your arm, that arm is then uncovered.

Take 5

Leave jewelry at home, or be ready to remove it (save wedding rings) prior to your massage. Be sure to go to the bathroom beforehand, too. You don't want anything to disturb or distract you.

Chill Out

You may be concerned about whether your massage therapist is licensed, certified, or otherwise trained and approved. If so, ask.

There are many varieties of massage. The more popular are the following:

➤ **Aromatherapy massage.** It uses massage oil made of fragrant essential oils for facial or body massage.

➤ **Deep-tissue massage.** This type gets into the heart of the muscles and connective tissue; it releases emotions and traumas that have been repressed and stored in the body.

➤ **Esalan massage.** This sensual experience is usually performed outside.

➤ **Hot rock massage.** This massage uses warm rocks instead of hands to massage the oil into the skin.

➤ **Reflexology.** This therapy uses firm pressure or massage on the appropriate area of your foot, hand, or ear to stimulate areas of stress or blockage for healing and relaxation.

➤ **Reiki** (pronounced *ray-kee*). This massage works with energy. Hands are placed at certain points corresponding to the chakras and the endocrine glands, which affect many aspects of your body and mind. The touch is held for a long time,

Take 5

Yoga is sometimes referred to as "internal massage" because the yoga movements do all that massage does in terms of opening chakras, compressing or releasing organs, and mobilizing energy.

usually three to five minutes, and it channels the universe's energy directly into your body.

➤ **Rolfing.** This deep-tissue massage realigns and changes the body's appearance to correct misalignments caused by bad habit and trauma.

➤ **Shiatsu.** The Japanese method of acupressure combines pressure, usually exerted with thumbs and fingers, with long massage strokes across the body's energy meridians.

➤ **Sports massage.** This form of Swedish massage is tailored to the athlete.

➤ **Structural integration.** This therapy moves the body back into alignment by manipulating muscles and connective tissue.

➤ **Swedish massage.** European technique of gentle manipulation of the muscles with the use of massage oils.

➤ **Trager.** Unlike the other forms of massage, the therapist talks to you constantly, telling you what your body is telling him. Trager works on the principle that pain, blockages, and all physical problems begin in the mind, and it accesses the subconscious mind through talking to permit healing of the body.

➤ **Trigger-point therapy.** This term refers to several therapies that use trigger points, or sensitive areas in tight muscles that cause pain in various parts of the body, that are pressed firmly until the tension releases.

Hydrotherapy

In Chapter 15, "Nature Calls!" we saw how water soothes and relaxes. It's no wonder then that water is used for therapy. Hydrotherapy comes in many forms, including baths, showers, saunas, ice and heat packs, hot tubs, and natural hot or cold springs. The different types of baths include mineral, salt, shallow hip, steam, and footbaths.

Etc., Etc.

Other services you'll probably find are wraps or masks, which I mentioned earlier. Masks may be facial or whole-body. Wraps and masks may be herbal, seaweed, or mud. They revive skin, soothe tired muscles, and absorb impurities from the skin.

Just for Men

Skin is skin, and massage is massage, no matter what the sex, but some spas do more to make the guy feel comfortable. For instance, they offer

➤ Male-only days, like Macho Mondays; even all-male spas and locker rooms.

➤ "Guy" drinks like beer instead of water.

➤ Male magazines (for example, *Sports Illustrated* and *GQ*).

➤ "Sport" manicures and "sport" pedicures (to make them sound more fitting for men).

If you're a guy and you're at all shy about trying a spa, begin with an all-male spa or go on male-only days.

Whether man or woman, your body, mind, and spirit need renewal, refreshment, and rejuvenation. Join the spa crowd and enjoy!

The Least You Need to Know

➤ Spas are not created equal, even though they all provide beauty and body treatments.

➤ With the diversity of experiences that are called spas, choose carefully to get the treatments and programs you want for your perfect escape.

➤ Larger spas, wellness centers, and resorts offer beauty treatments in their salon and body treatments in the spa area.

➤ Massages, hydrotherapy, and herbal wraps are wonderful gifts you can give your body, and most spas offer a range of each to choose from.

➤ Fellas, your bodies need nurturing and caring just as much as women's bodies do, and you can get both at men-only spas or on men-only days.

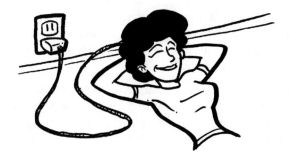

Chapter 19

Rejuvenating Retreats

In This Chapter

➤ Understanding the nature of retreats

➤ Deciding when to go on retreat

➤ Which type of retreat for you?

➤ How a retreat day might go

You want to make an important life decision and decide to spend a few days alone in the country. Workers get together over the weekend at a hotel to build team spirit. A study group ends its time together by camping overnight at a nearby park. A youth group attends a structured weekend at a retreat center as part of their religious program. All of these experiences have been called "retreats." No wonder there is such confusion about what the word means!

Today, the word *retreat* is used to mean almost any time away from your normal routine, whether it's a quiet weekend in the woods or a corporate team-building event. The heart of the retreat experience, no matter what the physical surroundings or stated goals, is a time set aside, out of the ordinary routine of life, to spend in review, reflection, and perhaps in prayer.

In this chapter, we'll look at the types of retreats available, and I'll help you decide which retreat might benefit you. I'll help you understand what you'll find when you get there, and what a typical day is like.

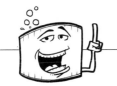

Jacuzzi Jive

For purposes of this book, a **retreat** is a place that, whether it uses physical activity or not, aids guests in reaching higher personal goals or spiritual renewal. The facility offers few or none of the services generally associated with spas.

Out of the Ordinary

To get anything of importance completed, you need to block out time and eliminate disruptions. A retreat does that. The amount may be as little as a few hours or as long as a week or more. It's up to you.

If you haven't gone on retreat before, you may want to start with a short amount of time, perhaps a day. It's better to leave feeling as though you wanted to stay longer than wish you were home already.

Use the time to clear your head—to find distance, values, and direction. Whatever your goal or reasons for going on retreat, listen to the voice from within that guides you. Put another way, we go on retreat to gain perspective, peace, and power over our lives. The special, secluded time allows us to examine ourselves and our life.

With New Eyes

Eyes are such an important part of us. As the saying goes, "The eyes are the windows of the soul." What do you see when you take time to look at yourself? Here is an exercise you can do to answer the question: Find a mirror and place it close enough to your face that you can see your face clearly. Look into your own eyes. What thoughts or images occur to you?

Of course, you cannot look into both eyes simultaneously, but it doesn't matter which eye receives your attention. Try not to decide; just let it happen. Look for as long as you can. It's kind of spooky and exciting at the same time to think you are looking into your own soul.

Chill Out

Don't go on retreat with a list of objectives. It is unlikely that you can address every concern adequately. Besides, you need to be open to the surprises that await you.

Regardless of whether you literally look into your eyes like this, you will probably be using your time on retreat to take a new look at yourself and gain a new perspective on your current situation or life circumstances. A retreat is a chance to step back and view yourself from the outside, as though you were a disinterested third party.

What in your life might benefit from some attention? Is your career not where you'd like it to be, or perhaps you have some undefined yearnings of something better or quite different? Perhaps there's a relationship that isn't as fulfilling as you'd like, or there isn't a relationship at all. Maybe you're feeling that it's time to give more attention to developing your spiritual side. Retreats are also great times to reward yourself and celebrate a major accomplishment or new beginning.

With New Comfort

You will find peace when you feel indecision, worries, or grief lessen, and you are instead cheered, calmed, or inspired with hope. The peace you gain from a retreat is a deep sense of calm, mixed with confidence that the sun is shining and will continue to shine on you and your decision.

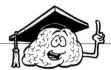

Mindful Moment

St. Ignatius of Loyola, the founder of the Jesuits, a Catholic order for men, is credited with beginning the first structured retreats. He called them "spiritual exercises." Available in book form, *The Spiritual Exercises of St. Ignatius,* a new translation by Louis J. Puhl, S.J. (Newman Press, 1959), details a program that is followed more often in a directed retreat setting. The program also includes a modified version for use at home.

With New Power

The kind of power I'm talking about is strength from within, a certainty and confidence in the correctness of your decision and the direction of the moment. You know you have the ability and control to carry out the decisions you made while on retreat and that you're determined to overcome any obstacles that might get in the way.

This kind of power allows you to be proud in your decisions and direction, regardless of what your friends, boss, or society think. These decisions may have you going against the flow, but you'll know that that's necessary. Great leaders, such as Gandhi, Dr. Martin Luther King Jr., and Mother Teresa, had such power and used it well.

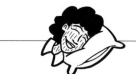

Take 5

A friend of mine used to have a poster on her wall with a quote by Frederick Douglass (1817–1895) that read in part: "You can't have crops without plowing the fields."

Reach for the Sky

The sky has been a metaphor for heaven or spiritual attainment throughout history and in all spiritual traditions. It is no wonder, then, that on retreats you "reach for that sky" with lofty desire and intentions. That is where your focus is and where it needs to be. Consequently, retreat time is not:

➤ Vacation time

➤ Work time

➤ Catch-up-on-sleep time

Although you don't have a specific agenda on retreat, you don't go without one, either. You make a commitment to reach for the best within yourself and then use your inner resources to influence your world, however large or small.

You Can't Go Wrong

You cannot fail, for even if you think you've learned nothing (which is unlikely), you will have succeeded in setting aside important time for yourself and your spirit, time for rest and renewal. Once you experience this renewal time, you just may decide that having such time on a regular basis is a necessary part of your life.

As my "Life Is a Dance" meditation/poem (see Chapter 6, "On the Road to Happiness") says, "expect no applause; accept roses graciously." This paradox describes the retreat experience. Your object is to *be*, not to *do*. Have no definite expectations because you'll need to be open to all that is and happens around you. You need to be a river, a river that accepts the fresh rain, the debris that the wind blows, and the contributions of other tributaries.

My husband recently chose a retreat because he knew and respected the retreat director. While there, he ran into an old acquaintance. He and this man spent much time together on the retreat, and he found that this man's counsel was more important to him than that of the director.

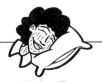

Take 5

Momentous changes may occur on retreat or in retreat-type moments, as these true stories show. One man who is not practicing a faith attends church one Easter, feels a remarkable pull, and is now a priest. A woman moving up the corporate career path leaves to become a massage therapist and open her own business. A grandfather, who as a young man gave up his heart's desire to become a priest, finally enters an order after he is widowed.

I, too, recently returned from a journey. I had no reservations, no fixed destinations, and no timetable other than beginning and ending dates. I left home consciously leaving my wanderings and welfare in the hands of the Other.

On the other hand, I did have some expectations, for why else would I go? I wanted to visit a shrine that is the oldest site of continuing pilgrimage in all of Great Britain. I also knew I wanted to get to the Irish Sea, from where, on a clear day, one can see 75 miles across the water to the Wicklow Mountains along the east coast of the Republic of Ireland.

I had expectations, but I didn't know why they would be important to me. This seeming contradiction of having no expectations and yet expecting something is the best description of the retreat experience.

Retreat Basics

Whether you use the language of religion or the language of metaphysics, the meaning is the same: You will be at the retreat where you were meant to be. You also will be helped and strengthened to face reality, not escape it, on retreat.

Sacred Spaces

Any experience occurs in relation to its environment, so your choice of retreat environment is important. The following are examples of retreat locations:

➤ *Monastery* or *convent*

➤ Conference center or hotel

➤ Retreat center or retreat house

➤ Chapel

➤ Private home

Spaces like monasteries and convents breathe spirituality in their structures and in their commitment to prayer, silence, and encounters with God. More secular surroundings such as conference centers, private homes, and some retreat houses are built without specific places reserved for prayer. The retreat organizers may, however, designate one room as a quiet room, in which all participants are expected to observe silence, conduct no business, and respect each other's prayer time.

Take 5

You may discover retreats in unexpected settings. Last year while on vacation, I found a church that held daily talks and worship services as part of a special weeklong program. I went on "retreat" for two hours each day by attending these sessions.

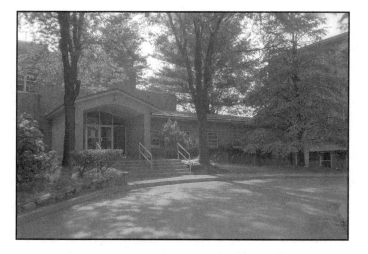

Not all retreat centers, even ones operated by religious congregations, look religious. Many retreats are held in less formal settings. (Photo of Mariandale Retreat and Conference Center, Ossining, NY; courtesy Linda Short)

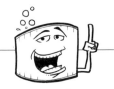

Jacuzzi Jive

A **monastery** is the building or group of buildings that houses monks, men who have withdrawn from the world for religious reasons. The residential house of a religious community of women is called a **convent.**

Often, retreat building(s) are located in quiet, natural settings so that nature can inspire reflection. Take time to look at trees and feel their bark. Invite the rain to wash over you. Taste a snowflake. Watch animals. Sit in the midst of the tall grasses and disappear. See the wonder and beauty of all that surrounds you.

Prayer Practices

Don't feel uncomfortable if you don't pray; you don't have to pray on retreat. Often there will be scheduled times for group or communal prayer, either in a chapel or in a space reserved for quiet. There might be full, formal worship, shorter prayer services, readings of sacred writings, or rituals created specifically to reflect the retreat's theme.

You are not required to attend any gathering, whether it's a prayer or lecture. If you are a pray-er, you may want to go to the community gatherings or pray alone at a time and place of your choosing.

Even if you don't pray, you can't escape the fact that going on retreat is a spiritual experience. It is a time of forming or revitalizing your spiritual journey. It is time away for your soul to stretch, blossom, and grow. It is a time for you to heal, rest, and renew.

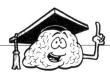

Mindful Moment

Indian poet Rabindranath Tagore (1861–1941), in a piece titled, "Thoughts from Rabindranath Tagore," wrote: "Religion is not a fractional thing that can be doled out in fixed weekly or daily measures as one among various subjects in the school syllabus. It is the truth of our complete being, the consciousness of our personal relationship with the infinite; it is the true center of gravity of our life."

If you feel the pull to begin to pray, or meditate, or focus, or center—practices that bring you closer to the Divine—give in. The important thing is that there is no "right" way to pray during a retreat or anytime. There is also no "right" place to pray.

As with anything, there will be times you may feel like praying, and times you won't. You can pray in a chapel, if you want. You can also pray while walking outside in nature, while journaling, while writing meditations, or while dancing.

You are praying when you sit in the sunshine and enjoy the warmth, peace, and safety of the moment, as though you are being held in the hands of the Holy One. Indeed, you're probably praying at times and don't realize it, or won't admit to it. Perhaps your retreat experience will encourage you to make some spiritual practice a regular part of your day.

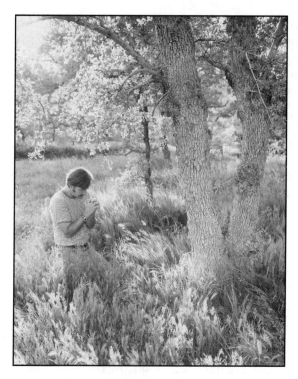

Retreat centers often have beautiful grounds that are conducive to reflection and spontaneous prayer. (Image © H. Armstrong Roberts)

Suitcases and Such

Forget fancy clothes. Leave your electronic anything at home. The facility will feed and house you well enough. You are not on retreat to impress anyone else.

The baggage you're looking at on retreat is what you carry around inside. If you are on retreat for the first time, you may be at a loss for how to describe what you're feeling and what you're carrying. It may be the first time you try to answer or even consider such a question as, "How's your soul?" That question is really at the heart of the common question, "How are you?" The retreat is your time to begin to assemble some images and words that describe the answer.

What's Your Type of Retreat?

Your day will be quite different depending upon the style of the retreat you are attending. Retreats can be:

➤ Directed or not

➤ Programmed or unstructured

➤ Silent

Directed or Not

As you continue to go on retreats, you may eventually undertake a *directed retreat*. During this kind of retreat, you have the opportunity to meet with an advisor who offers support, affirmation, and guidance on how God might be speaking to you, time to share what you are experiencing, feedback, a particular reading or appropriate passage, time for shared prayer, and/or help with personal problems. The primary purpose is support. The discussion, or interview as it might also be called, is yours to shape as you wish.

Outside of the interview, the rest of the retreat schedule is up to you. There are no lectures, no schedules other than meals and your meetings with the advisor, and no required readings or prayers. You aren't even required to meet with the advisor. Some people use the advisor frequently; others use the advisor seldom or not at all. It is entirely up to you to decide whether you want some private time with the advisor.

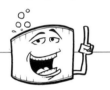

Jacuzzi Jive

A **directed retreat** is one that has a spiritual advisor. This advisor is a person who is available for individual conferences. A **non-directed retreat** is one where a spiritual advisor is not present or available.

You are in charge of your program. You read or pray or meditate when you wish and what you wish. Your contact with the advisor keeps you focused and challenged. Worship and meals are shared by all present at the retreat facility.

When spiritual direction in the form of individual scheduled interviews is not available, then you are attending a *non-directed retreat*. Many retreats, whether silent, programmed, or unstructured, are non-directed.

Programmed Retreats

Programmed retreats, also called guided or conducted retreats, adhere to a schedule that those on retreat follow. This kind of retreat may be a good choice for your first retreat because it provides a structure for the event, a framework for the experience, and guidance in putting all the facets of the retreat together.

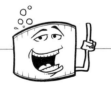

Jacuzzi Jive

A **programmed retreat** has a leader who takes the group through a set program schedule for the duration of the retreat.

A programmed retreat is usually centered around a theme and offers lectures at set times throughout the day, weekend, or week. The theme may, for example, be healthier living, dealing with addictions, choosing career paths, coping with loss, mindfulness, yoga, or meditation. Brochures are usually available describing the theme of the retreat and the schedule. Ask for details.

A Sample Day at a Programmed Retreat

My husband's retreat was programmed, silent, and at a religious retreat house. His daily schedule went something like this:

➤ Morning group prayer

➤ Breakfast

➤ Lecture

➤ Unstructured, individual time

➤ Lecture

➤ Individual time

➤ Lunch

➤ Communal prayer

➤ Lecture

➤ Individual time

➤ Dinner

➤ Recreation time (speaking permitted)

➤ Evening group prayer

The balance in such a schedule permits group and individual time, as well as prayer and unstructured time.

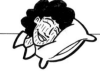

Take 5

Some retreat centers offer a series of lectures from which you choose those that suit you. Others may offer only one and expect all the participants to attend. Lectures may be announced beforehand or decided by the retreat leader after the group has arrived.

A retreat held at a conference center or nonreligious or nondenominational retreat center often follows about the same format, without the prayer times. Instead, the group lectures (or workshops, as they may be called) are alternated with individual time or small group sharing time. Interaction with others who share the same search is an appealing aspect of these kinds of retreats.

Unstructured Retreats

Unstructured retreats, sometimes called self-directed retreats, have no daily meetings with a director. You are entirely on your own to use the time and space as you feel led to do so. Facilities for these retreats welcome visitors but only offer lodging, meals, and solitude.

Some religious communities allot a small number of rooms for people for unstructured retreats. A spiritual advisor may or may not be available. This kind of retreat truly is one where "it is what you make of it."

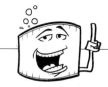

Jacuzzi Jive

You make an **unstructured retreat** by yourself and plan the entire time as you wish. The retreat facility may or may not have a spiritual advisor available.

Examine your motives and desire when you consider a self-directed retreat. It is certainly not something you'd want to do for your first retreat experience. You may never want to do one. An unstructured retreat could be an enriching experience, or it could be frightening, if you are unprepared. Without a guide, you might get lost.

Be sure it's not just an inexpensive Club God you want. Go to a hotel with a pool and hot tub for that. These precious few rooms are better reserved for individuals focused on their spiritual formation.

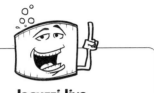

Jacuzzi Jive

During a **silent retreat,** everyone is expected to observe absolute silence at all times, or to speak only during specified times in permitted areas.

A **quiet day** follows a typical retreat day format but lasts only the one day, whereas a traditional retreat lasts at least three days.

Silence Is Golden

If you've never tried a *silent retreat,* perhaps you could for a short period. At my husband's silent retreat, he did not talk during meals, while outside walking the grounds, or during the lecture times. Participants were to speak only during the 45-minute recreation time set aside near the end of each day.

People who've not gone on a silent retreat before find that if they relax and settle into the silence, they come to tolerate it and sometimes even relish it. In a world filled with noise and chatter, it is never too early to learn the value of silence. Try it at least once.

Quiet Days

A traditional understanding of a retreat is a period of at least three days. The concept of a *quiet day* accommodates a busy lifestyle. These single days of quiet are often scheduled during certain times of the annual religious cycle. Quiet days are brief periods set apart that offer a restful pause or are used to reflect on the meaning of the season. These short but focused periods of time may provide you with some measure of respite in your hectic life.

Quiet days introduce you to the idea of retreat. However, they are limited:

➤ Although practical, a quiet day of six hours (which is typical) is short. You barely enter into the quiet, become accustomed to it, and begin to work with it when it is over.

➤ Lecture, address, or conference time is limited. Whatever time is spent listening is taken away from the already too-short time spent reflecting.

➤ If you experience an intense reaction to what you are hearing or doing, there may not be enough time for you to address it or to address it adequately.

Do not expect as much from a quiet day as from a full-length retreat. A typical quiet day schedule would be one of alternating periods of lecture and individual prayer with a meal in the middle of the day.

A quiet day can provide a good introduction to a particular area of spirituality. For example, the theme of one quiet day I recall was "The Call to Simplicity," designed for religious educators. As you can see, the content is appropriate for everyone. The handout used during the day and reproduced here with permission is a combination of material taken from an article, "Living Simply: Learning from Native Americans," with original material by Rev. Dick Rice, S.J. The left column is adapted from a "Living Simply" article; the adaptation and right column are by Rev. Dick Rice, S.J.

The Simple Life*	**The Complex Life**
We are humble and helpless—without our people and Creation's gift, we would be nothing. Every day we give thanks …	We claim most everything as our own accomplishment and we take everything else for granted.
Each person's spirit speaks in its own way. It is not for one person to tell another what should be done …	We claim the power to impose our own will on other's behavior.
We thank our visitors for coming to our lodges so we can share our gifts from the Creation with them …	We welcome no one to our homes, but we hope there is a motel in the vicinity.
Aunts, uncles, grandparents, sons, daughters, nieces, brothers, and sisters: We are one family …	We are dysfunctional and indirect in the ways we communicate in our families.
We are put on this earth to help each other. It is not our way for one person to leave their people behind. We cooperate together …	We compete with each other and, most of all, with ourselves. We always want to know the score and who is winning.
Creation shares with all it's creatures, giving us the privilege of sharing, in turn, with others …	We hoard as much as we can for ourselves and we build fences to keep others from getting what we have.
To be in harmony with the natural world, one must live within the cycles of life. Our spirit and those of the bird, bear, … plants, … stars, and sun must be in communication with each other …	We choose discord and so we do not respect the cycles of the year and month or night and day or the seasons of the year.
Our people believe and practice equality. Sex or age does not bar council. Among our people, it is said, "We are all the same height."	We blatantly practice inequality. Gender, age, and race determine who speaks, who is listened to, and who is silenced.
Our people respect our elders. We value their wisdom and guidance. We provide for them as they provided for us, their children …	We are trying to find ways to gracelessly eliminate our elders as they are in the way and are of considerable expense.
We walk parallel paths, each on her own road, but side by side in peace …	We claim the whole path and are willing to go to war to gain it.

Abridged from "Living Simply: Learning from Native Americans." Rising Dawn, Spring, 1987.

The Least You Need to Know

➤ A retreat, which may or may not be an actual place, is a precious time set apart to explore your life and its spiritual dimension.

➤ Retreats are not just for religious people; they're for anyone who seeks time away from the day to day.

➤ Because there are no goals or real expectations, you can't go wrong on retreat, so relax.

➤ Choose a structured retreat format for your first retreat.

➤ Attendance at community prayer times is optional, but some spiritual practice is advisable to integrate your reflections and your life.

➤ Attend a quiet day to experience a one-day retreat format on a topic of your choice, perhaps on an aspect of self-healing.

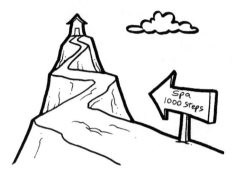

Chapter 20

Let's Go on a Pilgrimage

In This Chapter

➤ Defining pilgrimages and shrines

➤ Understanding their attraction

➤ Visiting a sampling of awe-ful sites

➤ Being a pilgrim without leaving home

Any schoolchild knows who the Pilgrims are. The children study them, dress up like them, and perhaps even have a Pilgrim Day around Thanksgiving. In this chapter, you'll find out more about another kind of pilgrim. These folks travel to places of extraordinary power and awe. Some places have hosted pilgrims for centuries; others are more recent. As you read about the variety of pilgrimages and their meaning for those who go, you'll understand in a small way the lure and life-changing nature of what it means to make a pilgrimage.

In Another's Footsteps

Pilgrims follow in the footsteps of all those who traveled that same journey before them. Years ago I read a book about Margery Kempe (b. circa 1373) that describes her pilgrimages to Jerusalem and Germany during the early fifteenth century. Perhaps my generalized account of her journey may help you understand the process of pilgrimage. In our search for self-healing, we are all pilgrims.

The pilgrim—each one of us—leaves home hopeful and happy. On the road, she meets many others, all going her way. She develops friendships, shares stories, and gains wisdom. As she nears the end of the journey, she experiences anticipation, perhaps anxiety. When she sees the shrine, she is overcome by emotion and weeps with joy and exhaustion.

When she finds herself upon the holy place, she is deeply aware of this being the same ground on which a Holy One walked. As she enters the shrine, she is in wonder that it is the same space in which the holy person touched, saw, moved, and breathed. It is truly awesome. She remains there for a long while, for surely the intervening years have been eclipsed and she is there just after the holy person has left. In prayer and stillness she passes the time.

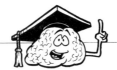

Mindful Moment

The Book of Margery Kempe, dictated in 1438 to her friend, is the story of Margery Kempe's trials and experiences on her spiritual journey. It is the first autobiography ever to be written in English. I read *Memoirs of a Medieval Woman: The Life and Times of Margery Kempe* by Louise Collins (Harper, 1964), based on *The Book of Margery Kempe.*

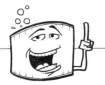

Jacuzzi Jive

A **pilgrim** might be described as a believer who looks beyond the local temple, mosque, church, or shrine, feels the call of some distant holy place, and answers the call by journeying there.

Take 5

The next Kumbha Mela will take place in 2001 in Allahabad, India.

Afterward, she gives offerings and then walks to see other smaller shrines. She may pick up a souvenir, but only a holy one, and then leaves. Her journey home is easy and energized. When she arrives, her family sees and feels the changes that have come over her.

The Call to Go

Pilgrims make up the largest gatherings of people on Earth. Tens of thousands of pilgrims arrive for Holy Week in Rome and Passover in Jerusalem. Over a million believers converge on Mecca each year from every part of the Islamic world. The Kumbha Mela, celebrated by Hindu pilgrims only every 12 years at the confluence of the rivers at Allahabad in India, attracts over 10 million people.

Why do they go? What do they seek? Why, across time and cultures, do people continue to sojourn to far off places? What about you? Isn't there a place, or places, that you long to see?

Everyone has a number of places they long to see. I do. I've scratched a few off my list, but whenever I complete a journey, I seem to uncover several more that I simply must make. It occurs to me as I write this that because I believe in a creator, God, who has created all things holy and good, my desire to experience lands and people is a desire to experience all parts of God's divine creation and, in experiencing them, to encounter God in all these manifestations. I'm not content to know only the tail or the ear or the leg of the elephant; I seek to know every part.

There are many reasons for going on pilgrimage:

➤ Responding to a personal need to answer an inner call, to reshape yourself or your lifestyle, or to come to terms with illness or death

➤ Awakening to the divine

➤ Expressing your faith as a sacred duty, visiting a sacred place, attending a religious event, or hoping for a miracle

➤ As an act of love, of forgiveness, of thanksgiving, or honoring a promise

➤ Connecting with one's heritage

➤ Being curious, seeking adventure, wanting a change

Outward Expression

A basic definition of *pilgrimage* is outer action that has inner meaning. The outer action may be

➤ A formal, organized journey by a large group.

➤ Commemorations of an important event.

➤ Private journeys.

These outer actions are as varied as the people who take them.

The outer action may not appear to have any religious content. Pilgrimages may be secular or patriotic, for example. In this country, people still flock to Graceland, home of Elvis Presley; President John F. Kennedy's grave in Washington, D.C.; Dr. Martin Luther King Jr.'s grave in Atlanta; the Vietnam War Memorial's Wall of Names; and Strawberry Fields in Central Park in New York City, just to name a few.

Many places in other countries attract pilgrims, too. Do you recall the men in their 70s and 80s

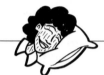

Take 5

Make a list of places you've always wanted to go. You may not understand why there is a longing inside you, but honor the yearning now. Give voice to whatever or whomever is calling you.

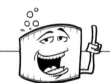

Jacuzzi Jive

A generalized definition that fits all varieties of **pilgrimage** is some outer action with inner meaning. Jean and Wallace Clift speak of pilgrimage in this way in their book *The Archetype of Pilgrimage* (Paulist Press, 1996). From a spiritual aspect, a pilgrimage is a journey taken to become closer to God or to touch the holy in life.

241

who felt compelled to parachute into France again to remember the fiftieth anniversary of the D-Day invasion of World War II? Individuals travel to Germany to see the former site of the Berlin Wall and to Egypt to see the pyramids.

Inner Meaning

Whatever the outer expression, even secular sites have some kind of inner meaning to them. A person might be said to plant her garden religiously, meaning that she does it with special care and attention because her garden has something of significance for her. Secular sites of pilgrimage also have special meanings for the people who visit them.

Other sites are obviously religious sites with religious meaning. According to the 1927 *Pilgrim's Manual* quoted at a pilgrimage site I visited while writing this book, a *pilgrimage* is a journey taken to become closer to God (whatever or whomever you believe that to be). It is a desire to touch the holy in life, when so much seems unholy. To balance the profane all around us, we seek the sacred.

Once you experience this profound inner meaning, you are changed. You may not be able to express what happened to you or within you. You may not wish to tell others, as though telling would diminish the experience. Indeed, "you had to be there" surely applies to a pilgrimage.

My Own Journey

For example, how could I make you understand how I got to Machu Picchu in Peru? I don't think it was ever on my "must go" list, yet after my sojourn to the Mayan sites on the Yucatan Peninsula of Mexico, I received all kinds of signs that led me to make the trip. Not only that, but I knew I had to make it on foot. Indeed, that was the only way I would go.

I found a small group that would hike four days on the Inca Trail to Machu Picchu. I could feel the energy building within me. As I approached the last series of stone steps leading to Intipunku, the Sun Gate, I remember asking my companions whether they could feel the energy, and then I flew up the steps, saw the ruins made so familiar in travel photos, and dissolved in a heap and in tears.

After a time, I rose and slowly began the last piece of the journey down to the city. I soon arrived at a place on the trail where I was overcome by the need to remove my boots and enter barefoot. I gave in to the compulsion. For the remainder of the day, a butterfly that landed on me as I entered the city stayed with me.

Those are the outer reactions I had. I cannot begin to relate what happened within me. It is, as Carl Jung wrote, "a great treasure, a thing that has become for [me] a source of life, meaning, and beauty, and that has given a new splendor to the world and to mankind."

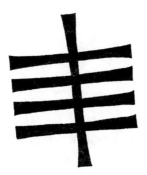

This is an Oriental symbol of the soul's pilgrimage through life. The horizontal lines signify the four worlds through which the soul must climb before being purified and passing from the darkness into the light.

Sacred Places

Not all pilgrimages occur outside ourselves to a distant land. For Hindu mystics and Sufis, for example, the sacred place is within themselves, a personal search within the mind and body. For others, the journey is only symbolic, as when Christians make the Way of the Cross or walk mazes on the floors of cathedrals.

Most pilgrims do make real journeys to a particular place. These places may be sacred landscapes such as Mont-Saint-Michel in France, a small island that is accessible only at low tide, or Croagh Patrick, considered the most sacred mountain in Ireland, which has been a pilgrimage place since 441 B.C.E., when St. Patrick spent the 40 days of Lent on its peak, fasting and meditating.

Shrines

Pilgrims also journey to *shrines,* even ones of only local significance. These shrines may be

➤ By the roadside where a loved one has died.

➤ On paths through woods or on mountainsides, as in Europe.

➤ A "spirit house" showing that the owners included the spiritual when planning their business, as in Asia.

➤ Where bottles of sake are left for Jizo, the spirit who protects travelers and children, in Japan.

Visiting these shrines and leaving offerings is a way to make a mini pilgrimage.

The shrine or holy place may have worldwide recognition. It may be where

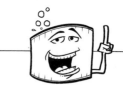

Jacuzzi Jive

Usually, the word **shrine** describes a fixed location that has strong associations with significant religious persons or events. It might house a sacred object, such as a relic, or stand at a sacred scene. A **relic** is an object associated with a saint, such as part of his or her physical remains or part of an article of clothing. Relics are used in prayer and for healing.

➤ Saints and prophets walked during their lifetimes.

➤ Holy people and saints are buried.

➤ *Relics* are kept.

➤ Miracles or visions occurred.

➤ Healing water has sprung up.

Shrines also may be secular, such as battle sites or war memorials. These places are sacred to persons who share those remembrances.

St. Winefride's Well

Some shrines are well marked, but others require the pilgrim to use faith and luck to discover their whereabouts. I visited the site of St. Winefride's Well in Holywell, Wales, also known as the Lourdes of Wales. This well-marked shrine has government-erected signs in both Welsh and English. The area garnered attention in the first half of the seventh century, and today St. Winefride's Well is the oldest, unbroken site of pilgrimage in Britain. A Pilgrim's Rest, operated by the Sisters of Charity of St. Paul, offers lodging and meals. Until recently, the crutches of persons who were healed as a result of bathing in the holy well lined the walls of the shrine.

Every holy place has its story. This well is famous because St. Beuno, Winefride's uncle, successfully placed her head back onto her body after it was severed by a disgruntled suitor. A well sprang up on the spot. The statues of St. Winefride show her with a thick, raised scar on her neck.

Pilgrims come to the well not only to bathe in the waters, but also to see her relic, half of one finger bone. This relic is all that is left after Henry VIII's dissolution of the monastery and destruction of her shrine and its relics. During certain times of the year, the relic is on display.

The bathing pool in front of St. Winefride's Well, Holywell, North Wales.

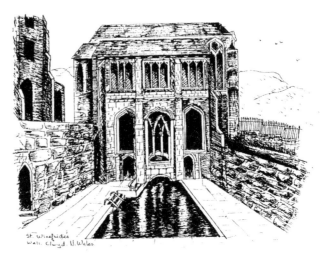

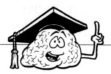

Relics were so nearly identical with the saints' living presence that pilgrims believed they would receive spiritual benefit by being near the relic. Pilgrims slept (the longer the better) near shrines to be showered by a kind of healing radiation from the relic, so they believed. Other faiths treasure relics. Relics of Buddha were distributed and placed in monuments known as stupas which became pilgrimage destinations.

How to Travel

When you go on pilgrimage, go lightly. Be able to carry easily what you bring. The journey is an inner one more than an outward one. When I entered the Pilgrim's Rest at Holywell, I had only one suitcase for my weeklong stay in Wales and England, but I felt embarrassed to be carrying even that much. I would have been more comfortable had I carried only a backpack.

Here are other considerations for your journey:

➤ Decide whether you are a solo or group traveler. Sometimes the decision depends on the safety of the location or the unfamiliarity of the customs and language.

➤ Prepare well, not just the passport and money stuff (prepare for contingencies and detours), but also with prayer, ritual washing, or other manners dictated by your conscience or faith. Christian tradition encourages use of meditation to instruct the mind, move the will, and warm the heart. Muslims must do nothing dishonest or unkind throughout their pilgrimage.

➤ Use special garments. Muslims traveling to Mecca, for instance, must wear an unstitched white cotton garment as a symbol of the equality of all Muslims. Bring a scarf or head covering, which is required in some areas. Women should bring modest dress. Clothing that does not cover the knees and leaves the arms bare is not permitted inside St. Peter's Basilica in Rome and in Muslim mosques and Jewish Orthodox holy places. At certain Islamic shrines, women must wear a floor-length veil. You do not have a choice here. Dress properly, or you don't enter.

➤ Follow the "pilgrim's way." For many sites, there are special paths that pilgrims have taken through the years. The way may be marked, decorated, or set apart. Using the ancient path is a connection with those who have gone before and a union with those who travel with you today.

➤ Think about those left behind. At home, address their fears and contact them while you are away. At the shrine, leave an offering, note, or prayer.

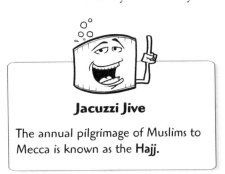

Jacuzzi Jive

The annual pilgrimage of Muslims to Mecca is known as the **Hajj.**

➤ Care for yourself. Contact local guides for advice on routes and religious customs. Do not offend anyone if you can help it. Record your encounters in a journal. Be willing and trusting. More important than caring for your well-used feet is caring about what happens in your heart and head.

➤ Take something home. Even if it's a blade of grass, collect something. The combination of the memory and the memento help recreate the original experience. Besides, if you have a home altar, you can use the memento there.

Muslim Pilgrimage

All Muslims must make the *Hajj,* or pilgrimage to Mecca, once in their adult lives if they are physically, mentally, and financially able. Muslims come from all over the world to Mecca and arrive dressed in a way that eliminates financial and social distinctions.

Muslims visit Mecca because they believe

➤ Creation began there.

➤ The father of the prophets, Abraham, built the first house of worship there, according to Muslim tradition.

➤ Mohammed was born there.

The city and its surrounding area is considered so sacred that non-Muslims are not permitted to enter.

Jewish Pilgrimage

Sacred writings dictated that all Jewish males go annually to the temple in Jerusalem on three festivals. The essence of the pilgrimage was the entry into the temple to worship. With the destruction of the Second Temple in 70 B.C.E., the Western Wall (formerly known as the Wailing Wall), the remaining part of the temple, became the focus of prayer and pilgrimage. Today, pilgrims push written prayers into the gaps between the stones. Following Orthodox Jewish tradition, men and women pray in separate enclosures.

Other sites, particularly the places where sages lived and were buried, are centers of Jewish pilgrimage. Still others relate to events and people spoken of in the sacred writings, for example, the tomb of Rachel, Jacob's wife, in Bethlehem and the tomb of King David in Jerusalem.

Buddhist Pilgrimage

In the Buddhist tradition, you make a pilgrimage to find traces of the Buddha in the world, and you meditate to find the Buddha nature within yourself. The internal journey brings you closer to *nirvana,* but a believer must acknowledge that the Buddha still exists in the world before he may follow the teachings.

For more than 2,000 years, Bodh Gaya has been the most important Buddhist pilgrimage site in India. This is the place where the Buddha attained enlightenment and is considered the birthplace of Buddhism. Buddhist pilgrims also travel to important shrines in Sri Lanka, which house the Buddha's footprints, or to Thailand, which stores Buddhist relics. For many pilgrims, the physical journey is not important, except as a way to turn their attention toward the Buddha. This initial step leads to the more important inner journey.

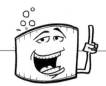

Jacuzzi Jive

Nirvana is the Buddhist state of perfect blessedness reached when the individual soul becomes one with the supreme spirit.

Tibetan Pilgrimage

In Tibet, it seems that almost everyone is moving all the time anyway, so pilgrimage is natural. A special feature of Tibetan pilgrimage is *circumambulation,* which comes from Indian Buddhism, where it is used to pay homage to a sacred person or object. While Tibetan pilgrims travel, they recite mantras, or sacred formulas.

Tibetans make many circumambulations of Mount Kailash, located at the western end of the Himalayas, from which four great rivers, including Karnali, a tributary of the holy Ganges, flow. All of the pilgrim routes cross at least one pass above 17,000 feet. Sometimes the pilgrims lie face down on the ground, and then rise and walk the length of their body, again falling to the ground. If they continue their pilgrimage in this way, it may take four weeks, instead of the usual three days, to cover the 30 miles around the mountain.

Take 5

The biggest Buddha in the western hemisphere sits at Chuang Yen Buddhist Monastery in Putnam County, New York. The 22-ton, 37-foot statue occupies the Great Buddha Hall, which is open to anyone who makes the pilgrimage. For information, contact Chuang Yen Monastery, RD13, Route 301, Carmel, NY 10512; 914-225-6117.

Hindu Pilgrimage

For more than 3,000 years Hindus have come from all over the world to Benares, India, to die. It is a strong Hindu belief that to die in the Ganges is to gain immediate

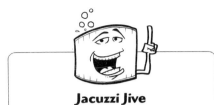

Jacuzzi Jive

In **circumambulation**, one walks in a circle around the object of their pilgrimage. This circular pilgrimage leads nowhere, and yet in the act itself of going, the old life is left behind and the pilgrim is renewed.

liberation from the wheel of rebirth. This river is their Holy of Holies, where the soul takes a warp-speed trip.

Hindus have other traditions. One is to travel the circle of the four dhamas, dwelling places of the gods. These four places, each facing in a different direction, are shown on the following map of India.

Many Hindu holy places are found near rivers or mountains. Varanasi, where the Ganges and Yamuna rivers meet, is especially sacred. Over four miles of temples stand along the Ganges in Varanasi, and hundreds of thousands of pilgrims visit this place each year.

Hindus travel in a circular pilgrimage to the home of the gods in the south, west, north, and east of India.

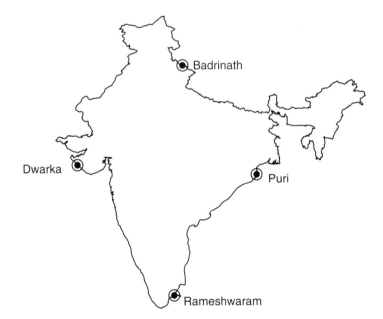

Christian Pilgrimage

Bethlehem, Galilee, and Jerusalem are all important destinations for Christians following in Jesus' footsteps. Rome, the center of the Roman Catholic Church, is an important place for Catholics. Many Christian sites are associated with Jesus, his mother Mary, or saints. The following pilgrimage sites, for example, are places where miracles or visions of the Virgin Mary occurred:

➤ Lourdes in France (1858)

➤ Fatima in Portugal (1917)

➤ Medjugorje, Bosnia (1981)

➤ Knock, Ireland (1878)

➤ Walsingham, England (1061)

➤ Our Lady of Guadalupe, Mexico (1531)

Christian Pilgrimage Sites in the United States

The United States has more than 100 pilgrimage shrines and places of miracles, for instance:

➤ The book, *Way Stations to Heaven* (Macmillan, 1996), lists 50 places around the country where people report they have seen weeping or bleeding statues and other extraordinary events.

➤ Colin Wilson's book, *The Atlas of Holy Places and Sacred Sites* (DK Publishing, 1996), lists more than 65 sites in the United States as well as many more worldwide, most of which are important to native peoples.

➤ The famous shrine at Chimayo, New Mexico, was established in the early nineteenth century to give thanks for health and prosperity. The shrine encloses a dry earth "well" that in earlier times was mud, reported to have healing properties. Today, pilgrims walk across mountain and desert to take away bags of soil from this hole or rub the soil directly on their bodies.

➤ Mother Cabrini, an Italian missionary nun, is honored at a site in the Rocky Mountain foothills near Denver, Colorado. Here, in 1912, it is said that she struck a rock with her staff and out came a spring of healing water.

➤ The Coronado Cross stands near Dodge City, Kansas, at a place on the Arkansas River. It remembers a Franciscan friar who was the first priest martyred in what is now the United States.

➤ Auriesville, New York, is the site of one of the three shrines to Blessed Kateri Tekakwith, known as the "Lily of the Mohawks." Born in 1656 to a Mohawk father and an Algonquin mother, Tekakwitha was baptized into the Catholic Church and given the baptismal name Kateri. The shrine at Fonda, New York, a few miles away, commemorates her baptism. The St. Francis-Xavier Mission on the river is where she is buried and is the only major place of pilgrimage on an Indian reservation.

Many religious orders have shrines and special places around the country. Just call one, or ask through your place of worship, and you'll probably discover more than you ever would have guessed.

Other important sites in this country are destinations, but not shrines, such as the Holocaust museums in New York City and Washington, D.C. The Trail of Tears, the name of the forced march removing most of the Cherokee nation from North Carolina to Oklahoma, is a walk waiting to happen.

Common Threads

There is so much to see and do, and we are a people wanting to see and do. St. Augustine wrote in his *Confessions,* "My heart is restless, oh Lord, until it rests in you."

Whatever our traditions, we respond to inner yearnings to search for self-healing near and far until we find what we seek and, finally, can rest and be at peace.

The Least You Need to Know

➤ All pilgrims share a search for and encounter with someone or something of significant meaning, especially holiness.

➤ Pilgrimages may be secular, historical, or patriotic places, but most often they are intertwined with a religious tradition. A true pilgrimage changes your life and changes you.

➤ There are more than 100 sites of pilgrimage in the United States.

➤ Because the interior journey is more important than the physical one, you may make symbolic, yet real, pilgrimages by participating in maze walks or The Way of the Cross or by living a life of care and concern for yourself and others.

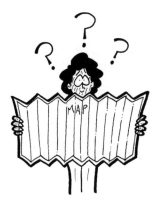

Chapter 21

Finding Your Way at a Spa or Retreat

In This Chapter

➤ Determining what kind of experience you want

➤ Surveying the services

➤ Asking the right questions

➤ Making your decision

Going to a spa or on retreat that a friend told you is great or that is recommended in a book or magazine might have been just wonderful for someone else, but only by going will you know whether it's great for you, too. Look at the lists of spas in Appendix A, "The Spa Finder Directory of Spa Retreats and Spa Resorts," and descriptions of some spiritual retreats in Chapter 22, "A Sampling of Retreats." These lists are just a small sampling of the places you can choose from. There's an ocean of possibilities, and in this chapter you'll look at

➤ What you want.

➤ The services you wish were there.

➤ Where in the world to get it all.

You can't begin too soon! Ready to take the plunge?

Getting Your Toes Wet

I wouldn't be surprised if, as you read along in the pages that follow, you feel a little overwhelmed with all the choices open to you. Don't get hung up here. Take the spa search a step at a time. Review the following checklist to test the water.

When you inquire at spas or retreats that catch your eye, ask questions and carefully consider and compare the answers you get. Then trust and be open to guidance, from without and from within. Look for signs that point you in a general direction or to a particular place. Relax, and remember: If the one you pick isn't a good fit, there are hundreds of other places to try next time. More likely, you will rejoice at your choice and wonder how you'll ever manage to get to any of the others.

Checklist for Making Your Big Decision

Item	Matters Much	Little	None
Spa-type beauty treatments	❏	❏	❏
Fitness activities	❏	❏	❏
Retreat-type programs/classes	❏	❏	❏
Vacation	❏	❏	❏
Use of at-home spa	❏	❏	❏
Day spa	❏	❏	❏
Vacation spa	❏	❏	❏
People			
Single	❏	❏	❏
Married	❏	❏	❏
Couples	❏	❏	❏
Divorced	❏	❏	❏
Widowed	❏	❏	❏
Family	❏	❏	❏
Men only	❏	❏	❏
Women only	❏	❏	❏
Size			
Less than 20 guests	❏	❏	❏
21 to 50 guests	❏	❏	❏
More than 51 guests	❏	❏	❏
Staff-to-guest ratio	❏	❏	❏
Personal trainer	❏	❏	❏
Lodging			
Private	❏	❏	❏
Semi-private	❏	❏	❏
Dormitory	❏	❏	❏
Cabin	❏	❏	❏
Camping	❏	❏	❏
Motel	❏	❏	❏
Shared bath	❏	❏	❏

Item	Matters Much	Little	None
Meals			
Scheduled	❏	❏	❏
Flexible	❏	❏	❏
Sufficient	❏	❏	❏
Special diet	❏	❏	❏
Atmosphere/Setting			
Country	❏	❏	❏
City	❏	❏	❏
Grounds	❏	❏	❏
Structured stay	❏	❏	❏
Free time	❏	❏	❏
Religious	❏	❏	❏
Relaxed, casual	❏	❏	❏
Near other attractions	❏	❏	❏
Affiliations			
Religious	❏	❏	❏
Otherwise	❏	❏	❏
Spiritual advisor	❏	❏	❏
Communal prayer	❏	❏	❏
Nondenominational chapel	❏	❏	❏
Silence	❏	❏	❏
Geographic Location			
Outside/within United States	❏	❏	❏
Mountains/desert/forest/water	❏	❏	❏
Weather	❏	❏	❏
Medical Considerations			
Physical condition	❏	❏	❏
Special equipment	❏	❏	❏
Medication	❏	❏	❏
Personal Considerations			
Clothing requirements	❏	❏	❏
Electronic needs	❏	❏	❏
Schedule	❏	❏	❏
Hermitage	❏	❏	❏
Length of stay	❏	❏	❏
Timing	❏	❏	❏
Legalities	❏	❏	❏
Cost	❏	❏	❏

Chill Out

If you want specific kinds of services, ask specific questions. No two spas are created the same. The title *spa* does not a guarantee a particular set of services, fitness activities, or classes. If you want a quieter experience, don't rely simply on the word *retreat*. Be specific about what you want, and ask for it. If you don't like the answers, go somewhere else. There are plenty of other choices.

What Kind of Experience Do You Want?

You know by now that the words *spa* and *retreat* have as many different meanings as the facilities that provide such programs and services. Ask yourself where you want your focus. Are you looking for

➤ A total spa with focus on spa activities for a weeklong stay?

➤ A spa attached to a resort or hotel offering vacation options and sports for you or the family?

➤ Lifestyle changes?

➤ Quiet time for introspection?

➤ A mix of possibilities?

This main question is, of course, only the beginning. From people and atmosphere to lodging and weather, lots of factors contribute to your spa or retreat experience.

A retreat doesn't have to be religious. Art activities, for example, may be the basis of artist retreats or used as a healing therapy for all persons, including families and those with physical or developmental disabilities.
(Photo courtesy Linda Short)

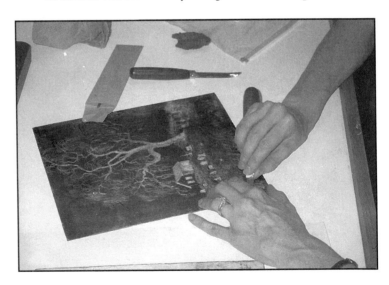

Who's There?

Are you single, married or otherwise attached, divorced, or widowed? Are you looking for a location that caters to one of these groups? Do you want an adult-only experience? Or do you want a spa for women only or men only?

Are you going alone or with a spouse, family member, or friend? Are you going with the entire family? Some facilities are especially delighted to see families and have separate, parallel, age-appropriate activities for children.

Size

What size program do you want? Some are intimate, with only 8 to 12 guests per rotation. Others house hundreds and look and feel more like vacation resorts. Is there a busy season? When do greater—and fewer—numbers of guests arrive? What's the staff-to-guest ratio? Is the staff licensed or certified? Will you have a *personal trainer?*

Lodging

You will want to ask whether the accommodations are private, semi-private, or dormitory style. If you are traveling with others, ask if you may room together. Rooming together is particularly important if you are a family or an unmarried couple.

Are the rooms in a main building, an outbuilding, or in cabins? Is lodging provided in tents or trailers or must you bring your own? Are clean but spartan facilities acceptable, or do you need room service? Are you willing to share a bath? Are you willing to have a roommate not of your choosing?

Are the rooms heated or air-conditioned, as needed? If the sleeping rooms are, what about the rest of the building? I once stayed at a facility built around an open-air courtyard. When it rained, you got wet. When it was cold outside, you were cold. Are there smoking and nonsmoking rooms?

Is the facility undergoing renovations? With the booming business, centers continue to accept guests while they expand or renovate. If you don't mind, fine. Just know what you're getting into.

Meals

Know which meals are included in your stay. Do you want table service, or is cafeteria-style okay? Ask whether meals are served at set times. If you miss a meal, know whether you can snoop in the fridge or get a doggie bag. Can you keep snacks in your room? Is a room refrigerator available?

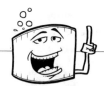

Jacuzzi Jive

A **personal trainer** is an individual who works with you to create a personal fitness routine.

Take 5

Ask whether you will need to keep your own room tidy or whether a cleaning service is available. Some facilities also ask you to strip the bed and make it up for the next guest upon your departure.

Chill Out

If you know you need room service, pick a facility that has it. Don't sabotage your experience, waste your money, give yourself a headache, and have a less-than-wonderful time because you weren't honest with yourself.

255

Even when meals are included, not all meals are created equal. If your spa or retreat experience is located in a resort hotel or conference center, for example, you may take meals in a main dining room, but be permitted to order only certain items. You may be given a voucher for use in the main dining room, with excess charges being your responsibility.

Will you like the food? Ask for sample menus if you are uncertain. If you have food allergies or dietary restrictions, make these known before you book a stay. It isn't fair to show up and then demand special foods.

If you don't like the food, can the spa serve you something in its place? If you feel you need more food than is being served, is the spa flexible enough to give you more? I remember a guest on a weight-loss diet who felt that her breakfast, a glass of juice and a potassium pill, wasn't sufficient for how she was feeling that morning. She asked for an egg and got it.

Take 5

If you have problems with the food for whatever reason, ask whether you can bring in your own and get a discount on the cost of your stay. It can't hurt. The worst the spa can do is say no.

Atmosphere, Setting

Do you prefer a country or city setting? Do you want beautiful grounds to walk in, lie in, and gaze upon? Schedules or none? Lots, some, or little free time? Other people around, or almost none? Do you want the setting and the buildings to suggest "God is here" or do you prefer no obvious expression of anything spiritual?

Do you want to be near other sites and attractions? (For example, Bethany Springs Retreat House in Kentucky is within walking distance of the monastery where Thomas Merton resided. Guests at Bethany Springs are welcome to attend prayer with the monks; see Chapter 22.) Or will you be like a hermit and stay oblivious to the world outside your door?

Do you want a relaxed, casual setting where you can wear jeans all day? Or do you prefer a structured, more formal setting where you dress up a bit for dinner?

Chill Out

Even programs designed for weight loss may be too strenuous for some, especially during the transition time. If you think you're getting weak or uncomfortably hungry, ask for more or different food. You will be leaving soon enough and will need to maintain a fit lifestyle at home on your own anyway. One extra piece of toast, glass of juice, or slice of cheese won't make or break the day.

Affiliation

Is the religious, civic, business, or professional affiliation or lack thereof a factor for you?

Are you looking for a program where there's a spiritual advisor or communal prayer available, even if you may not participate every time? Would you like a quiet room? Is a chapel important?

Do you want silence or talk or opportunities to socialize and meet people?

Geographic Location

Is this a tourist-pilgrim combination trip? A 20-year late honeymoon combined with a yoga retreat trip? Do you yearn to see a special physical or spiritual site? Do you want to be by the desert, mountains, forest, or water? Should physical challenges (such as hiking, aerobics, or horseback riding) be part of your program?

What about the weather? Could it be too hot, too cold, too rainy when you go? Will you be inside or outside during your stay? If the outdoors is used for programs and activities, what are the alternatives in bad weather? Do you like what's planned? Will you need special clothing or shoes to protect you during harsh weather?

Medical Considerations

If you have a physical condition requiring special equipment or access, be sure you ask whether you can be accommodated. If something breaks, can you get a repair or replacement? If you take medication that needs special handling, is it available? If you have any special needs, explain them to the facility you're considering and be sure it can accommodate you.

If you become injured, what then? If it's blisters and such from too much hiking or too-new shoes, do you bring along the bandages and such or are they provided? If you pull or strain a muscle or break something from too many weights, who pays for your treatment? If you experience an adverse reaction to a facial or body product or a new food or treatment, what can you expect from your hosts?

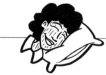

Take 5

Encourage the person you speak with to be honest with you about your needs and the facility's ability to meet them. It's better for both of you.

Clothing

Especially if this is your first time at a spa, you may prefer a facility that provides standard clothing to all guests. You save some extra bucks and can be sure that you'll be appropriately dressed for the activities and atmosphere of the center. On the other hand, shorts, T-shirts, and sweats are always in fashion. Of course, if you're a fashion plate, you may have your own ideas about dress and want a place with more style.

Hermitages

If you wish to be a hermit, ask whether there is a place set apart and how you will receive your meals so that you can avoid all (or almost all) human contact. (For more on hermitages, see Chapter 22.)

Length of Stay

Is the length of stay flexible, with guests arriving for as many or as few days as they want? Does the facility provide a set program that begins and ends the same time each week? How are early or late arrivals handled?

Take 5

When making your list of spa requirements, include every service or program you're interested in, even if you're not absolutely positive you will do it. Remember, this is your ideal, your perfect getaway. Later, you may have to give and take to find suitable matches.

Schedules

Do you want to get up early, on a set schedule? Or do you want to sleep late because you were up until all hours meditating, writing, or socializing? If you are staying at a religious community, do you wish to participate in daily activities?

Services for the Asking

Know what services and programs you want and whether they are included in the overall fee or come at extra cost. Spas and retreats usually have written information they can send you and/or a Web site you can visit that lists all their services and programs and the charges for each. But before you look for this information, review these lists of questions that you'll want to keep in mind.

Beauty and Body Treatments

If beauty treatments are your main reason for getting away—and even if they aren't—begin asking questions such as

➤ What services and treatments are available? (Ask for descriptions of unfamiliar ones.)

➤ Which services, and how many of each type, are included in the base price?

➤ If I want more of something I'm already getting, what is the cost of additional treatments?

➤ Is there a difference in price or availability depending upon the location of the service? For example, is a massage in my room different from one given in the gym or salon?

➤ Must I make appointments in advance? How far?

➤ During what time of the day are appointments available?

➤ Is there a service charge or tax added to the list price of a service?

➤ If a confirmed booking is cancelled, am I charged a cancellation fee? May I reschedule instead?

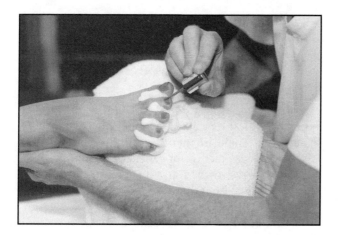

Try an unfamiliar body treatment as well as the customary pedicure. Have fun and enjoy a variety of treatments and services. (Photo © Artemis Picture Research)

Fitness Activities

Physical activity is another matter. If the program uses physical activity as a benefit in itself, or is required to access your interior space, are you fit enough? Ask whether there are beginner, intermediate, and advanced activities for participants' different fitness levels. If not, ask for descriptions of what's planned and an assessment as to whether you will be comfortable or challenged. If water activities are planned, can you swim or are you afraid of the water? If you are hiking, do you have foot or leg problems? How difficult is the terrain?

If you are especially interested in a particular type of physical activity, be sure it is offered during your stay. Sometimes classes are held only at certain times, or instructors take time off. You don't want to show up for yoga and find out that yoga doesn't meet that week. Similarly, if you become attached to a particular instructor, be sure he or she is teaching the week you're there.

If you are interested in fitness activities, ask for the class schedule. Note the time of your classes and whether they conflict with anything else you want to do. Are the fitness activities included in the price, or are you charged by the class or by the hour?

Programs or Lectures

Think about what you expect to gain most from this experience. Do you want, for example

- ➤ Stress reduction?
- ➤ Spiritual development?
- ➤ Peace and solitude?
- ➤ Advice for a healthier lifestyle?
- ➤ Fitter figure?
- ➤ A hot springs cure?
- ➤ Relationship work?
- ➤ Your addictions healed?
- ➤ Career goal assessment?
- ➤ To learn new skills?

259

Time at a spa or retreat is time to forget your daily obligations so that you can devote yourself to rest, beautification, renewal, and celebration.

Near Home Sweet Home

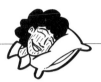

Take 5

If you are visiting a retreat site sponsored by a faith different from your own, be sure to ask for guidance on dress and behavior.

Appendix A has a sampling of spas around the United States, Chapter 22 a sampling of retreats, and throughout this book, as well as in Appendix C, "Further Reading," there are mentions of directories and Web sites you can refer to for others. But what if you don't want to leave town? Can you get a spa and retreat experience close to home? Most likely, yes. It probably isn't going to be the total experience you'd get by staying at a spa or retreat center, but then again, it may be all that you need and at a price you can afford.

You can assemble your own package of services and classes by using local, individual providers of massage, reflexology, manicures, facials, pedicures, meditation, and yoga classes. Check out

➤ Your mall and large department stores, where beauty treatments are often connected with the cosmetic department.

➤ Large hotels.

➤ Hospital wellness centers.

➤ Gyms and health clubs.

➤ Continuing education programs through town or county recreation departments and colleges and high schools.

➤ Local houses of worship and their regional, state, or national offices.

➤ Library-sponsored workshops, study groups, and classes.

Nuts and Bolts

Chill Out

Many spiritual retreat houses will not permit, or strongly discourage, their guests to make and receive calls. You are on retreat to take a break from them, remember? Emergencies are different, of course.

You're not quite ready to leave yet; there are some other things you have to think about. Although you've narrowed down the choices or chosen your ideal getaway, there are still some details to consider.

Length of the Stay

Did you make arrangements for family and work left behind? Can you get your unfinished business to a point where it can sit until you return?

If your visit seems short, can you extend your stay another day or so? If the visit is dragging, can you leave early and get a refund? Does the facility have a structured program that always lasts from Sunday to Saturday, for example, or are you able to show up whenever you need to, to fit your timetable?

The Timing

How far in advance do you need to book a reservation? Are there last-minute booking options? What are the consequences if you cancel? Re-schedule? If you cannot get in on the dates you want, is there a waiting list?

Don't forget to time your trip in light of weather conditions, festivals, religious observances, and any other special timing considerations.

Legalities

If you're traveling outside the country, do you have a valid passport? The necessary immunizations? Local currency?

Cost

I don't know about you, but I don't like finding out later that there are hidden, fine-print charges. They tend to run the bill up rather quickly. Here are some cost items you need to be clear on:

1. Are there different weekend and weekday rates? If so, would you change your timing to take advantage of lower rates?

2. Are there any special holiday or other package deals being advertised? How long will they be available?

3. Are there discounts for members of certain groups, like auto club members and seniors?

4. Is the price any different depending upon whether you book directly with the facility or go through an agency?

5. How much extra will you pay for the additional services you want to enjoy during your stay?

6. Will service fees or taxes be added?

7. Will you be expected to leave tips for each service employee, for example, the manicurist, masseuse, or cook?

8. Will you want to leave an offering if you've stayed at a religious center?

9. Did you bring along extra money if you wish to leave earlier or later than originally planned?

10. Concerning transfers from ground or air transportation to your destination: Is the cost included? Is the transportation by private car, van, bus? Are gratuities expected, included? How are early or late arrivals handled? Is there an extra fee, even if transfers are normally included in the cost?

To get a total cost of your adventure, don't forget to add transportation costs, additional meals and lodging, and incidentals.

I've taken you through the steps to find a getaway that is right for you. The only steps left are to choose one and to make your reservation. And to go, of course!

The Least You Need to Know

➤ Use the checklist in this chapter to organize your thinking about the kind of experience you want to have and understand the kinds of information you need.

➤ Ask yourself where you want the focus to be: How much coddling or challenge do you want? Is this trip for a lifestyle change or just a vacation?

➤ Consider where you want to be geographically.

➤ In the end, the decision is easy: Be true to your heart.

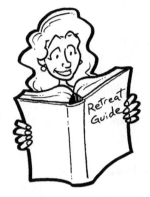

Chapter 22

A Sampling of Retreats

In This Chapter

➤ The many meanings of the word *retreat*

➤ Types of retreats: artist, writer, family, single sex, religious, and more

➤ The hermit's life

➤ Stories from the field

A retreat doesn't necessarily mean a place for worship. There is an incredible variety of retreat houses and facilities, both religious and non-religious. Do you want to be alone or with a crowd? Do you seek guidance from others or only from within yourself? Do you want a retreat that focuses on a specific interest?

One article in *Modern Maturity* (September–October 1998) by Lori Erickson titled "For the Peace of the Soul," reports more than 1,400 retreat facilities in the United States alone. They include ones hosted by or housed in monasteries, abbeys, and religious congregations, as well as private and nondenominational centers across the country. This chapter provides a sampling of the available retreats.

Different Retreats for Different Folks

Many retreat centers are designed to create an environment that meets the special needs of artists, musicians, writers, followers of yoga, families, and people with physical or developmental disabilities. This section will show you what's available in special-interest retreats.

Art Retreats

The Alliance of Artists' Communities is a national service organization that supports artists' communities and residency programs. The communities are professionally run organizations that provide time, space, and support for artists' creative research in nurturing environments, both in cities and in the country. The word *art* is defined broadly and includes any creative endeavor, from painters, photographers, and composers to storytellers, architects, and choreographers. To learn more about this organization, check out the Artists' Alliance Web site at www.teleport.com/~aac/main.html.

Take 5

Find listings in the United States and abroad for retreat and residency facilities for artists at http://dir.yahoo.com/arts/organizations/artists_retreats_and_colonies/. Check Yahoo! (www.yahoo.com) and search under (what else?) "artists retreats" for more information.

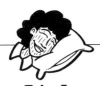

Take 5

The restored home and studio of Aaron Copland, composer of such well-known pieces as *Appalachian Spring* and *Billy the Kid* is located in Westchester County, New York. His home is now available for sabbaticals, upon application, for serious musicians who want time to create new compositions. To apply, visit www.coplandhouse.org.

9 Mountain Retreat

The 9 Mountain facility in western Massachusetts is not a retreat for artists per se, but it uses art, dance, and music in a weekend holistic health retreat. Yoga, meditation, massage, hypnotherapy, and vegetarian cuisine are available as well.

A day at one of its retreat weekends might begin with meditation and yoga, followed by your choice of art classes during the day. During breaks and after dinner, you have time for hiking, playing the drums, or soaking in a hot tub. No formal art experience is necessary, although the facility has professional artists on staff. The retreat, located on 45 acres of woodlands, is limited to 15 people.

You can contact this retreat at 9 Mountain Street, Plainfield, Massachusetts 01070; 888-NINE-MTN; e-mail: mail@ninemtn.com; or check out its Web site: www.ninemtn.com.

Writing Retreats

Writers have many options for ways to work on their craft: writers' conferences, workshops, courses, seminars, festivals, residencies, retreats, colonies, organizations, and publications. Check out these Web sites for information on writers' retreats:

➤ Pikes Peak Writers Retreat Resources at cotlanza@ix.netcom.com

➤ www.dataconnections.com/writersretreat for reservations to live and write in mountain lodgings

➤ A woman's writing retreat at www.prairieden.com

You can find other writers' retreats by using any online search engine, such as Yahoo! and Alta Vista, and searching for "writers retreats."

Music and Dance Listings

You won't find many retreat listings for music and dance, but there are a few (use an Internet search engine to search for "music retreats"). Note though that some of the previously mentioned artist retreats include musicians as participants.

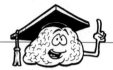

Mindful Moment

If you are looking for something to do and someplace to go, check out this Web site: www.shawguides.com. It lists all kinds of programs: art and craft workshops, cooking schools, educational travel, golf schools and camps, language vacations, photography schools, workshops, and tours, tennis schools and camps, water sports schools and camps, and writers conferences.

For Those with Special Needs

Camp Hebron in Pennsylvania is one place that has specific programs for adults who are physically handicapped or developmentally disabled. Situated on 300 acres north of Harrisburg, it offers retreat, vacation, and camping experiences in tents, cabins, motel-like rooms, and private cottages. Camp Hebron hosts many family retreats as well, particularly during the summer months. To contact Camp Hebron, write 957 Camp Hebron Road, Halifax, Pennsylvania 17032; e-mail: hebron@camphebron.org; or check out its Web site at www.camphebron.org.

A very different setting is the Mercy Center, which is an international spiritual and conference center operated by the Sisters of Mercy of the Americas and located in Burlingame, California. Retreatants enjoy 40 acres of lovely grounds, with a chapel and meditation room and lodgings that include four rooms with handicapped access. Women and men are welcome to make personal retreats of a day, a weekend, or longer. For more information, write 2300 Adeline Drive, Burlingame, California 94010; phone: 650-340-7474; fax: 650-340-1299; e-mail: mc@mercy-center.org; or visit its Web site at www.mercy-center.org.

Family Retreats

Family retreat? Isn't this an oxymoron? Fortunately, there are places that want to prove that you can combine a family vacation with something a bit more, particularly some built-in structured time to communicate meaningfully and get through to the core of things, rather than just breezing past each other in the hall.

Large, park-like settings such as Camp Hebron are possibilities. There are also many church camps for families around the country, for example, the MiVoden Summer Camp and Retreat Center in Coeur d'Alene, Idaho (visit www.mivoden.com).

Take 5

To find camps and retreats for children with Attention Deficient Disorder, go to www.kidscamp-retreats.com.

A similar setting but with a decidedly nondenominational flavor is Peace Valley Retreat Center in the Ouachita National Forest of southwest Arkansas. Located on 70 acres crossed by trails, this center offers personal retreats, setting for family time, and vacation activities. There are hayrides, swimming, sports, animals on the property, fishing, canoeing, and digging for crystals in the nearby mountains. Workshops such as Native American medicine wheel teachings are offered, and there are Lakota teepees and a sweat lodge on the grounds. Write to HC 65, Box 73B, Caddo Gap, Arkansas 71935; 501-356-2908; e-mail: pvnet@cswnet.com; or visit its Web site at www.cswnet.com/~pvnet/.

The Marianist Family Programs are led by teams of families and priests or nuns. The program that began in Cape May Point, New Jersey, has expanded over the years to other locations to accommodate the many families who wish to participate. The structured program lasts one week.

A typical day looks like this:

➤ Morning meeting and prayer, followed by breakfast

➤ Skit geared for all age groups

➤ Peer group discussions about skit's message

➤ Family group project about skit

➤ Worship followed by lunch

➤ Free afternoon to swim, travel, and socialize

➤ Gathering prayer followed by dinner

➤ Activities and social time before night prayer and bed

Marianist Family Programs have a Catholic focus and are designed to provide a time of community and understanding in an atmosphere of fun and acceptance at an affordable price. Although the cost varies with the location, there is a cap for large families.

Marianist family retreat programs are available in these states:

Alfred, Maine	603-742-9617
Baltimore, Maryland	410-668-0963
Cape May Point, New Jersey	609-884-3829

New York (programs are held in Massachusetts)	914-621-7000
North Topsail Beach, North Carolina	910-328-1584
Governor's Island, Ohio	937-842-4902

New programs are being set up in California and Texas; contact the main office for information: 609-884-3829.

For Other Specific Groups

When you browse the Web, you'll find other possibilities for retreats, including:

➤ Adventure Health Travel, which includes listings for spas, retreats, and ecofitness: www.adventurehealthtravel.com.

➤ Spirit Journeys, specializing in retreats for the gay community: www.spiritjourneys.com.

➤ Crystal Creek Wellness Adventures, for backcountry wilderness retreats for women to stimulate the body, mind, and spirit: www.jacksonholenet.com/crystal.

➤ Sacred Journeys, for women's retreats, pilgrimages, tours, and workshops: www.sacredjourneys.com.

➤ Physician Wellness Foundation, which gives conferences and retreats for physicians and health care professionals and for physician couples to renew relationships strained by the demands of practice: www.physicianwellness.com.

➤ Filoha Meadows in Colorado offers retreats for physicians and their spouses: 800-227-8906.

➤ Modern Life Guide, a site devoted to "robust living," which includes information on holistic medicine; hundreds of listings for spas, resorts, fitness centers, and natural hot springs in 38 countries; a gift store; and links to other health sites: www.modlife.com.

Spiritual Retreats

When most people think of a retreat experience, they think of a time for spiritual renewal. Centers that offer such an experience vary widely.

Jewish Experiences

Elat Chayyim is a project of ALEPH, an organization dedicated to advancing Judaism that is "deeply spiritual, environmentally conscious, and politically engaged." Its Elat Chayyim Center for Healing and Renewal is located in upstate New York. Contact the Elat Chayyim Center at 99 Mill Hook Road, Accord, New York 12404; phone: 800-398-2630; fax: 914-626-2037; e-mail: generalinfo@elatchayyim.org; or visit its Web site: www.elatchayyim.org.

267

Take 5

I love Elat Chayyim's motto: "Blessed are You Who has given us life, lifted us up, and enabled us to reach this season."

ALEPH also has the following resources:

➤ The Jewish Renewal Life Center, which offers weekends and residential programs

➤ The Spiritual Eldering Institute

➤ The Institute of Contemporary Midrash, supporting clergy, educators, and artists in using the arts to interpret sacred texts

➤ *New Menorah*, a quarterly journal

You can contact ALEPH at 7318 Germantown Avenue, Philadelphia, Pennsylvania 19119; phone: 215-247-9700; fax: 215-247-9703; e-mail: alephAJR@aol.com; or see its Web site: www.aleph.org.

Eastern Experiences

If you are interested in Buddhist retreats, definitely check out *The Complete Guide to Buddhist America,* edited by Don Morreale (Shambhala Publishing, 1998). It lists Buddhist centers and retreats around the country.

One site mentioned in the book is the Providence Zen Center in Rhode Island, which is free and open daily for practice and to hear talks. Beginners are welcome. There are monthly retreats lasting from one to seven days, including Buddhist-Christian retreats. For more information, contact the center at 99 Pound Road, Cumberland, Rhode Island 02864; phone: 401-658-1464; fax: 401-658-1188; e-mail: kwanumzen@aol.com; Web site: www.kwanumzen.com/pzc/index.html.

The Satchidananda Ashram-Yogaville in the foothills of the Blue Ridge Mountains of Virginia is a 1,000-acre ashram. At the center is the Light of Truth Universal Shrine, a lotus-shaped structure situated on a 16-acre lake with views of the surrounding mountains. Most programs emphasize the spiritual and physical healing benefits of yoga. Located 40 miles southwest of Charlottesville, guests stay in motel, dormitories, or camping sites. Write them at Buckingham, Virginia 23921; phone: 800-858-9642; or on the Web at www.yogaville.org.

Protestant Experiences

You can find many Protestant retreat centers that look like vacation destinations. There is an abundance of land, swimming and sporting activities, and perhaps even summer camp. There may be indoor or outdoor chapels. Often, the centers do not present their own programs but are used by groups offering programmed retreats. The centers do accommodate individuals making non-directed, unstructured retreats.

Disciples of Christ

Located in a rural setting of 350 acres, the Tall Oaks Conference Center offers year-round retreat facilities. It has two interesting features. First, a Lakota area, which is used by local Native Americans and which is open to visitors. Second, use of an equestrian program to teach lessons applicable to daily life. Contact them at 12797 189th Street, Linwood, Kansas 66052; phone: 800-617-1484; or visit their Web site: www.talloaks.org.

Lutheran

The Carol Joy Holling Conference and Retreat Center is located halfway between Omaha and Lincoln, Nebraska. Their land borders a state park, and offers a lake, lots of trees, swimming, canoeing, volleyball, hiking, and both outdoor worship sites and a chapel room. Hotel-like lodging or cabins and buffet meals are available year-round. Sponsored by the Nebraska Lutheran Outdoor Ministries, reach them at 27416 Ranch Road, Ashland, Nebraska 68003; phone: 888-656-6254; e-mail: info@nlom.org; or Web site: www.nlom.org.

Methodist

In western North Carolina, the Lake Junaluska Assembly Conference and Retreat Center offers educational seminars, church religion programs, retreats, and family vacations. This complex includes two hotels, lodges, apartments, and a campground as well as private cottages. Set on 1,200 acres with a 200-acre lake and 18-hole golf course, the center is 26 miles west of Asheville. Write Box 67, 759 Lakeshore Drive, Lake Junaluska, North Carolina 28745; phone: 800-222-4930; e-mail: info@lakejunaluska.com; Web site: www.lakejunaluska.com.

Presbyterian

Makemie Woods is a camp and conference center owned and operated by the Presbyterian Church and supported by the United Methodist Church. Available for individuals and families from August through June on 275 forested acres, Makemie Woods offers recreational activities and an outdoor chapel. Cabins are available for private and family retreats and vacations. Find them at Box 39, Barhamsville, Virginia 23011; phone: 800-566-1496; e-mail: makwoods@makwoods.org.

The Vanderkamp Center is a joint mission of the Presbyterian Church and the Evangelical Lutheran Church in America. Located in upstate New York near Syracuse, the center is situated on 1,100 acres of forest and meadows with a 48-acre lake and walking trails. Lodges and cabins are available. Write RD1, Box 50, Martin Road, Cleveland, New York 13042; phone: 315-675-3651; Web site: www.vk.org.

Chill Out

Most, but not all, denominations welcome persons of other faith traditions to their retreat and conference centers. All my samples welcome everyone.

Religious Orders

The retreat centers listed in this section describe those that are operated by religious orders of Anglican or Catholic monks, priests, or nuns. Sometimes the center is a building that does not cry out "religious place." In other instances, the orders use their monasteries and convents, for example, to house the retreats. Some centers offer programmed retreats; others unstructured, individual ones. When you look for your retreat house, choose the surroundings that make you comfortable.

Monasteries

Holy Cross Monastery, located on the Hudson River in West Park, New York, is a Benedictine community of men within the Anglican (Episcopal) Church. There are two guest houses: the monastic enclosure and the church of St. Augustine. The buildings are historic sites registered with the National Historic Register. The work of the monastery is guest ministry, which means that its primary purpose is to schedule retreats for guests throughout the year, as well as provide space for individual and group retreats. (A writer friend of mine visits here frequently for unstructured retreats to get work done.)

Scheduled retreats vary in their purpose. One five-day silent retreat is spent in prayer and reflection. A personal director meets each day with his or her assigned retreatants. Participants are asked to provide a brief synopsis of their spiritual journey to date and a statement of their hopes for the retreat.

Another retreat explores the Benedictine experience and is a weeklong retreat. Participants join the monks in their daily prayers and meditations, lecture/discussion meetings, afternoon work periods, and evening gatherings for group reflection. Emphasis is given to the dilemma of how to live a more balanced life within the chaos of day-to-day living.

Other scheduled retreats may include shadow work (looking at the repressed, unknown, and unintegrated part of the psyche), centering prayer, or meditation instruction and practice. Contact this Benedictine community at The Guesthouse, Holy Cross Monastery, Box 99, West Park, New York 12493; phone: 914-384-6660; fax: 914-384-6031; e-mail: guesthouse@idsi.net; Web site: www.idsi.net/holycross.

Jesuit Retreat Houses

Themotto of the Jesuit Retreat House on Lake Winnebago in Oshkosh, Wisconsin, is "gateway to serenity." It sounds like a great place to dump your stress-filled body and get a spiritual tune-up.

This Jesuit-run center is, as most retreat houses are, open to anyone of any persuasion. Located on the grounds of the former *novitiate,* it offers retreats year 'round, including ones based on the spiritual exercises of St. Ignatius, founder of the Jesuits. This center has a long history but is less outwardly religious than the Holy Cross Monastery, for example. The expansive grounds and lake offer natural places for walking and focused meditation.

Check out the current retreat schedule by contacting Jesuit Retreat House, 4800 Farmwald Road, Oshkosh, Wisconsin 54901; phone: 920-231-9060; fax: 920-231-9094; e-mail: jrhouse@execpc.com; Web site: www.wju.edu/jesuits/centers.html. There are many Jesuit retreat houses nationwide, and they offer men-only, women-only, and couples retreats.

Religious Communities of Women

Mariandale Retreat and Conference Center is a retreat facility located on the grounds of a women's religious congregation. The Dominican Sisters of Hope, organized about four years ago when several congregations experiencing declining numbers joined together to form a new congregation, offer a rich variety of classes, workshops, and retreats.

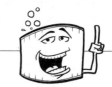

Jacuzzi Jive

In religious orders, the **novitiate** houses the novices, who are individuals beginning their study in the order and who have not taken final vows to become full members.

Get the center's catalog to see all that is available, including massage, praying with clay (they have a pottery studio on the grounds and a master potter among their sisters), couples work, certification as a spiritual advisor, extended retreats celebrating different times of the Christian church calendar, and a day learning about and living the life of woman saints.

The grounds are on the Hudson River, with spaces for walking and viewing the river. The main building is brick and looks much like a dormitory. You'll find friendliness around every corner. If you are interested in this type of experience, contact Mariandale Retreat and Conference Center, 299 Highland Avenue (Route 9), Ossining, New York 10562; 914-941-4455; e-mail: jmcgorry@ophope.org.

A similar experience is available at Kordes Enrichment Center located on the grounds of a monastery in southern Indiana. Contact Kordes at 841 E. 14th Street, Ferdinand, Indiana 47532; phone: 812-367-2777; toll-free: 800-880-2777; fax: 812-367-2313; e-mail: kordes@thedome.org; Web site: www.thedome.org. Lodging here is college dormitory style. Meals are served in common, or you bring your own. Workshop and weekend retreat rates are in the $50 to $150 range.

Another retreat is Linwood Spiritual Center, 139 S. Mill Road, Rhinebeck, New York 12572; 914-876-4178, which is a residence for retired nuns that provides year-round weekend programs for spiritual renewal, regardless of your religious focus. Request the brochure listing programs for the coming year.

Sinsinawa Mound on rolling, wooded countryside in southwest Wisconsin has a Native American setting and flavor even though it is home to a Catholic order of Dominican nuns. Guests stay in dormitory-style lodging and retreat topics include Dream Journeying, Christian-Buddhist dialogue, and The Feminine Face of God. Meditate in the modern, circular chapel with 37 stained glass windows or hike on trails that wind around the wooded mound, once a Native American sacred site. Phone: 608-748-4411, ext. 811.

Farmhouse Retreats

Bethany Spring calls itself "a place to be." Sponsored by the Sisters of Charity of Nazareth, it's a six-bedroom farmhouse in the country on rolling hills in Kentucky, south of Louisville. Located one mile from the Abbey of Gethsemani where Thomas Merton stayed, Bethany Spring offers "an informal and personal approach to prayer, solitude, and spiritual direction." Retreatants are free to walk the road to the abbey to join the monks in prayer.

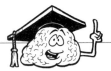

Mindful Moment

Thomas Merton (1915–1968) was a Roman Catholic monk, author, and poet, whose life followed three distinct phases: secular, monastic, and public. This last phase is marked by an intense involvement in Asian spirituality. Perhaps his most famous book is *Seven Storey Mountain,* an autobiography.

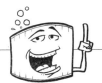

Jacuzzi Jive

A **hermitage** is a place set apart for its occupant to experience not only silence but also solitude. Try this living arrangement if you want to spend time completely alone.

Bethany Spring is a place where men and women of all faiths come to "do their own thing" on unstructured retreats. You plan your schedule. If you want a session with a spiritual director, that may be arranged. The stocked kitchen is yours to cook breakfast and lunch whenever you wish. The dinner meal is taken in common. For guests who want more solitude, there is only one *hermitage,* which is booked a year in advance. Fees are low in order to make retreats available to as many persons as possible. At the time of this writing, the suggested donation is $35 per night. For more information, write 115 Dee Head Road, New Haven, Kentucky 40051; or call 502-549-8277.

Hermitages

Hermitages are available throughout the United States. Often they are an adjunct to a retreat center. By their nature, they accommodate one person at a time and therefore may be in short supply in your area. Waiting lists of up to a year are not uncommon.

You can find additional hermitages attached to retreat facilities in Iowa at The Ark; visit its Web site at www.theark1.com. In Mississippi, there's the Dwelling Place House of Hospitality and Prayer: phone: 601-738-5348; fax: 601-738-5345; e-mail: dwellpl@tilc.com; Web site: www.dwellingplace.com/.

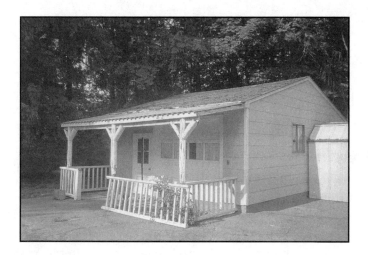

Your hermitage may be as simple as this one-room dwelling. Situated away from others, your simple lifestyle of a weekend, a week, or longer is directed at your inner furnishings. (Photo courtesy Linda Short)

Our Lady of Solitude

At Our Lady of Solitude House of Prayer, you live alone in the desert as did Anthony (251–356 A.D.), credited with beginning the monastic way of life in northern Africa. This special desert experience may be the only one of its kind in the United States. Although it is sponsored by a religious community, no one is on site except a caretaker. Three hermitages offer contemplation and absolute solitude (unless you request a spiritual director) in this desert and mountain area 40 miles north of Phoenix.

You have a key to the meditation chapel and free access to miles and miles of Sonoran Desert and mountains for walking. Retreatants are advised to bring sturdy walking shoes. A library offers more than 1,400 volumes to help pass the time. In this hermitage, you have your own little shelter to live in the middle of nowhere. Here, the hermitage is a self-contained unit with bed, desk, bath, prayer porch, and small kitchen. Food is whatever you bring with you.

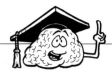

Mindful Moment

How do you read the word *nowhere?* Most of us see it as "no where." We can't find our place because we are no where to be found. But there is another way to read it, a way that is always true. That way is "now here." Isn't that a wonderful way to see where you are? You are never no where; you are always here, where you are now. Don't dwell on the past or the future; appreciate where you are, now here.

Admittedly, not everyone is ready for the hermitage experience. Initially you may feel lost in such surroundings. After all, there's no one you need to answer to, wait on, or yell at (even if you wanted to!). You create whatever schedule you want. You may come for as short or as long a time as you'd like, up to a year, in fact.

Contact Our Lady of Solitude House of Prayer at Box 1140, Black Canyon City, Arizona 85324; or call 623-374-9204 between 9 A.M. and 12 P.M. Arizona time. (There is no fax, no e-mail, and no Web site. This is a place of technological solitude as well.)

Desert House of Prayer

The Desert House of Prayer is similar in setting and style to Our Lady of Solitude, but it provides a community of people to talk to and friends for the journey. Located in northwest Tucson, Desert House accommodates up to 15 retreatants.

Desert House is situated on 31 acres of desert, just below Safford Peak in the Tucson Mountains and adjoining Saguaro National Monument. Lodging may be in the main building, each wing of which houses six private rooms and a chapel. In addition, three self-contained hermitages and two travel-trailer hermitages are set at a considerable distance from the other buildings. Meals are taken in common, and retreatants are asked to help with cleanup after dinner.

The daily schedule is quite different from some other retreat facilities. The emphasis here is on prayer, contemplation, and meditation. It provides opportunity for all those who, most often because of work, have had too little time to cultivate a life, either physical, psychological, or spiritual. The Desert House is a place of integration, a place to adjust living to include not only activity but also contemplation.

Each day, retreatants may join in

➤ Morning prayer.

➤ Formal church service.

➤ An hour session of group-centering prayer (meditation).

➤ Walking meditation outside.

➤ Evening prayer.

In addition, retreatants are encouraged to use their free time to read, reflect, and pray. Every Wednesday evening a peace and justice forum is held. Either one of the members of the religious community or an outside expert working in the field of social justice gives a talk.

The library contains more than 10,000 volumes. Each week, a film is scheduled for viewing and discussion. Recently, artists and writers have begun to come to Desert House to create their work while keeping to the prayer schedule.

Anyone is welcome, provided you are serious about making a retreat. This is not a place to bunk while you sightsee in the area. (But then that applies to any of these retreat facilities.) For reservations, contact Desert House of Prayer, Box 570, Cortaro, Arizona 85652; phone: 520-744-3825; fax: 520-744-0774.

Programmed Retreats

You may be seeking personal or even social transformation in community with others rather than on individual retreats. In these instances, you may turn to centers that offer workshops or courses of study in a retreat setting. The emphasis here is on change through interaction with others. When reviewing these options, notice that some centers also offer space for individual, private retreats and for family gatherings.

Kirkridge

Kirkridge Retreat and Study Center is located on 270 acres on the Kittatinny Ridge of the Appalachian Mountains. It's a nonprofit corporation supported by fees and contributions whose facilities are available for individual, family, and group retreats and host many scheduled workshops, classes, and forums. To obtain a catalog, contact Kirkridge at 2495 Fox Gap Road, Bangor, Pennsylvania 18013; phone: 610-588-1793; fax: 610-588-8510; Web site: www.kirkridge.org.

Take 5

Make an online retreat by visiting the Web site: www.creighton.edu/collaborativeministry/r–how.html. Sponsored by the Jesuit order, the site is valuable for persons who can't get away for a retreat, or want resources and a structure to follow for making a retreat at home. Read or download 34 weekly guides to consider, pray about, or meditate over during the week. The site also offers tips for prayer in everyday life.

The private retreat houses for individuals or families have their own kitchens and baths. There are many hiking trails, including the Appalachian Trail, which cuts through the property. The neighbors at the private Columcille Megalith Park, designed as a miniature Stonehenge, welcome Kirkridge guests to the Columcille stone chapel and park (locate them on the Web at www.columcille.com).

In addition, Kirkridge offers weekend programmed retreats around an array of topics, including a regularly scheduled Sabbath experience. If you want guidance in how to enjoy some silence and use quiet time in the company of others, Kirkridge might be for you. Past weekend programs have included

- ➤ The feminine soul.
- ➤ Mysticism.
- ➤ Writing.
- ➤ Buddhism.
- ➤ Preaching.
- ➤ Interfaith dialogues.

Other special workshops include men-only recovery weekends and sessions for the gay and lesbian community and for advocates and helpers who work with victims of sexual assault and abuse.

Lama

The Lama Foundation also presents diverse practices tied to many spiritual traditions, including Tibetan, Sufi, and Hindu. Summer retreats (May through September) last one to two weeks at their center in the mountains of northern New Mexico overlooking the Rio Grande valley. Write to the Lama Foundation at Box 240, San Cristobal, New Mexico 87564; 505-586-1269; e-mail: lama@compuserve.com; or visit the Web site: www.taosnet.com/lama.

Oregon House

The grounds of the Oregon House overlook the Pacific Ocean. The grounds include several forested acres and trails, as well as access to a creek and secluded beach with tidepools and caves. A meditation and healing room is available at the modest house there. You are welcome to reserve a room for a private retreat and are within easy reach of recreational and sightseeing venues.

Staff also offer day or overnight workshops on topics ranging from living simply to your aura and music for health. Massage and some healing treatments are available during your stay. The House accommodates a maximum of 25 guests. Contact Oregon House at 94288 Highway 101, Yachats Oregon 97498; phone: 541-547-3329; fax: 541-547-3754; e-mail: metatoh@pioneer.net; Web site: www.oregonhouse.com.

Just for a Day

There may be times when you can't afford to take off even for a weekend, but you'd like to get out of your daily routine for the day. Perhaps you need a respite from the office (or the children!). You're not interested in traveling very far, but you'd like a place to hang out. Maybe you'd like a room (a view would be great, too) or just a quiet place to be alone. There are locations that offer solace for the day retreatant.

Our Lady of Divine Providence

The Our Lady of Divine Providence House of Prayer, near the water in Florida, is one such daytime retreat house. It was recommended to me by a friend who visited after the death of her husband. Located on the north shore of Old Tampa Bay on 12 acres of land, 20 minutes from Tampa, Florida, this house of prayer is "for all peoples." It is open for individual prayer and quiet reflection on weekdays from 10 A.M. to 3 P.M. Walk the grounds and visit the rose garden to clear your head and delight your senses. There is a tape- and book-lending library on the premises.

On weekends, the house is used by groups for renewal and days of quiet reflection. Twice a year there is a weekend retreat open to the public. There is an additional twice-yearly retreat for men and a monthly men's prayer group.

The Cenacle of Our Lady of Divine Providence School of Spirituality, also at this location, is affiliated with the Franciscan University of Steubenville, Ohio. Retreat houses on the grounds provide lodging for those participating in these classes or Ignatian Retreats. Contact the school at 702 South Bayview Avenue, Clearwater, Florida 33759; phone: 727-724-9505; fax: 727-724-9421; e-mail: thecenacle@juno.com; or visit the Web site: www.LHLA.org.

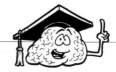

Mindful Moment

Today more lay men and women attend spiritual and seminary–type college courses than professed religious men and women.

Bethany Retreat House

Even in the city, you can find quiet, tucked-away places. Some are sponsored by religious congregations, such as the Catholic-sponsored Bethany Retreat House in East Chicago. Bethany offers no talks or discussion, but it does offer private time, a chapel, and a library with videos, tapes, and meditation music as well as books. It encourages guests to "befriend your inner self, renew your energy for life." Enjoy the calming energy of nature in the backyard garden, a nearby park, or Lake Michigan, which is a short drive away.

Longer stays are possible, and spiritual direction is available upon request. Contact Bethany at 219-398-5047; e-mail: bethanyrh@sprynet.com; or see the Web site: www.bethanyretreathouse.org.

The Path Retreat Center

Located in northern Minnesota in the Lake District, the Path Retreat Center is a private house offering rooms for hours or days to individuals and small groups and is a secular retreat facility. The schedule is yours to make. There isn't a separate chapel or meditation room. It's simply a place for a quiet time away.

The owner is a consultant and gives workshops on the topic of finding your path, which she presents both on- and off-site. Address inquiries to Rt.1, Box 193A, Detroit Lakes, Minnesota 56501; phone: 800-650-5074; fax: 218-532-7436; e-mail: kmarcil@hotmail.com; Web site: www.kathymarcil.com.

These sample listings are a mere fraction of the retreat possibilities waiting for you to discover. Seek and ye shall find. In whatever setting, enjoy and treasure the moments you spend on retreat.

The Least You Need to Know

➤ There are retreats for individuals, groups, families, and persons with special needs.

➤ When you want a traditional-looking religious place operated by a particular faith tradition, you can find it.

➤ When you want a nondenominational or very secular-looking center offering retreat and workshop topics (including self-healing, of course), you can find one.

➤ When you want silence and solitude and an unstructured retreat, accommodations are available.

➤ Whatever the setting and whatever your time commitment (one day, one weekend, one week, or an entire year) there is a retreat waiting for you.

➤ Search for additional retreat possibilities by checking with your place of worship, your friends, and Appendix C.

Part 7
Following the Spirit

Sometimes it's a no-brainer: An opportunity arises, and you take advantage of it. Other times the decision is agonizing, and even after you've made it, you're not sure you've decided correctly. Be happy; don't worry. You followed your heart (or your doctor's or therapist's advice) and stand at the threshold of a potentially life-changing experience at a wonderful spa or retreat.

Part 7 will help make your stay there a pleasant and satisfying one. It offers an array of guidelines for when you arrive and how to make the very most of your stay. Perhaps more important, you'll need to make adjustments when you return home. I'll help you deal with your out-of-sync feelings and suggest ways to nurture the new you.

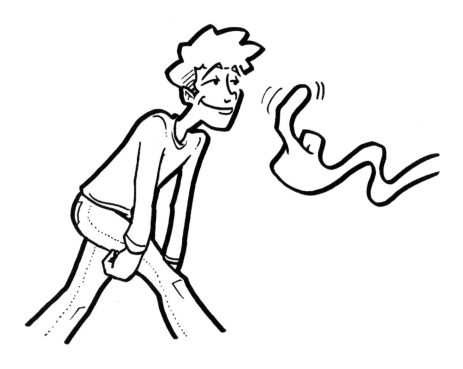

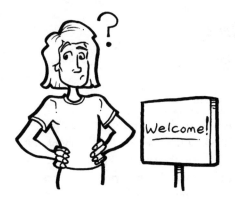

Chapter 23

I'm on Retreat, Now What?

> **In This Chapter**
>
> ➤ Equipping yourself for a retreat
>
> ➤ Making yourself feel comfortable
>
> ➤ Respecting your limits
>
> ➤ Listening to your inner wisdom
>
> ➤ Knowing when to call it quits

Your reservations are made, your bags are packed, and your plants are watered; the moment has arrived. You're ready to walk out one door and go through another. This door is unfamiliar, unsettling, and a bit uncomfortable, but it won't be for long. Close the door behind you, and get on with the adventure ahead! Your journey of self-healing has begun.

Crossing the Threshold

Crossing a threshold is a marvelous symbol of transition. The threshold separates what came before from what is now. That's where you are now, on the threshold.

Just as taking the first steps on the moon were so momentous, so also are your first steps over your thresholds. You do not know what awaits you, where you will end up, who will accompany you, or how you will be changed. Such important events must be noticed, celebrated, and identified in some special way.

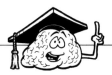

Mindful Moment

The Old Testament of the Bible tells of worshippers who are careful not to step on the threshold of a temple. Pilgrims in Syria think it is unlucky if they step on the threshold of a saint's shrine or of a mosque. Marco Polo, a thirteenth-century traveler, reported that guards were stationed at every doorway of the palace of Kubla Khan to prevent visitors from stepping on the threshold. In India, the threshold is the home of a goddess named Lakshmi. Today people may protect their doorways with horseshoes for luck, with blessings on the new year, or with a *mezuzah*, a small case of religious texts used by Jews.

Leaving in Style

Planning something special to signal your new beginning is important. It helps you

➤ Leave behind what came before, including your old selves.

➤ Become ready to accept whatever lies ahead.

➤ Become mindful, conscious, and alert to your new state.

➤ Focus your attention on new experiences and opportunities.

Some actions are better done before leaving home. Others can be taken as you prepare to cross the new threshold.

Small Actions Speak Volumes

How would you mark your crossing? What might you do to show yourself and the world that there is a separation between your normal, ordinary, daily life and the step across the threshold that you are poised to make?

Your ritual might be to

➤ Leave behind all jewelry (save, perhaps, a wedding ring), timepieces, and electronic gadgets.

➤ Wear or bring certain articles of clothing.

➤ Purchase a new journal and a new pen (and don't forget to pack them).

➤ Bring a special book, candle, an item that holds personal meaning, or an object that symbolizes your journey, your hopes, and your new beginning.

➤ Pray, meditate, or listen to a particular piece of music.

➤ Bless your doorway as you leave and when you return.

➤ Bless your new, temporary home.

What sets these actions apart and creates the separation between the old and the new, the familiar and the future, is that you're doing them deliberately, intentionally, and with your entire focus.

Advice upon Arrival

When I was a kid, my last name began with the letter A, so my desk was first in the row. Small wonder, then, that all the words that flashed into my mind for my first bits of advice also begin with the letter A. As you take your first steps in new surroundings, these advisory words may make your stay that much more agreeable. (There I go again!)

Attention!

You don't need to stand up straight and salute, just pay attention. You were aware of your leave-taking and your new beginning. Just because you made it to the retreat doesn't mean you can collapse. You can release the burdens of your ordinary life, but make sure you take in all that is around you.

Notice the sky, the sun, or lack of it. Notice the colors of wood, which are not uniform throughout its surface. Notice the people, the way they carry themselves, the twinkle in their eyes. Sense their feelings. Coming here was your decision. This is your life. Live it.

Take 5

I hope you brought along a journal and pen; you will want to record some impressions. Notice especially what you might normally ignore. Paying attention has itself made changes in you.

Acceptance

A pilgrimage is about receiving whatever is there, all of it, as part of the total experience. Because you are now paying closer attention, there will be even more to receive. Take a walkabout. Orient yourself to your new surroundings.

There is a way to understand your experiences that can help you accept what is happening. The process goes by different names, but it is essentially asking yourself two questions:

1. What was really good, enjoyable, the best about today?

2. What was the worst, the saddest, angriest, most uncomfortable moment?

Take 5

Here's a tip from Thich Nhat Hanh, a Vietnamese Zen Buddhist monk living in France: "A look filled with understanding, an accepting smile, a loving word, a meal shared in warmth and awareness are the things which create happiness in the present moment."

You may use other words, but you get the idea. Having the answers, you next offer thanks and request understanding and acceptance of the answers. In that acceptance, a new person will go back home.

Attitude

Attitude is your key to success, however you define that word. And your attitude is under *your* control. Look on this experience with enjoyment and expectation. Be in wonder and in awe of where you are, how you got there, and where you might be going. Expect that the best awaits you here and hereafter.

Adventure

See yourself as that first person to set sail from a distant shore when no land was in sight. Throw off your schedules, timetables, and date books. (At the least, save some room each day for surprises.) Being open to adventure is a freeing, truly liberating experience. Living to tell the tale is even more exciting.

Adventures—unusual, stirring, at times daring, experiences—add so much to life. Even more, they show that you are able and willing to accept what the universe wants to give you. See life itself as an adventure and enjoy!

Activity

A familiar Shaker hymn says, "To turn, turn, will be our delight/Till by turning, turning, we come round right." The hymn suggests you keep turning and moving until you "come round right." What is right? Muslims move and face Mecca throughout the day during their prayer. When people meditate, they move inside themselves to access a greater power.

Even while you're active, draw your attention to "coming round right." Rest in the moment and use it to

➤ Give thanks.

➤ Meditate.

➤ Review your life's journey until now.

➤ Consider changes.

➤ Celebrate.

Do not be distracted by the blur around you or by all the stuff you brought with you. On all pilgrimage roads, the secular and the sacred are intertwined. Use wisely the moments you are given, so you, too, may "come round right."

Dealing with Disappointments

You know how important the shape, style, and size of your bed are to a good night's rest. On a recent trip, I had a lovely room but a substandard bed. The mattress had too many raised springs, which I couldn't seem to avoid. The bed also had both a head-board and footboard, which is bad news unless you are short enough to fit between the two, which I'm not. (At least being alone meant I could sleep diagonally!)

Like any traveler, you may find conditions that do not suit you. You may be in a semi-private room with a stranger who snores and is either too messy or too neat for you. You may find yourself in a private room that is next door to a lounge that attracts too many people too late into the night.

In some cultures, hardship is welcomed. It adds merit to the journey. Somehow, I don't think you'll be satisfied with extra merit. You expected a comfortable stay. So what should you do? You know your choices. You can

> ➤ Leave.
> ➤ Scream.
> ➤ Sulk.
> ➤ Be reasonable.

Try this last approach. If there's a way to fix or alter whatever it is that has gotten under your skin, fine. (Remember to ask nicely and calmly.) If it can't be fixed, then let me share some words of wisdom from one of my teachers: Look for the lesson in any circumstance. Focus on the incident and on your reaction. Ask, "What do I need to learn from this? What do I learn about myself?"

Chill Out

You will have enough mental and emotional baggage for several stays. Take this opportunity to unload some of it.

Learn and Make the Most of It

Learning from others you meet is part of the spiritual path worldwide. These are people you need to meet. They enrich you and help you explain the patterns unfolding around you.

I always notice, quite dramatically, the mild, level way one of my friends speaks with her children. It reminds me to monitor my tone, even when my words are good. Listen to others you meet and grow from them.

Take 5

As you begin each day, ask the universe what it is you are to learn that day. Then pay attention to the answers.

Then relax. Remember your attitude. If you are staying, accept, enjoy, and expect the best. Consider it part of the adventure.

What If I Don't Wanna?

As a child, the world influenced you. If Mom said you were going to school, or to bed, more than likely that's where you went. You listened to and learned from family, friends, school, your place of worship, and the media. The outer environment was your primary influence then.

But as an adult, you influence the world. Your inner environment becomes the force that compels you to look at life differently. You revisit and question all that came before. You choose what you want to keep and use it as you look outward.

Carl Jung, in The Stages of Life, *divided life into two halves. During the first half of life, the forces affecting us are from the outside. During the second half of life, they originate within us and extend outward.*

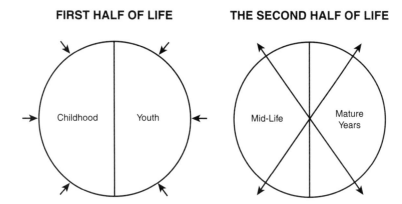

FIRST HALF OF LIFE

Childhood | Youth

THE SECOND HALF OF LIFE

Mid-Life | Mature Years

Keep Your Eyes on the Prize

After being on retreat a while, you settle into some kind of routine. There is a balance and flow between waking and retiring, resting and activity. You move throughout your day easily. It is now when, perhaps midway into your stay or journey, you arrive at a time as critical as when you first crossed the threshold. Hindus call it *tirtha*.

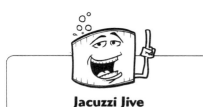

Jacuzzi Jive

Tirtha is the Hindu word for "pilgrimage," but it means a sacred crossing and may apply to many different aspects of an individual's life. Tirtha is the middle place you move across to reach a more ideal state.

Essentially, this is the point where you have done some personal traveling, enough to perhaps give you an inkling of where you are going and will end up or what you will have to change or become. It's your last-ditch bail-out point. It's the sign that says "Last exit before crossing the bridge" or "Last exit before paying the toll."

Cross the Bridge, Pay the Toll

You cross a real bridge as you move from the beginning across a midline that leads you toward completion. And you do pay a real toll when you stick it out. The toll is recommitting to whatever ideal you held up, whatever purpose you had in front of you, when you began. You need to refocus your energy on the prize.

I remember a very overweight woman about my age who was participating in a program that included hikes that increased in length daily. She was slow. Her breathing was labored. She was always last on the trail. Every day, at some point in her journey, she met tirtha. Every day, at that point, she needed to gather her reserves and focus to recommit to her goal.

When you are into your journey, the decision to continue may not be difficult. After all, you've come this far already. But if and when the road is difficult, look to

> ➤ The preparatory work you did.
>
> ➤ What you have done already physically.
>
> ➤ How far you have come spiritually.

Remember your grand purpose. Revisit the longing you felt and the original decision you made to set out on this path. Then take another step forward for self-healing.

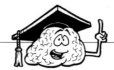

Mindful Moment

Sometimes you will never see the prize for which you strive. It's like waiting to harvest a date. It takes 80 years from the time you plant a date seed to when you can harvest any fruit (if you live to be older than 80). That's why it's important to have your purpose clear. Believing in what you're doing is more important than seeing the results.

If You Want to Leave

You must decide. That's not to say that you must finish everything you begin. Sometimes your task is finished in a different way (like perhaps leaving the date harvest to others yet to come). Sometimes you become distracted, but you realize that the journey allowed you to reach this distraction, which now needs your attention more. Sometimes, perhaps, you weren't meant to make the journey after all.

Now would be a good time to get out your journal. If you have been using it to record your observations, feelings, and musings, it will give you answers (and not just a litany of your daily schedule!). Reread what you wrote. I find it fascinating to go back and read my journals from years ago. I have forgotten so much. I sound different. They record the changes in experience and mood.

Your journal will tell you the same. Your time may not be as difficult as you believe. Perhaps it's only one little thorn that's getting to you, but overall, you read and remember the joy and discovery and your growing comfort with your space and your place in it.

On the other hand, your journal may be a litany of complaints. Maybe it describes you as still unsettled, afraid, and worried. What is keeping you this way? Probably you yourself.

Don't Shortchange Yourself

I remember a particular retreat. I went only because my husband did not want to go alone this first time. I didn't think I was grousing about the experience, but I wasn't sure I wanted to be there, either. Then at lunch, as the group were gathered together around one table, the leader began talking about something, but I wasn't listening. That is, I wasn't listening until I heard her say, "Take Linda, for example. She hasn't yet decided to join us." She was correct, of course. After I changed my attitude and got with the program, I left with some life-changing experiences.

If your decision is to leave or quit an activity, spend some time reflecting on your decision:

➤ Are outside influences or inner forces motivating you?

➤ Are you fearful or doubting?

➤ Is your goal still the same?

You may discover that your goal has changed or that you had a different purpose altogether in mind when you set out. If your goal is intact, and your motives still true, perhaps fear is blocking your channels of energy.

I wrote this once upon a time:

> This is not working for me
>> but my life-giving breath is
>> my care-giving heart is
>> my strong, decisive voice is
>> my straight, tall back is
>> my sturdy, flexible leg is
>
> This is not working for me
>> for I have forgotten the source of all life
>> I have ignored the source of my energy
>> I have separated from the source of my life
>
> This *is* working for me
>> taking time to sit quietly
>> to feel my breath
>> to hear my heartbeat
>> to see the divine energy like a river rushing through me
>> And then giving thanks.

Clear your head. Take a walk, pray, meditate, do some yoga, dance. Do what calms you, energizes you, and focuses you.

You may not be 100 percent certain. After all, we often don't know whether we've made the right decision except in hindsight, if then. In the end, access your inner wisdom. Be still and listen closely. Then accept and learn from your response.

The Least You Need to Know

➤ Mark the beginning of your personal journey in some way to symbolize and separate it from the rest of your life.

➤ Bring along your attention, acceptance, positive attitude, sense of adventure, and right activity.

➤ Despite what others say or think, respect your limits and honor your boundaries.

➤ If you encounter difficulties, focus, keep your purpose foremost in front of you, and listen to your inner wisdom.

➤ In every situation, look for lessons you may learn.

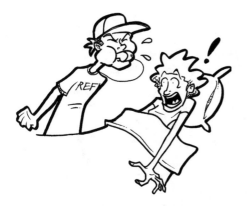

Chapter 24

Rules for Your Rest

In This Chapter

➤ Getting the most from your stay at a spa or retreat

➤ Keeping your foot out of your mouth

➤ Understanding your place

➤ Avoiding faux pas

Are you having fun yet on your little adventure? You haven't done any irreparable damage to yourself or to someone else. You haven't made any mistakes that you know of. Ah, but have you read the rule book? Ignorance is bliss, but it is also the stuff of which faux pas are made.

These rules were not handed down to me from any mountain. I haven't read them anywhere else. But I've done quite a bit of research about spa and retreat experiences, and I've defined some areas that I believe need your attention. Here, then, are my 10 C's for self-healing.

1. Commitment

According to one's actions, according to one's conduct, so one becomes—the doer of good becomes good, the doer of evil becomes evil.

Now they say further that this Person is made up of desire alone: as he desires so he resolves, as he resolves so he acts, as he acts so he becomes.

—*The Upanishads*, circa 900–600 B.C.E.

The 10 C's according to Short.

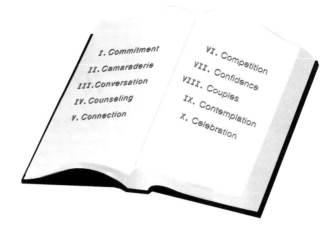

I. Commitment
II. Camaraderie
III. Conversation
IV. Counseling
V. Connection

VI. Competition
VII. Confidence
VIII. Couples
IX. Contemplation
X. Celebration

Immerse Yourself

You are where you wanted to be. This is your special place for the few days or week or longer that you are here. This is the place on which you fixed your heart. Give yourself to the place, the people, and the program. Don't let it be observed of you that "you haven't decided yet to join us."

Use Your Time

You may only have a few hours in the grand scheme of things to be here. You have only these few hours to move along your path toward the fulfillment of your purpose here. You have only these few hours to renew, reflect, and refresh yourself. Use your time wisely and well.

Persevere

Take your experience slow and easy. Remember, this is new to you, or at a new facility. The environment may be different from what you expected. Don't give up so readily. Ease into the routine, ask questions, take breaks.

More important than finishing is giving yourself, honestly, to the experience. Accept the surprises and difficulties. Meet the challenges. Work through them all. Be able to look back on your stay with no regrets.

2. Camaraderie

You cannot hope to build a better world without improving the individual. To that end each of us must work for his own improvement, and at the same time share a general responsibility for all humanity, our particular duty being to aid those to whom we think we can be most useful.

—Marie Curie (1867–1934)

Offer Silently

Many of us have difficulty accepting help. It's okay if we can give it, because then we are in control. There is at least one way you can offer help to someone without calling attention to the need and without therefore requiring that person to acknowledge their momentary weakness: Provide help silently simply by being present.

The first morning my retreat group and I hiked what was known as "the fire trail." It was a loose dirt and rock path, at places more like a channel for runoff, and it went straight up. It was difficult, but nothing I couldn't handle.

Not so for another woman in the group. At times she was slipping, holding on to anything to keep from sliding down the hill. She was going slowly, and we soon caught up to her. Rather than pass, we remained behind with her. We didn't ask her if she needed help, which would have increased her anxiety and her guilt at holding us back. We freely made our decision and offered her silent support and conversation that distracted her from the challenge at hand until we reached the top.

Join In

Everyone has different rhythms, and sometimes you just need to be alone. But the other folks with you made the same decision you made: to come to this place at this time. Perhaps you have other things in common as well. If you avoid them the entire time, you won't know. If you always stay in your room or shun the small talk before and after workouts, you won't gain the knowledge or the lessons that may be yours for the taking.

Chill Out

I'm not saying you have to spend every waking moment with the group. When you do want to be alone, assert your boundary and be courteous about it. Find your balance.

Choose Well

Will Rogers said, "I never met a man I didn't like." Regardless of whether that statement is true for you, it is true that we all get along better with some folks than with others.

If you find a person you really get along with, great. Others may just rub you the wrong way. As you come to know the people staying with you, you'll notice which ones are easier on you than others. You don't need to avoid anyone deliberately. Enjoy your stay by enjoying the company you keep.

3. Conversation

Speak your truth quietly and clearly and listen to others, even the dull and ignorant; they too have their story.

—*Desiderata* by Max Ehrmann

Keep Confidences

Anyone who has ever participated in a group process of any kind knows that the first rule is confidentiality. Remarks are not prefaced by, "Please don't tell anyone else but …," and they shouldn't have to be. Whatever anyone else tells you beyond their name, rank, and serial number is for your ears only. If they want to spread the news, let them do it themselves.

Chill Out

Confidentiality applies to discussions with your spouse or friend who came with you, too. To the speaker, your spouse or friend is just another member of the party. So be it. Use that imaginary key to lock your mouth. Others' stories are not for your analysis or food for the gossip mill.

Take 5

If you want to speak with someone but he or she is involved with someone else, keep your distance. Don't eavesdrop, and don't intrude. Wait your turn.

Be Civil; Be Courteous

You may not like what you are hearing from someone else. You may not appreciate the tone, language, or ideas. Maybe you disagree strongly with whatever it is that person said. Register your disagreement courteously. Remember, "speak your truth quietly and clearly." You don't need to get involved in arguments about politics or religion.

Finally, don't exclude anyone arbitrarily. Don't assume because of the job a person has or how that person looks, dresses, or acts that he can't offer anything. Listen to everyone. You may be given useful words of wisdom in return.

No True Confessions

There are times when we need to dump on someone. We are so overloaded with worry, anxiety, frustration, or pain that we have to get rid of it. It's times like these when we tend to corner someone and unload. We may also be swollen with pride or success, and then we want to share the details of our triumph.

Either way, it puts a burden on the listener. Does she want to be under your cloud? Is she worrying enough about her own situation? Will your successes make her feel small? You've come together for a short time with motivations as diverse as your personalities. Does she really want to know this about you? Probably not. If you need someone to listen to you, seek out a professional.

4. Counseling

For the Lord God will help me; therefore shall I not be disgraced: therefore I set my face like flint, and I know that I shall not be put to shame.

—Isaiah 50:7

You Weren't Asked

Some people presume to know the answers to everything. They've read it, heard it, or experienced it all. They begin their sentences with, "If you ask me …" The point is, you weren't asked, so don't advise.

Even if you are asked, keep your own counsel. You can't know all the factors involved, and it isn't your place to find out. Don't be an armchair psychiatrist. Besides, you're supposed to be working on yourself. Don't use someone else as a distraction.

No "Shoulds"

I had a wonderful teacher who was very careful with her language. She would suggest something or invite you to consider something. She never presumed to know the right answer to your dilemma. She believed that we're all capable of finding our own answers by tapping into our inner wisdom, our higher selves, or what some would call our divine nature.

Take 5

If you want to share some experience that relates to the conversation, go ahead. But do so without comment. Allow the listener to make connections and draw his own conclusions.

No Appointments

Even if you happen to be a professional in a helping field, a retreat is not the time for you to be making appointments for a time during the stay or afterward. Folks didn't come here to see you anyway (well, probably not). This is not the proper forum to drum up business; no ambulance chasers are allowed. Mind your own business, and let others mind theirs.

If you believe you have something to offer someone, send that person a note and your business card later on. It might be a word of greeting to keep in touch if you had a cordial relationship during your stay. If he isn't interested, it will be easier for him to say no, and you will not have intruded during his stay.

5. Connection

Our lives are but fine weavings that God and we prepare
Each life becomes a fabric planned and fashioned in His care.
We may not always see just how the weavings intertwine,
… For He can view the pattern upon the upper side
While we must look from underneath …"

—Greeting card verse, unattributed

Remain Detached

Remember from Chapter 15, "Nature Calls!" how you laid on your back on the grass and watched the clouds drift by? You noticed their patterns, named them, or created stories about them. Then you let them recede from your sight as you shifted your gaze to focus on the next entry in the jetstream.

The movement of the heavens is a metaphor for your connection with your fellow travelers. You are supportive, interested, and caring, but you're not invested in them, their situations, or their continuing presence in your life. You remain detached.

At a couples retreat, my husband and I entered into a prayerful exercise. The women formed an inner circle, and the men formed an outer one. As we moved from person to person, we were instructed to share or pray in different ways with that person. On this occasion, the women were asked to place our hands near the man's heart, without touching him. We were not to speak, but we were to feel and send unconditional love.

As I did this, the man I was with began to shiver, then convulse, and finally sob. When the time ended, we rotated and began a different practice with new partners. I did not seek out this man or ask about his experience. I honored his space and what had happened. Wherever you are, realize it is a special albeit somewhat artificial situation. Receive what is offered. Return home content with what you have given or received.

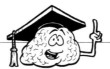

Mindful Moment

St. Ignatius of Loyola, who founded the Jesuits, gave this example of detachment from his life: When asked what he would do if the religious order he created, built up, and devoted his life to were to be expunged, Ignatius replied, "I would pray 15 minutes, then turn to something else."

Don't Presume

Your spa or retreat experience is giving you just what you need. You are relaxed and feeling good. You are brimming over with helpfulness and concern for everyone you meet.

But be careful. Your concern may be misdirected, unwanted, or intrusive. For example, when a woman was crying while sharing her story with a group, someone else presumed she needed a tissue and slid a box across the carpet. She returned the box swiftly and sharply. Don't presume you know what someone else needs.

Break Cleanly

If you have been practicing detachment, then making a clean break from your retreat group or spa friends will be easy. Unlike St. Ignatius, most of us harbor some attachment to an object or a person. But when you tear a thread in two, the ends are left uneven and frayed. A swift, deliberate snip with a pair of scissors does a neater job. You will know whether it is appropriate to keep in touch.

Don't ask for addresses

➤ Unless it's clear to you that you've made a connection that might continue for a time.

➤ For business purposes.

➤ To be polite.

➤ If it's a superficial overture like "let's do lunch some time."

Instead, thank the participants, especially those with whom you spent some time. Perhaps offer a word that indicates how they have touched your life. Celebrate the shared moments. You will always have them.

6. Competition

> … I tell everyone among you not to think of himself more highly than one ought to think, but to think soberly … For as in one body we have many parts, and all the parts do not have the same function, so we, though many, are one body … and individually parts of one another. Since we have gifts that differ according to the grace given to us, let us exercise them ….
>
> —Romans 12:3–6

Don't Keep Score

This spa or retreat experience isn't a game. You're not on a team that is trying to beat "the opposition." It doesn't matter if you do only two laps and John does five. It doesn't matter if your skin isn't quite as smooth or glowing as Sally's. It doesn't matter if you feel as though you are in, as St. John of the Cross called it, the dark night of the soul, and everyone else is bright and merry. (They might be faking it, not totally honest, afraid to admit their disappointments, or they might really be bright and merry.)

Compete against yourself. Do you feel healthier? Are you more peaceful, relaxed? Are you more patient and kinder to others? If you must compete, how about keeping track of:

➤ How often you smile

➤ How many compliments you give

➤ How generous you are

Chill Out

If you pay attention, you will feel the competitive energy generated by others. Don't let that energy excite your own competitive spirit. Keep yourself under control, regardless.

Take 5

The Velveteen Rabbit reminds us to look to what is real. Separate the short-lived from the lasting.

Better to focus your attention and energy on values such as these, and on yourself.

Find Your Place

You're not fighting the world, just trying to find your place within it. Having found your place, you're working on being content with it and with doing your best. Remember, we each have been given gifts. If yours is to repair shoes, do your task well. If it is to arrange walking tours, be attentive to the places, the people, and their desires.

The reading from Paul's Letter to the Romans that opened this section uses the body as a metaphor for the differing talents of people. It asks, if every part were an eye, how would we hear? If every part were an ear, how would we see? If every part were a stomach, how would we think? We are complete and functioning people because we are made of different, specialized parts, all of which are necessary for our being.

Recognize that only you can use the gifts you have been given. You have them to fulfill a purpose, whether you are completely mindful of it or not. One gift is not any better than another, despite what some people might say. You need to come to terms with that.

7. Confidence

Like a lion which fears not noises, unobstructed like the wind whistling through a net, not touching anything like the lotus leaf untouched by water, let one walk alone like a rhinoceros.

—A disciple of Buddha, sixth century B.C.E.

Appearances

You've probably heard the saying, "clothes make the man." I suppose to some extent that is true. We dress up on holidays, and the dressing up and the new clothes make us feel great and be confident that we look great.

But don't fail to pay attention to what you wear inside. As you prepare to leave for the spa or retreat, buying a few new duds may be part of your separation ritual, your crossing the threshold (see Chapter 23, "I'm on Retreat, Now What?"). It could very well make you feel better about yourself and more able to cope at your yet-unseen destination. However, even a suit of armor cannot give you inner strength. Look to what is lasting, not to ephemeral fads. Be who you are, even away from home.

Be Not Afraid

What is there to fear? The staff is paid to be cordial. Some guests might be off-putting, but you'll be in a controlled situation. Are you afraid of people not liking you? So what? You'll go home and never see those people again. Are you afraid of getting hurt? It's just what you must work through. If you believe in karma, then work through it now before the problem escalates to the point where you can't avoid it.

Stand Tall

To stand tall means throwing off your burdens. There is often a change in body posture from the beginning to the end of a time away. Look closely. People arrive with stooped shoulders and rounded backs, heads hanging. As they relax and exercise and stretch, their spine returns to its natural erect alignment.

Standing tall tells your body how to be, and your body tells your brain, "Oh, she's standing tall. She must feel good. She must be confident about this adventure and about the next." What's exciting is that your body gets used to this straight, tall, uplifting way of standing. When you aren't standing tall, your body reminds you.

Show the world how good you feel. You know there is a difference in your mood when you hunch and when you sit up. Exhibit confidence: Stand tall and expect that good will come to you.

8. Couples

> ... let there be spaces in your togetherness,
> And let the winds of the heavens dance between you.
> ... Fill each other's cup but drink not from the same cup.
>
> —Kahlil Gibran, "On Marriage"

Do Your Thing

My husband has always wanted to go to Greece. I went to Mexico and Peru. We both want to go to Jerusalem. He loves tennis at high noon, sweat pouring off his brow. I prefer a fast game in the early morning or late afternoon out of the sun's rays.

You know what each of you enjoys and hates. Just as in other parts of your life, you may find fulfillment in different kinds of spa or retreat experiences. If the purpose meets your needs and contributes to the strength and vitality of your union, then go your separate ways for a time.

Chill Out

If you go on retreat or to a spa together, don't keep tabs on each other. It creates suspicion, arguments, and distraction from your own work.

Together but Apart

The more difficult experience may be when the two of you make reservations at the same center. Be aware especially of competition issues. You will need to work through your needs for togetherness and separateness. Must you always eat together, keep similar hours, associate with the same people, or attend the same classes?

If the answers are yes, then you are acting as though you have identical interests and needs. I hate to break it to you, but I bet it ain't so. If your answers are no, then you still must discuss how much togetherness you expect and how much separation you will tolerate.

Sometimes the nature of the program will give you the answers. One retreat my husband and I attended was specifically for couples. We knew we would spend the structured retreat time together. During meal and stretch breaks, we decided to mix with others.

At another retreat, we agreed that we'd go our own ways because the program was better suited to it. We also considered the comfort level of other guests at this retreat. We were the only married people who attended as a couple. Consequently, we didn't sit together at meals or grab spaces next to each other during activities. However, we weren't strangers to each other either. We shared a room, spoke, and occasionally spent short stretches of time together. Make your own adjustments to meet the circumstances and your needs.

When you attend a spa or retreat, decide whether to attend with or without your partner. How much closeness do you want? (Image © H. Armstrong Roberts)

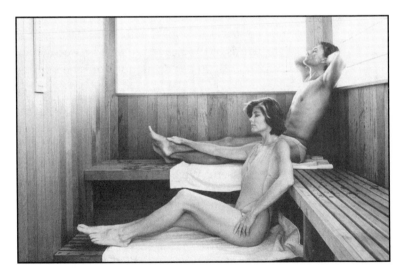

Reunion

Whether you and your partner have gone away together or separately, have a reunion when you return home. Don't let yourself believe that you like being apart, especially

if you tend toward more solo trips than togeth
ones. Recognize that you each may have had
experiences that you

> ➤ Never want to share.
> ➤ Want to share but not yet.
> ➤ Cannot find the words to share.
> ➤ Need to understand yourself.

Let the experience settle. Celebrate the
road and then the return.

Part 7

Following the S

10. Celebrati

The dawn
another
We ar
feel
bra

9. Contemplation

In order to understand the world, one has to turn away
order to serve men better, one has to hold them at a distance to
the solitude necessary to vigor, the deep breath in which the mind co
and courage gauges its strength(.)

—Albert Camus (1913–1960)

Don't Run

I don't mean running as in jogging and exercise and activity. I mean keeping a fast
pace throughout the day, running from the quiet and running from any interior issues.
Getting distracted is easy to do. If you are attending a scheduled program, it's one
session after another. Your activity blends with your massage blends with your meal
blends with a lecture. Then there are the interesting people, the evening plans, the
discussions that go on into the night.

Don't fill up every free moment. You may not be ready for any heavy-duty interior
work, and that's okay. But a bit of journaling, prayer, meditation, or just sitting still
won't hurt. It just might open up something that's been waiting to see the light of day.

Use the Quiet

In every part of every day there are opportunities, however brief, for moments of
contemplation. Find them while you are in the shower, getting dressed, or having a
manicure. Be alert to the moments as they present themselves and treasure them. Use
them to offer one-word prayers. Use them to ask a question of the universe. Use them
to just still your mind and listen with your soul.

Unite Body and Spirit

Consider how you might integrate this getaway experience. Notice how being away
from your daily routine has affected your behavior and your attitudes. What have you
gained? What have you lost (besides maybe some weight)? How will you move forward?

...on

...ng of a new day needn't begin at dawn. It begins whenever we have ...clear divine insight about ourselves, and our connectedness to the One. ...part of the perfection of God if we but permit ourselves to know it, we can ...he truth of it. We are perfect, for we are spirit. We are perfect, for we are a ...nch of the perfect vine. We are perfect, for we are love. We are perfect, for we ...e one with Father Mother God. Isn't the day glorious?

—Linda Short, 1994

Celebrate your leaving. Celebrate your journey. Celebrate your coming home. Celebrate you.

The Least You Need to Know

➤ Decide to commit yourself to the process, avoid giving advice even when asked, and compete only against yourself.

➤ If you are part of a couple, you need to decide whether you want to travel together but follow your own star at your destination or travel to separate locations. Whatever you decide, schedule a reunion upon your return.

➤ Wherever you find it, and in however minute a quantity, cherish and use the quiet.

➤ Celebrate all of it and all of you.

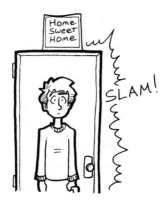

Chapter 25

Back Home Again

In This Chapter

➤ Coping with re-entry

➤ Staying free of old patterns

➤ Committing yourself to peace and relaxation

➤ Celebrating who you are

A satisfying spa or retreat experience always has the potential for being life-changing. Regardless of whether you feel that momentous "a-ha" this time, you come home to a very different routine when you walk back through your front door. You are more aware and more fully alive; things have changed, in your eyes and in those who know you well. Yet it's the same home, the same job, and the same friends. You can feel, as the saying goes, like a fish out of water. Stay with me for one more chapter, and I'll help you get back into the swim of things. Ready? Dive!

Wow! What Happened?

That's what I'd like to know. Everyone, and I do mean *everyone,* who knows you went will want to know what it was like and how you did (it's that *doing* instead of *being* again). They may even beg you to "please tell me all about it, and don't leave anything out." Even worse, they may want to see pictures.

This is the time to sit back and not rush into tales. You'll probably need to hop right into your old routine with work and family and activities and such, but don't wait too long to reflect—all by yourself—about what happened. It's always a good idea to review your life regularly anyway. Many people do this around New Year's Day or at birthdays. Look at where you used to be emotionally, physically, spiritually, and financially.

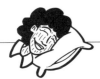

Take 5

Bring back a brochure, perhaps with a photo, and offer that to inquisitive folks as explanation while you take the time to come to a clearer understanding for yourself about your stay and its implications.

Chill Out

If you wait too long to think about what happened, you'll do more than simply forget; you'll give your psyche the message that you don't want to remember, perhaps that something happened or didn't happen that was unsettling. Examine your feelings (sit down and do a scan) about the experience. What do they tell you?

Review your history of relationships, friendships, employment, outside activities, and worship. You can offer thanks and celebrate all of it, the down times and the up times. In hindsight, look at what good the down times brought you. (It's there, if you look with eyes that see.)

Think back to this spa or retreat experience you completed. Remember:

➤ How you came to go in the first place

➤ Why you chose that particular place

➤ How you felt upon leaving home and how you felt when you arrived there

➤ Who you met during your stay and what you learned from others

➤ What surprises awaited you

➤ What the worst moment was; what the best was

➤ How you changed from the first day to the last

➤ What you want to carry with you

If you kept a journal, read it and see what was important to you in that moment. Do you remember the incidents you describe?

When I came back from a trip I took to Mexico, I wrote a narrative of what happened. I used my journal and my recollections. I sent my story to a couple whom I had met and befriended on that journey. Neither of them could recall anymore many of the events that I'd written about. If you intend to remember, do it soon.

Re-Entry Reactions

As momentous as takeoff is, re-entry and splashdown are even more so. You've survived, accomplished, experienced, and returned safely. Like old Rip van Winkle discovered, however, re-entry can be a bit traumatic!

People Are Strange

Some people may be different, but you are the one who has changed. You are the strange one. Your energy is different now. It's been stirred up and massaged; you've been energized. You feel supercharged. You may be bouncing off walls and ceilings with an outer glow and excitement you haven't shown in years—or ever. People will see, feel, and know the difference.

On the other hand, you may come away from your stay feeling unsettled or out-of-sync. Know that this feeling will pass. In the meantime, allow yourself to feel that way. After all, feeling that way is normal. You've just come from an environment where your only responsibilities were to get to your massage, decide when or if to meditate while you walk, and enjoy a lovely meal. You have been waited on hand and foot (literally, if you were at the spa). Now you return to real life. It makes sense that you can't adjust in a split second or even a week.

If you had a revelation of some kind, your adjustment will take longer. Don't fight it; it won't help. Respect what happened to you. You will come to terms with yourself before long.

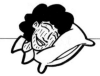

Take 5

Tell friends and family if you feel out of sorts and need time to process your experience. They'll understand better and give you some quiet instead of many questions.

New Old Routines

There is a story in sacred writings about putting new wine into old wineskins. It's like losing 50 pounds but continuing to wear your old, now quite baggy and unshapely clothes. Or getting married to someone you love but wearing a constant frown. Your new condition demands a change.

Very likely, you'll want to make some changes, even if they're only little ones. Perhaps you've decided to change the way you eat or take walks during lunch. Maybe you'll spend more time with your family or do more volunteer work and put in less overtime at work. Maybe you've decided to refrain from gossip and to compliment one person each day. Whatever it is, someone will notice.

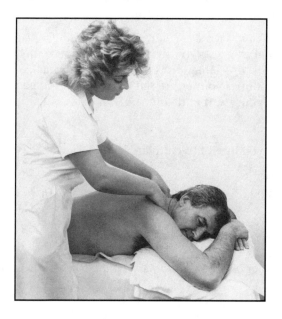

You don't need to go to a spa to get a tension-relieving massage. Look for certified massage therapists near your home and continue to enjoy the health benefits year 'round. (Image © H. Armstrong Roberts)

Moving Forward

Now is your moment: Do you want to move forward and grow or to cling to the familiar?

The Harbor or the Sea

The decision you make is akin to either remaining in the harbor or moving out to sea. The harbor is your protected inlet, your former ways of moving and being. You feel safe and confident when you are surrounded by what you know and when there are no surprises.

Now you've had a satisfying spa or retreat experience. Your ocean, or the view of it, has changed. However small or insignificant it may appear to you now, your new awareness and energy are leading you beyond the harbor. The question is, will you sail out to sea?

Turn your "I wishes" into "I wants" or "I dids." Don't add to your list of past regrets. Go for it. Pull up anchor.

Back-Sliding

You promised yourself you wouldn't eat any more greasy, salty potato chips, but you decide to "have just one." Unfortunately, you bought the brand that doesn't allow you to eat just one. You promised yourself you would exercise daily, use nightly all those skin-care products you purchased, and find a few moments of quiet. Instead, your only exercise is climbing the stairs to bed, your skin care consists of giving your face a gentle rub as your head sinks into your pillow, and the quiet you find only comes when you're sleeping. We've all done it. It's the stuff of which broken New Year's resolutions are made. We slide backward as often as we step forward.

Dr. Edward Taub, author of *The Wellness Rx: Dr. Taub's 7 Day Program for Radiant Health & Energy* (Prentice Hall, 1994) suggests you sign a proclamation to help keep your new path before you. Writing a proclamation is one way to personalize your promises. Adding your signature notifies your entire self that this is a sacred promise, one that you intend to fulfil with your heart and your soul.

If you want to use this idea:

➤ Write down what behaviors you intend to cultivate

➤ What attitudes you will keep

➤ A closing line about promising on your honor

➤ Sign and date it

➤ Post it where it is visible

The proclamation will be a reminder of the steps you are taking to enjoy health and renewal on a daily basis.

Being Realistic

Remember earlier in this chapter when I encouraged you to review your experience and think about what you want to take from it and keep with you? You may have listed everything from walking slowly and speaking gently to eating well and meditating. That's great, but let's get real here. Will you make every change overnight? Is it physically possible?

Some of us do have *epiphanies*. In a blink of an eye, everything suddenly becomes clear. Some of us immediately change as a result. We come home from our experience, and voilà! we change behaviors and attitudes.

Then again, most of us need time, encouragement, and support when we challenge ourselves to take on a new role. (That's the reason for the success of programs like Weight Watchers and 12-step groups.) When you are looking to change something about yourself, look to these steps:

1. **Identify one new habit.** Nature abhors a vacuum, so be sure to replace an unwanted habit with a desired one. If you don't, the unwanted habit will come back. For example, fill a candy dish with coins instead, or float flowers. Keep the fridge stocked with snack-size veggies instead of the pantry stocked with salty, fatty tidbits.

2. **Make the new habit a healthy habit.** You know the stories about people who are addicted to smoking. They cut back or quit, but they replace smoking with eating. Now they have a new series of complaints and a new habit to deal with.

3. **Forgive yourself.** If you give your attention to each and every instance of back-sliding (I only ran 15 minutes instead of 30. I only lost two pounds instead of three. I wanted to meditate 20 minutes but only did 19.), you're focusing on the negative. Remember that whatever you give your attention to grows. If you attend to your faults, they will multiply, expand as yeast does in dough, and take over your mind, attitude, and will. Forget the missteps. Keep your focus on the positive.

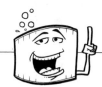

Jacuzzi Jive

Epiphany is a moment of sudden intuitive understanding, a flash of insight. For example, "I know why my feet are killing me! My shoes are too small." (But more often epiphanies are associated with more significant realizations!)

Chill Out

Certain people may be your bad habit. Be honest and ask yourself which you want more: their friendship or your new path. Besides, you will meet new people who support and share your new passion.

Making major changes to you and your environment after your spa experience may mean adding a hot tub to your deck or backyard.
(Image © Camerique Stock Photos)

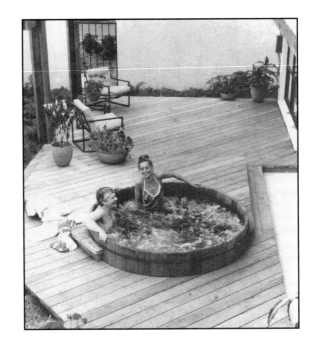

4. **Understand.** Sit in quiet. Go inside and understand what benefit you derive from this way of living. It must give you something, or you wouldn't continue with the behavior. When you more fully understand the reasons behind your actions, you can let go of them more easily and embrace a more joyous existence.

5. **Celebrate your achievements.** You can't celebrate unless you know how you're progressing. Focus on your triumphs, however small. Perhaps your triumph is a smile to someone with whom you don't relate well. Maybe your triumph is biting your tongue so that you don't have the last word again (this is *really* difficult when you're dealing with teenagers!). Keep track. Write down these successes.

Take 5

Just as you put a list of grocery needs on your fridge or bulletin board, keep a running list of accomplishments and of gains in realizing the new you.

6. **Give yourself time.** Significant changes may occur overnight, like a springtime blizzard. More often, though, some span of time and distance is needed. While you move forward, begin with a single step:

   ➤ Make only one change at a time.

   ➤ Live with that one change for a week.

   ➤ Add a second benefit the next week.

   ➤ Expect it to take about two months for new habits to take hold.

You finish a meal by taking one bite at a time. You begin a journey of 100 miles by taking one step. Sacred writings teach that the race is not to the swift, but to those who persevere. Emulate the tortoise.

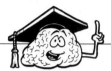

Mindful Moment

On the Inca Trail in the Andes Mountains of Peru, the highest pass is Warmiwanusqu, at about 13,000 feet, and I recall my ascent vividly. A few of the group I was in were like the hare: Beginning quickly, they became fatigued and fell back as the rest of us went by. We found a rhythm and kept with it: 1, 2, ... 99, 100 steps, rest, 1, 2. Because the end point seemed difficult, we focused on what we could accomplish easily, that is, putting together 100 steps. Persevere and celebrate the individual steps on your way.

Little Things Mean a Lot

When two people do not like each other, you know it by the little things. They don't look at each other, they speak in unfriendly tones, or perhaps one turns away when the other approaches. Similarly, when two people enjoy each other's company, it shows in a glance met, a word, a touch, or laughter.

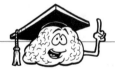

Mindful Moment

"We cannot all do great things, but we can do small things with great love."

—Mother Teresa

Whether you went away on retreat or to a spa or enjoyed some spa benefits in your own home, you may be ready to become an even better person to yourself and to others. You don't need a major overhaul to begin. The seemingly little things will make a big difference.

Listen to Your Language

Words are powerful. They reflect what we know and what we hide inside in our attitudes. When you articulate something, such as a feeling or a belief, you strengthen that feeling or belief.

What you say and how you say it comes back to you. Is life confusing? Too short? A puzzle? A celebration? How you describe it reflects your attitude. If you believe in the law of attraction, your words will bring to you whatever you say. If you say life is confusing, you'll get a big ball of confusion.

Many of us say, "I have to go to work." What do we really mean when we say that? We may be saying:

➤ I don't want to go.

➤ I don't like my job.

➤ I don't like the people.

➤ I have no choice.

➤ I can't find another job.

➤ I can't pay my bills any other way.

➤ I have a passion for this particular position.

When our choice of words hides how we feel, our unconscious notices, even if we don't. If day after day we feel "I have to go to work," then we may become

➤ Despondent because we see no other possibilities.

➤ Resentful that we have no choice.

➤ Anxious about any rumored workplace reorganization.

➤ Doubtful about our abilities.

Monitor your words. Make them expressions of hope and well-being, excitement even. Why not say

➤ I can't wait to get to work today!

➤ I wonder what I will learn today.

➤ I'd better get going so I can use my talents to help others.

Isn't this a better way of looking at the place of work in your life?

When you make changes in your lifestyle, monitor your language here, too. Do you choose to eat healthier foods "to lose weight" or to "live longer"? If your expressed reason is to lose weight, you'll have no basis for continuing your healthier choice after you lose the weight. If your reason is to live longer, then your reason will never go out of style.

Notice your language. Choose words that are beneficial, positive, and hopeful. When you first speak, you may not mean what you say. But after a while, your new words will take root. Soon you will believe them as well.

Lighten Up

How often do you smile in a day? How often do you laugh? How often do your eyes tear and your sides hurt from laughing hard? Laughter is passion without words. We cry until we laugh, laugh until we cry. Are you depressed? Laugh yourself silly and get back on the road to health.

Here's something to laugh about: *Stressed* backward spells *desserts*. That's a discovery I love. (May I have seconds?) Try these suggestions to lighten up your life:

➤ Do a smiling meditation: Peaceful people smile.

➤ Lighten your steps: Twirl, skip, do the *Wizard of Oz* Yellow Brick Road dance, or take dance classes.

➤ Fire up your prayer or meditations and count your blessings.

➤ Give up trying to do everything: Allow others to give you the gift of doing.

➤ Use lighter words: Forget the whining and naysaying.

➤ Delight yourself each day: Make time for one of your favorite activities.

➤ Be a light to others: Lose yourself in service and compassion for others.

➤ Schedule playtime, a humor night, a humor meal, or humorous movies.

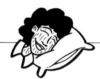

Take 5

Victor Borge once said that the shortest distance between two people is a smile. Build bridges of peace and friendship between one another with something as simple as a smile.

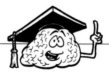

Mindful Moment

In one scene of Mel Brooks's film *Silent Movie*, the characters are dressed in suits of armor. The actors enter the cafeteria, still in armor, and try to negotiate trays and chairs and food. My husband found the scene so hilarious that he was sliding out of his seat and nearly fell on the floor of the theater. Has anything grabbed your funny bone in such a complete way?

Remember the Sabbath

If you do nothing else, take this one step: Set aside hallowed time to enjoy and celebrate what is beautiful and good. Use the time to refresh and nourish yourself and those you love. You might:

➤ Light candles, sing songs, and worship.

➤ Tell stories, laugh, and play.

➤ Bless children and each other.

➤ Give thanks.

➤ Take a nap or soak in a tub of bubbles.

➤ Share meals.

➤ Walk in the woods, sit and daydream, or pursue other afternoon delights.

Make this time sacred. Don't be concerned about your work; powerful forces are taking care of you and the world while you rest. Trust them during the holy day, afternoon, or hour that you spend in life-renewing pursuits. Be still, and know who gives you life.

Celebrate Who You Are

Individually, one moment at a time, you have the power to fashion a better world and reaffirm the specialness of all of life. Follow these guidelines:

➤ Care for yourself. This caring is not self-indulgence, but self-preservation. You can't give to others what you don't have.

➤ Get support when you need it.

➤ Accept yourself. Say, "I accept myself unconditionally as I am," twice a day for the next month. Say it out loud.

➤ Give yourself peace and love. Place your hand over your heart. For 30 seconds, think of someone or something that you love unconditionally.

➤ Care for your thoughts. Reject negativity. Don't blame; forgive. Remember your blessings.

➤ Embrace your potential for healing and health for yourself and for others. List your accomplishments and be aware of the good and life-affirming actions you do take.

Final Thoughts

All this talk about satisfying experiences, spas at home, epiphanies, and regular retreats may leave you throwing up your hands in despair, wondering where to begin. I suggest you begin by looking closely at yourself and your life and see how awe-filled it already is.

You don't need an earth-shattering, life-transforming makeover. You are a good person (and you know it). Even the good can be a bit better, however, so plan each day with time to:

➤ Smile

➤ Rest

➤ Pray

➤ Do a good deed

Whenever you are able, include a more intense and a more relaxing experience for yourself, wherever that may be.

A Sanskrit proverb says it this way: "Yesterday is but a dream, tomorrow is but a vision. But today well-lived makes every yesterday a dream of happiness and every tomorrow a vision of hope. Look well, therefore, to this day." Celebrate life, one day at a time. Namaste. Shalom. Peace be with you.

Take 5

Doing the heart exercise will lower your stress level, balance out your body, and regulate your heart rhythm. Indeed, it's also a great exercise to give love to a partner: Place your hand on his heart while he places his hand on yours. Feel and send only love and acceptance.

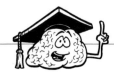

Mindful Moment

The Lakota language has no words for love or for hate; it does have a word for peace that means "all is in harmony."

The Least You Need to Know

➤ Bask in the glow of your spa or retreat experience. Remember it, re-live it, and rejoice over it.

➤ Understand that out-of-sync feelings upon returning home are normal; take time to re-orient yourself.

➤ Focus on only one change at a time, and recognize that back-sliding is normal. Focus instead on your new direction, and realize that it takes about two months before new behaviors become habits.

➤ Add a time of rest, prayer, laughter, and service to every day.

➤ Happiness and contentment come from knowing that your corner of the world is better because you walked there.

➤ You are called to be only who you are. Celebrate life; celebrate yourself.

The Spa Finder Directory of Spa Retreats and Spa Resorts

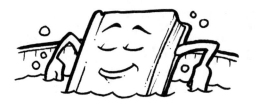

To plan your spa vacation or to find the latest information on programs and prices, contact Spa Finder reservations at 800-ALL-SPAS or 800-255-7727. In New York City, call 212-924-6800. Visit Spa Finder on the Web at spafinders.com. (Note: For more information on spas and retreats outside the United States, contact Spa Finder.)

Key:

A	Adventure hiking	M	Mind-Body-Spirit
D	Detoxification	R	Relaxation
F	Fitness	S	Stress management program
H	Healing	Sp	Sports facilities and programs
L	Luxury	W	Weight management

Price Key:

$	Less than $150 per day per person double occupancy
$$	$150 to $250 per day
$$$	$250 to $400 per day
$$$$	Over $400 per day

Spa Retreats

East Coast

Green Mountain at Fox Run, Vermont
$$
W F S R

Green Mountain at Fox Run has been teaching women how to lose weight without dieting for nearly 25 years. Clients learn how to create a personal lifestyle that integrates the best principles of nutrition, exercise, behavior, eating management, stress management, and wellness. With additional workshops on binge eating, food cravings, stress management, dining in restaurants, and relapse prevention, clients begin to enjoy eating again without stress or guilt.

Under the guidance of certified exercise physiologists, guests develop personalized, enjoyable exercise programs that include aerobics, walking, stationary biking, hiking, body conditioning, swimming, stretching, relaxation, and weight training.

Accommodations are comfortable in a country lodge on 20 acres in the Green Mountains of Vermont. A staff of nutritionists, psychologists, exercise physiologists, physical therapists, a physician, and eating management specialists is on hand. This women-only spa accomodates only 42 women at a time. The atmosphere is casual and friendly.

Contact Green Mountain at Fox Run at 802-228-8885 or 800-448-8106.

New Life Fitness Vacations, Vermont
$$
A F W R Sp

The New Life Fitness program offered at the Inn of the Six Mountains is the creation of Jimmy Le Sage, the popular motivation and lifestyle consultant and one of the pioneers of spa cuisine. Activities at the Inn include hiking, fitness classes, weight training, tennis, swimming, water aerobics, yoga, and bicycling. Golf and horseback riding are available nearby. Massage, a full line of skin-care treatments, and fitness profiles are featured.

New Life's healthy, low-fat meals are designed to help guests lose pounds or maintain their present weight. The Inn's atmosphere is casual with an emphasis on warm, friendly group experiences.

New Line Fitness Vacations can be reached at 800-228-4676.

Northern Pines Health Resort, Maine
$
D H M R

A warm and caring environment, clear air, pure water, and wholesome food are all part of the attraction at this beautiful lakeside resort on 70 acres of pine forests in southern Maine. Owner Marlee Turner co-founded Northern Pines in 1980 on precepts she followed during her battle with thyroid cancer.

Because the number of guests is small—30 in summer and 18 in winter—the supportive staff is able to offer personal guidance to every guest. Activities include stretching, yoga, swimming, boating, hiking, and cross-country skiing in winter.

The vegetarian cuisine is delicious and varied. A choice of accommodations is offered, ranging from cabins with fireplaces and private baths, to an authentic yurt (a circular, domed tent), to cozy rooms by the lake with adjacent modern facilities.

Contact Northern Pines at 207-655-7624.

The Spa at Grand Lake, Connecticut
$
F W R

Life at The Spa at Grand Lake begins each morning with a brisk walk through the spa's gardens and lawns, out over rural byways, past farms and crystal clear lakes, and into an ancient New England forest. The walks are followed by low-impact aerobics, stretching, and aquathinics in the large indoor or outdoor pools. In the course of the day, guests also enjoy a free massage and three deliciously satisfying meals.

An exercise gym and tennis courts are on the premises, and excellent golf facilities are nearby (as is a casino). When you want a little pampering, manicures, pedicures, body treatments, and facials are all available. Evening entertainment features music, a video, or a lecture.

Rooms are comfortably furnished, each with private bath, television, telephone, and air conditioning. The atmosphere is casual and friendly.

The Spa at Grand Lake can be reached at 800-843-7721.

Vatra Natural Weight Loss Spa, New York
$$
F W D R Sp

Tucked away in the beautiful Catskill Mountains is the surprisingly inexpensive Vatra Natural Weight Loss Spa. Although the Vatra Mountain weight-loss and fitness program is active and fun, high value is also placed on relaxing on the porch with a good book and just breathing in the country air.

New hiking programs have been added to the established fare of pace walks, aerobics classes, aquatic workouts, sculpting and strengthening exercises, toning, stretching, dancing, and yoga. Tennis clinics are offered in the summer, and cross-country skiing is offered in the winter. Downhill skiing is moments away at the Hunter Mountain slopes.

Healthy, low-calorie, vegetarian meals are served. Pampering massage treatments are included in the various packages, and a wide choice of other skin-care and body treatments are available.

Phone 800-232-2772 for more information.

New Age Health Spa, New York
$
F M W D R A

Situated on 160 acres of rolling hills in the Catskill Mountains, just a two-hour drive from New York City, New Age Health Spa prides itself on both its wide array of fitness activities and its holistic philosophy.

The normal spa day begins with a sunrise meditation and ends with after-dinner speakers who present talks on wellness topics. Hikes, water aerobics, low-impact aerobics, cross-country skiing, yoga, and tai chi are some of the other daily activities. The spa is equipped with two tennis courts, indoor and outdoor pools, a new fitness center, and an alpine tower complete with rope courses.

New Age Health Spa also offers a wide range of health consultations and beauty treatments and special meal plans for weight loss or weight control. Guest accommodations are rustic, with beautiful views of the woods, hills, and mountains.

Call 800-682-4348 for information.

317

Deerfield Manor Spa, Pennsylvania
$
F W R A

This charming country spa is located in the Pocono Mountains of Pennsylvania, an easy drive from New York City, Philadelphia, Pittsburgh, and Washington, D.C. Friendly, intimate, and a good value, Deerfield Manor accommodates only 33 guests at a time in its seasonal fitness and weight-loss programs.

A full range of fitness classes is offered in the Manor's new, high-tech gym. Hikes, swimming, tennis, yoga, and tai chi are just some of the other activities. Horseback riding is available nearby.

Delicious, low-calorie meals are served in the cozy dining room; guest rooms are decorated in Laura Ashley prints and fabrics; and all furnishings are country-style.

A full range of salon and body treatments is available in the spa, including Swedish, shiatsu, and reflexology massage, seaweed body masques, aromatherapy, paraffin treatments, manicures, pedicures, facials, and cosmetic arts lessons.

Reach the spa at 800-852-4494.

Structure House, North Carolina
$$
W S F R

The Structure House program, with its emphasis on maintaining weight loss, was developed 20 years ago by its director, clinical psychologist Dr. Gerard Musante. Guests work with counselors in focus groups and in one-on-one sessions to uncover and resolve the emotional roots of their eating problem. A supportive staff of physicians, nurses, psychologists, nutritionists, dietitians, behavioral educators, exercise physiologists, trainers, and massage therapists is on hand.

The 21-acre campus houses a fitness center, comfortable private apartments (some handicapped-accessible), seated dining service, indoor and outdoor pools, and a woodland walking trail. The immediate area has three universities and offers a rich choice of music, dance, theater, and sports activities.

Contact 800-553-0052.

Westglow Spa, North Carolina
$$$
F R W A

Located in the Blue Ridge Mountains of North Carolina, this beautiful plantation house has all the amenities of a first-class spa. Every room has been faithfully decorated with vintage furniture so that guests can experience the elegant living of a bygone time. The only difference is that the beautifully prepared meals served in the dining room are designed to assist in weight management.

If losing weight is a special objective, Westglow's weight-management program, a comprehensive regimen including nutrition, exercise, and behavioral components, is a safe and easy way to melt away pounds. During the summer months at Westglow, a special hiking and outdoor adventure program is offered. In the winter months, many guests enjoy skiing along with the regular spa activities. Guests are spoiled with massage, facials, soothing herbal body wraps, Parisian body polishes, manicures, pedicures, and reflexology.

Westglow can be reached at 800-562-0807.

Hilton Head Health Institute, South Carolina
$$$
W F S R Sp

The Hilton Head Health Institute has developed an international reputation for success in the fields of weight control and rejuvenation under the guidance of its director and founder, Dr. Peter M. Miller. A clinical psychologist, Dr. Miller is the author of nine books, including *The Hilton Head Metabolism Diet.* The Institute offers one- to four-week programs and refresher courses specializing in weight control, fitness, smoking cessation, stress management, and other behavior modification areas.

The Institute is located on semitropical Hilton Head Island where guests can enjoy 12 miles of white sandy beaches, walking trails, nature preserves, world-famous golf courses, and tennis facilities. Participants stay in Shipyard Plantation's comfortable cottage villas within easy walking distance of the Institute.

Call 800-292-2440 for more information.

Hippocrates Life Change Center, Florida
$$$
D H R S

The Hippocrates Life Change Center's 30-acre, subtropical, wooded estate is the setting for a serious health program that emphasizes revitalization through a comprehensive detoxification and nutrition process. Considered radical when it began 40 years ago, the Center's program, stressing the role of nutrition in the process of healing, is now widely accepted.

The one- to three-week programs, under the supervision of holistic health caregivers, combine Dr. Ann Wigmore's concept of living foods with nonstressful exercise sessions, health analysis, counseling, massage therapies, and daily lectures. A diet of raw foods plus wheatgrass juice helps cleanse and detoxify the digestive system. Breathing unpolluted air, drinking pure water, and releasing stress from the mind and body are integral parts of the Hippocrates Health Institute's approach to healthful living.

Phone 800-842-2125 for more on the Hippocrates Life Change Center.

Spa Atlantis Oceanfront Health Resort and Spa, Florida
$
D W R S

SpaAtlantis offers a comprehensive program of health education, weight loss, exercise, and stress management in a fun-filled, relaxed atmosphere. Daily health education lectures and classes in vegetarian food preparation enable guests to take home what they learn in the Fit For Life program. Special courses address addictions to overeating, nicotine, and caffeine and other unhealthy habits.

Walks on the beach, yoga, low-impact step and water aerobics, and movement classes are all daily activities. The fitness center has treadmills, stationary bikes, step machines, and free weights. Snorkeling and sailing are other popular water activities.

Eight treatment rooms provide the setting for facials, massage, herbal wraps, manicures, pedicures, reflexology, seaweed and cellulite wraps, aromatherapy, and neuro-muscular massage. Gourmet vegetarian meals are served. Rooms are spacious with private baths, a balcony or patio, and views of the ocean, pool, or garden.

Contact Spa Atlantis at 800-583-3500.

The Regency House, Florida
$
D W S R

Located on a sandy beach in southern Florida, The Regency House is dedicated to the concept of holistic living. Guests are shown not only how to lose weight and be fit, but also how to cultivate a peaceful mind and a positive attitude.

Activities include low-impact aerobics, aqua exercises, stretching and toning, power walking, and yoga with meditation. An outdoor heated pool and the ocean provide opportunities for swimming; other amenities include a whirlpool, sauna, and a gym with Nautilus equipment. Lectures on topics such as health and disease, psychology, stress reduction, behavior modification, and hypnotherapy are offered daily.

Guests can choose from a menu of restorative spa treatments, featuring massage, lymph drainage, reflexology, facials, and body scrubs. Meals at The Regency House are vegetarian and feature a gourmet entree every day.

For more information call 800-454-0003.

Central

Birdwing Spa, Minnesota
$$
F W R

The northernmost spa in the Midwest and an hour's drive from Minneapolis, Birdwing is located on 300 acres of wooded property adjacent to Star Lake. The main lodge, a Tudor-style chalet, houses the elegant guest rooms, dining room, and the spa treatment facilities.

Although the atmosphere is tranquil, high-geared workouts in aerobics, stretching, toning, and weight training are options, as are nature hikes, cross-country skiing, biking, and pool activities. Sitting by the open fire with a good book is also encouraged, and a wide array of luxurious European-style spa treatments is available. Evenings are spent in the company of dynamic speakers and entertainers.

The chef at Birdwing uses only natural ingredients in preparing the international spa cuisine. If long-term weight loss is your goal, Birdwing offers sound nutritional counseling. Breakfast is served in bed at any hour the guest chooses.

Phone Birdwing at 320-693-6064.

The Raj, Iowa
$$$$
D H M R S L

The Raj offers programs based on the works of Maharishi Ayur Veda, the world's oldest comprehensive system of preventive health care. In an atmosphere of quiet elegance in the Iowa countryside, The Raj offers both traditional Ayurveda Panchakarma (rejuvenation therapies) and lifestyle modification programs. Panchakarma treatments use herbs, massage oils, and other natural methods to reduce stress and toxins and to stimulate the body's natural rejuvenating abilities.

A typical day at The Raj might start with group yoga followed by two hours of treatments. A treatment may incorporate a special two-technician massage, herbal steam bath, primordial sound, or purification therapies. After lunch, health-enhancement classes are available to teach the diet, exercise, and daily routines appropriate to each guest's mind/body type. The evening offers more classes and lectures.

The dress code is workout casual. The cuisine, based on Ayurvedic principles, is vegetarian.

Call 800-248-9050.

The Heartland Spa, Illinois
$$$
F W S R

Located on beautiful lakefront property within easy reach of Chicago, The Heartland Spa offers both a fitness program and an environment that's made for unwinding. The emphasis is on self-improvement, rejuvenation, and fun. This is accomplished through a wellness program that combines physical fitness training with educational sessions. All Heartland's packages also include spa treatments, such as massages and facials.

Challenging outdoor activities feature a par course with a quarter-mile track, hiking, cross-country skiing, boating, and tennis. Indoor facilities include a large pool, exercise equipment, saunas, whirlpools, and steam rooms.

The spa's registered dietitian and the spa chef design a menu of vegetarian dishes that are low in salt, sugar, and fat and are supplemented by occasional servings of fish. Generally, a day's meals contain 1,200 calories for women and 1,500 calories for men.

Reach The Heartland Spa at 800-545-4853.

The Kerr House, Ohio
$$$$
F M S W R L

The Kerr House is one woman's vision of what a spa experience should be. This Victorian manor accommodates just six to eight women at a time. (A few weeks and weekends are for men or are co-ed.) The ratio of staff to guests is three to one. Every amenity is provided—from robes to tank suits to beauty products.

Meals are calorie- and fat-controlled and are prepared using natural ingredients. Breakfast is served in bed on a wicker tray with fresh flowers. Dinner is celebrated in the oak dining room and is served by candlelight and accompanied by the gentle chords of a harp.

Laurie Hostetler, owner of The Kerr House, is a Hatha Yoga instructor. She teaches the two daily yoga classes. Aerobic exercise is performed on rebounders to avoid jolts to the weight-bearing joints. Daily treatments by the staff and walks along the towpath of the Maumee River are other popular activities.

Phone 419-832-1733 for more information.

Tennessee Fitness Spa, Tennessee
$
F W A R

The formula at the Tennessee Fitness Spa is simple: beautiful scenery, fun activities, good food, and an opportunity to lose weight and get in shape, all at a low price. Hiking in the Tennessee countryside and classes in aquarobics, low-impact aerobics, stretching, and toning help restore shape and vigor. Delicious, healthy meals that are low in fat, sugar, and salt eliminate pounds. Massages soothe the aches of the day.

Accommodations are simple but clean and functional. A long-term vacation is decidedly inexpensive, and sharing a room can make it even more so.

Call 800-235-8365.

The Greenhouse, Texas
$$$$
L F W R S

At this luxury spa, with its exclusive women-only program, the gracious living is apparent as soon as you enter your tastefully decorated guest room. The room opens onto the glass-enclosed pool area that boasts a three-story atrium and domed skylight.

A day at The Greenhouse starts with breakfast delivered to your room, complete with a personalized daily schedule. The day is then dedicated to movement, pleasure, and beauty. All exercise programs include a fitness evaluation with the spa's resident physiologist. Expert beauticians and color technicians are available to help you achieve your own sense of beauty and style.

In the dining room, imaginative table settings change each evening to complement the gourmet food. After dinner, an evening program is presented that might include a discussion of contemporary women's issues, a noted guest speaker, or a fashion show.

Contact The Greenhouse at 817-640-4000.

Lake Austin Spa Resort, Texas
$$$
F W S A M Sp

This charming spa is situated alongside rolling evergreen hills on the shores of tranquil Lake Austin. Each luxurious guest room offers views of the lake and hills. Near the lake, hammocks, swings, docks, and decks provide ample locations for relaxation.

Guests at Lake Austin plan their own day; however, there are structured programs focusing on body image, stress management, nutrition, and body care. Activities include massage, yoga, meditation, NIA, cardiovascular movement, boxing, hiking, biking, lakeside tai chi, muscular strengthening, canoeing, and sculling.

Featured treatments run the gamut from massage, aromatherapy, acupressure, and therapeutic touch to the spa's own special menu of offerings, such as the honey mango scrub.

Call 800-847-5637 for more information.

Shoshoni Yoga Spa, Colorado
$
M S D

TheShoshoni Yoga Retreat combines the serenity of a Rocky Mountain hideaway with the physical nurturing of a holistic health spa. The emphasis at Shoshoni is on yoga and meditation with a unique form of Shambhava Yoga inspired by Shambhavananda Yogi, founder of the Shoshoni retreat. Daily pranayama classes teach yogic breathing techniques for relaxation and stress reduction.

Massage therapy, herbal body scrubs, aromatherapy facials, and foot massage are enhanced by the practice of ancient yogic healing mantras. Spa facilities include a hot tub and herbal sauna.

The food is vegetarian, low in fat, and delicious. Guests are accommodated in log cabins nestled in the pines. The newly renovated cabins are spacious and contain all the comforts of home.

Phone 303-642-0116.

Red Mountain Spa, Utah
$
F W A S R Sp

The Red Mountain Spa is located amid the spectacular scenery of southwestern Utah in a desert climate that is perfect for hiking and mountain biking. This ultramodern retreat offers tennis, aerobics, racquetball, and weight-training facilities, as well as professional massage and beauty treatments.

The spa's special fitness and weight-loss programs are affordable, even for extended stays. A professional staff guides guests through a program that include such topics as stress control, time management, and nutrition. Guests can order either vegetarian meals or a modified diet that includes poultry and fish.

Red Mountain Spa can be reached at 800-407-3002.

Green Valley Fitness Resort and Spa, Utah
$$$
F A W S R M Sp L

Located in red rock canyon country, Green Valley features a fitness program that takes full advantage of some of the most extraordinary scenery in the country. Each morning begins with a hike through the magnificent nature of nearby parks and red rock canyon areas. Afterward, guests return to the fitness center for water aerobics, aerobics, or other activities. Green Valley also features a golf program and a tennis college.

The spa offers a full slate of aromatic water treatments, massage, facial and upper-body treatments, pedicures, and reflexology, as well as programs featuring Native American rituals. Each guest has a luxurious private bedroom and bath in the newly built Coyote Inn. Green Valley dining features natural cooking, prepared without added salt, sugar, or fat.

Call 800-237-1068 for more information.

Miraval, Life In Balance, Arizona
$$$$
M S L R F Sp

Miraval is what might be termed a "next-generation spa," because its emphasis is more on stress reduction, self-discovery, and mind-body interaction than on diet, fitness, and traditional therapies. However, nothing has been sacrificed in the pampering department or in the range of activities.

Miraval has three swimming pools, riding stables, a fitness center, tennis courts, volleyball courts, hiking trails, mountain and biking paths, a Jacuzzi, a sauna, Zen garden, croquet lawn, desert botanical garden, and 400-seat auditorium. Rock climbing and a challenging athletic program called Quantum Leap are also offered, and the Personal Service Center provides skin care, facials, massage, and body and relaxation treatments.

The food is fresh, healthy, and appetizing. Care for roast loin of black buck antelope with sun-dried cherries or rotisserie pintail pheasant glazed with pure maple syrup and pecans? Definitely not your mother's spa cuisine! Miraval accommodates 200 guests, housed in 106 casita-style rooms and suites.

Contact Miraval at 800-232-3969.

West Coast

Mountain Trek Fitness Retreat and Health Spa, British Columbia, Canada
$$
A F R

Hiking is the raison d'etre of this adventure spa founded by Wendy Pope, a former financial analyst, who decided to create a more fulfilling lifestyle for herself in British Columbia's majestic Kootenay Mountains. The food at Mountain Trek is hearty vegetarian fare (although there are plans to add some chicken and fish dishes), high in complex carbohydrates, low in fats, and free of liquor and caffeine. Throughout the season (April through the last week in October) certain weeks are set aside for supervised fasting programs, "value spa weeks," and weeks for gentle hiking and expert hiking.

Call 800-255-7727 for more information.

The Ashram, California
$$$
A F D R

This spa is not for people who are looking for luxury, the latest pampering technique, or a hot new piece of exercise equipment. But it is a place for those who like a serious physical challenge and wish to renew their spirits.

The Ashram accommodates only 12 guests at a time. There are no private rooms, private bathrooms, or gourmet spa meals. In fact, The Ashram has often been compared to a monastery. So what brings people back again and again to this spartan spa? The answers are a strong focus on weight loss, a challenging fitness program, and the opportunity to shed one's persona. The low-calorie diet is designed to purify the body, mind, and spirit. The Ashram is also known for its massages, its hiking program, and its yoga and meditation instruction.

Contact The Ashram at 818-222-6900.

Cal-A-Vie, California
$$$$
L F W R M A Sp

This elegant spa retreat in the hills north of San Diego resembles a small village in Provence, France. Days at Cal-A-Vie start with a hike through verdant hills followed by a nutritious breakfast. Fitness programs in the morning include aerobics, body shaping, weight training, step classes, water classes, stretching, yoga, and tai chi. After lunch by the spa pond, the next several hours are spent in a regimen of cleansing, balancing, revitalizing, soothing, polishing, and beautifying treatments.

Guests reside in Cal-A-Vie's 24 private cottages, decorated with flowered chintzes and filled with carved wood furnishings. All of Cal-A-Vie's weeklong programs run Sunday to Sunday. The majority of the weeks are co-ed, with one or two women's weeks each month. Recreational activities include tennis, golf, hiking, and boating.

Phone 619-945-2055.

Golden Door, California
$$$$
L F W D R S M Sp

Created 39 years ago, the Golden Door's 377-acre site was selected by its founder, Deborah Szekely, for its perfect year-round climate and undisturbed natural beauty. The Golden Door replicates a Japanese Honjin Inn, with its centuries-old tradition of thoughtful care and renewal for the traveler. Formal Japanese gardens, a natural meandering brook, gentle splashing waterfalls, and ponds of darting fish are part of the tranquil setting Ms. Szekely created. Fresh flowers, museum-quality art, and antiques decorate every room. Occupancy is limited to 39 guests who are cared for by a staff of 160.

Each guest's level of fitness and range of motion is assessed so that a customized training program can be implemented and taken home. A continuous blend of movement, massage, yoga, and other therapies are designed to eliminate tension and emphasize the interdependence of mind and body. For most of the year, the Golden Door offers its weeklong program exclusively for women, but there are special men's and co-ed weeks.

Call 800-424-0777.

The Lodge at Skylonda, California
$$$$
A F R M L

Built of ponderosa logs and river rock, this secluded retreat is as well known for its majestic scenery as it is for its spa program. Skylonda's facilities include massage and facial studios, saunas, steam rooms, Jacuzzis, an aerobics and exercise complex, and a glass-enclosed, ozone-purified swimming pool.

Hiking among the oldest trees on earth provides the cornerstone of Skylonda's outdoor recreational program. The many trails vary in difficulty, from casual walks—some along sandy beaches—to rigorous climbs that challenge experienced hikers. Yoga, aquatic exercises, and a circuit-training course in the new Cybex gym are some of the other activities offered.

Meals in the Skylonda dining room contain less than 20 percent fat. Chef Sue Chapman's specialties include local seafood, roasts, ragouts, breads, extravagant salads, tarts, sorbets, and custards.

For more information call 800-851-2222.

The Oaks at Ojai, California
$$
F W R

Located an hour and a half north of Los Angeles, The Oaks offers 18 fitness classes daily, low-calorie gourmet cuisine, entertainment, and evening seminars. Spa facilities include massage, facials, body wraps, aromatherapy, body scrubs, hair and nail treatments, and makeup and color analysis. Expert advice and training are also available through private fitness consultations, restorative yoga sessions, and one-on-one nutritional counseling.

As the name implies, The Oaks buildings and recreational facilities are located on beautiful grounds in the shade of old oak trees. Accommodations are available in the main lodge or in spacious cottages around the pool area.

The Oaks is located in the heart of the Ojai Valley, home to a lively arts colony famous for the Ojai Music Festival and Folk Dance Festival and to the Ojai Tennis Tournament. Golf, tennis, and shopping are minutes away.

Contact The Oaks at 800-753-6257.

We Care Health Retreat, California
$$
D R

The We Care Health Retreat teaches the principles of holistic health to just eight guests at a time, ensuring individual guidance while cleansing body, mind, and spirit. The revitalization program offers the synergistic action of fasting, colon hygiene, lymphatic exercises, yoga, and meditation, as well as shiatsu, reflexology, facials, mud baths, herbal wraps, and hot mineral waters. The private retreat is located in a small canyon at the foot of the San Jacinto Mountains, easily accessible from San Diego and Los Angeles.

Phone 800-888-2523 for more information.

The Caribbean and Mexico

La Casa de Vida Natural, Puerto Rico
$
D A S

La Casa de Vida Natural is perched atop a foothill in El Yunque, the national rainforest park, commanding a view of the ocean and within an easy drive to five beaches. The 10-acre property offers vacations for eight guests at a time who share an interest in natural living.

Who needs step machines when there is a mountain trail, or a flotation tank when there is an ocean, or a therapy tub when there is a sparkling mountain waterfall? Even the mud used in the mud pack treatments is collected from El Yunque, the seaweed is harvested on a remote beach, and the herbs are gathered only minutes before use.

La Casa offers five-day workshops featuring massage therapy, natural foods, movement, tai chi, acupuncture, and more. You may even come to La Casa as an overnight guest. Accommodations are modest but comfortable. Some rooms have private baths.

Call Spa Finder at 800-255-7727 for more details.

Jackie's On The Reef, Jamaica
$
M S

The ambiance at Jackie's On The Reef is relaxed, unstructured, elegant, and spiritual. Float in a coral pool hewn out of rock; meditate in an American Indian teepee; or enjoy the bird aviary where parrots, parakeets, and nightingales are at home in nature. On the seaside, watch blue herons fish and dolphins swim.

Workshops and seminars are offered for spiritual development, while the body is nurtured with wraps, massages, reflexology, and facials. Activities include hiking, tennis, horseback riding, biking, and boating.

Guests stay in cottages handmade from limestone. Meals are healthy with much of the produce grown in Jackie's own gardens.

Phone 800-255-7727 for more information on Jackie's On The Reef.

Rancho La Puerta, Baja California, Mexico
$$
F S M R D A Sp

Rancho La Puerta opened in 1940 when a week's stay cost $17.50—but you had to bring your own tent. Today, the Rancho La Puerta, with its romantic Spanish Colonial architecture, occupies 3,000 acres of lush oasis surrounded by unspoiled countryside. Up to 150 guests per week are accommodated in 83 cottages and served by a staff of 300.

Rancho La Puerta has nine gyms for aerobic and restorative classes, plus three more for weight training. Other facilities include four tennis courts, three pools, hot tubs, saunas, and steam rooms. Separate men's and women's health centers provide massages, facials, and herbal wraps. The resort also provides a beauty salon, arts and crafts center, public lounges, a library, and a center reserved for classes in yoga, tai chi, and meditation.

Mount Kuchumaa, sacred to Native Americans, overlooks the resort and provides the inspirational focus. On its slopes, guests enjoy hiking on several thousand acres of rugged terrain. The vegetarian cuisine features produce grown in Rancho La Puerta's own organic garden. All programs last a week, from Saturday to Saturday.

For more information contact Spa Finder at 800-255-7727.

Punta Serena, Jalisco, Mexico
$
D S M

Punta Serena is a holistic retreat on a mountainside overlooking Tenacatita Bay on Mexico's west coast. A blend of emotional, physical, and nutritional guidance is offered here in a natural, lush setting.

Guests can refresh their spirits with yoga, tai chi, chi kung, and chakra. Also offered are fitness programs, behavioral counseling, psychotherapy, shamanism, guided daily meditation sessions, massage therapies, and sessions in the Temazcal native Mexican sweat lodge.

Facilities include horseback riding, tennis, a private beach where swimsuits are optional, swimming pool, and a hot tub. Meals are vegetarian. Punta Serena has only 26 rooms, all with balconies or terraces and beautiful views.

Call 800-255-7727 for more information.

Resort Spas

East Coast

Topnotch at Stowe, Vermont
$$
F R Sp M

Located in the ski capital of the east, this 120-acre resort and spa features New England friendliness, fine accommodations, spectacular views, gourmet meals, and plenty to do throughout the year. Topnotch's 92 rooms and suites have been individually designed with selected furnishings, antiques, and amenities. Also available are two- and three-bedroom townhouses with fireplaces, saunas, whirlpools, and sun decks.

The spa features a 60-foot indoor pool, a 12-foot whirlpool with cascading hydro-massage waterfalls, and three fully equipped fitness studios. Guests are offered a wide range of personal services, including massages, facials, fitness assessments, and nutritional consultations.

In spring, summer, and fall guests can hike to the summit of Mount Mansfield, bicycle through the countryside, fish for trout in nearby streams, or play tennis on Topnotch's courts.

Phone 800-451-8686.

Norwich Inn and Spa, Connecticut
$$$
F R Sp

The Norwich Inn is a private retreat with cozy rooms, country antiques, and a modern, full-service spa offering a blend of fitness, nutrition, and beauty and body treatments. Guests stay in the historic, full-service inn itself, which was built in the 1920s, or in one of the more recently constructed private villas nestled in the woods. Each villa has a wood-burning fireplace, balcony, and compact kitchen. Activities at the inn include golf, tennis, horseback riding, and biking.

Phone Norwich Inn and Spa at 800-275-4772.

Gurney's Inn Resort and Spa, New York
$$$
R F M

Gurney's Inn, located on a beautiful private stretch of beach on Long Island, is the only year-round marino-therapeutic spa in the United States. The International Health and Beauty Spa uses the curative resources of the sea, combining spa treatments and traditions with healthful exercise and nutrition. General facilities include a heated indoor seawater pool overlooking the Atlantic Ocean, seawater Roman baths, Finnish saunas, Russian steam rooms, Swiss showers, and an oceanview fitness center with cardiovascular and weight-training equipment.

Aquatic exercise, aerobics, yoga, tai chi, daily beach walks, and hiking in the "Walking Dunes" are integral parts of the total spa program. Attached to the spa is a full-service Salon de Beaute for facials and hair and nail care, using the Yonka skin-care line and Phytologie hair products. Spa cuisine is served in the dining room overlooking the ocean. Accommodations are either oceanview or oceanfront.

Gurney's Inn can be reached at 800-445-8062.

Nemacolin Woodlands Spa, Pennsylvania
$$$
R F Sp L

Nemacolin Woodlands Spa is located in the scenic Laurel Mountains of Western Pennsylvania, only a short distance from Frank Lloyd Wright's famous Fallingwater house. The main hotel building, Chateau Lafayette, was inspired by the classic hotels of Europe, with its sparkling neoclassical facade, two-story Paladian windows, and elegant rooms with marble baths.

More than 60 treatments and services are offered at the Woodlands Spa, which recently underwent a $6.5-million restoration and expansion. The 32,000-square-foot facility includes a new spa restaurant called Sante and a state-of-the-art fitness center.

Nemacolin is famous for its Equestrian Center, which has a polo field and indoor and outdoor arenas. A championship golf course, five swimming pools, four tennis courts, and a 50-foot climbing wall round out the recreational facilities. There's also boating, canoeing, trout fishing, and skiing at Mystic Mountain.

Call 800-422-2736 for more information.

The Greenbrier, West Virginia
$$$$
R Sp L

Afternoon tea, dinner dances, and chamber music concerts are all part of the Old World elegance of this grand hotel set on 6,500 acres in West Virginia's Allegheny

Mountains. For over 200 years, guests have traveled here to experience the ambiance of The Greenbrier and the benefits of its natural sulfur waters.

Today, guests also come to enjoy the three golf courses, including one designed by Jack Nicklaus; the 20 championship tennis courts; and the new multi-million-dollar spa. The natural sulfur water treatments have been incorporated into a modern spa program, along with skin and body therapies, massage, hydrotherapy, fitness profiles, and beauty treatments.

Phone 800-624-6070.

Chateau Elan, Georgia
$$$$
R L Sp

Chateau Elan began life as a vineyard in the rich soil of Georgia just 30 minutes north of Atlanta. Soon, however, people began visiting for more than the award-winning wines. The lush gardens, the sixteenth-century French-style chateau, the excellent food, the recreational facilities, and the spa also became attractions.

Today, Chateau Elan has 3,100 acres of softly rolling land, 63 holes of golf, and seven restaurants, including an authentic Irish pub. The Spa at Chateau Elan is a full-service, European-style facility offering guests instruction in restorative stress management, preventive health care, and responsible body maintenance. It features an extensive menu of relaxation, body, and skin-care treatments performed by highly trained therapists. The Spa has its own restaurant, Fleur-de-Lis, which specializes in gourmet cooking for the health-conscious guest.

Contact 770-271-6064 for information.

Sea Island Spa at The Cloister, Georgia
$$$
R Sp F L

The Spanish Mediterranean-style Cloister Hotel is located on beautiful Sea Island, just off the coast of Georgia, 70 miles south of Savannah. Golf is foremost at Sea Island, with much of the landscape devoted to the game. There are 36 holes at the Sea Island Club and another 18 at the adjacent St. Simons Island Club. Sea Island also has an excellent Golf Learning Center.

Other recreational facilities include 18 tennis courts, skeet and trap shooting, horse-back riding on the beach, deep-sea fishing, swimming, biking, lawn sports, ballroom dancing, marsh walks, and turtle expeditions. The Sea Island Spa offers soothing aromatherapy, seaweed or moor mud treatments, therapeutic massage, facials, Swiss showers, reflexology, skin care, and beauty services.

Sea Island Spa can be reached at 800-732-4752.

Eden Roc, Florida
$$$
F R Sp

If a vacation combining a spa and the beach is what you're looking for, Miami Beach's 350-room Eden Roc Resort, a lovingly restored masterpiece of Art Deco Florida architecture, is an ideal destination. The 55,000-square-foot beachfront Spa of Eden offers Swedish, shiatsu, deep tissue, reflexology, and aromatherapy massages and sports treatments in the spa itself, in your room, or on the beach. Body treatments include algae body masks, Dead Sea mud body and scalp treatments, sea fango paste, seaweed and salt body polishes, and herbal body wraps.

329

Eden Roc has a state-of-the-art weight-training center and cardiovascular theater, plus boating and water sports, racquetball, squash, basketball, and rock climbing in the indoor pavilion. A full slate of aerobics, yoga, ballet, and boxing aerobics classes is offered daily. Spa cuisine is served in the restaurants, rooms feature ocean views, and Eden Roc is a stone's throw from trendy South Beach.

Call 888-333-6762 for more information.

PGA National Resort and Spa, Florida
$$$
Sp F R

The PGA National Resort is a perfect place to vacation if sports and spas are your passions. The seven-year-old, 14,500-square-foot spa has 31 private treatment rooms for massage, hydrotherapy, and other salon services. The main attraction of the spa is the Waters of the World collection of six outdoor therapy pools, each serving a different purpose.

The resort boasts five world-class tournament golf courses, 19 tennis courts, a heated five-lane lap pool, a seven-mile trail for walking or jogging, and a championship croquet facility. Indoors, an expansive fitness center houses racquetball courts, Nautilus equipment, and dance and aerobic studios.

PGA guests have their choice of seven dining rooms and lounges, including a spa restaurant. The resort has 339 rooms and suites and 80 cottage apartments, all newly renovated.

Contact 561-627-3111.

Safety Harbor Resort, Florida
$$
F R S Sp

While searching for the fountain of youth in 1536, Hernando de Soto landed on the site of this full-service spa a little too early! Safety Harbor has a Clarins Institute De Beaute on the premises, offering all-natural skin and body treatments from France. Also available are expert body massages, deep-cleansing facials, reflexology, herbal wraps, loofah scrubs, mineral baths, and more.

Safety Harbor's fitness center houses 50,000 square feet of exercise space and cardiovascular and weight-training equipment. Classes are offered in aerobics, aquatics, stretch, relaxation, strength training, sports training, boxercise, hip-hop dancing, swimming, tai chi, and yoga.

If tennis is your game, there are seven Har-Tru clay courts and two hard courts. Expert instruction for every level is offered in clinics for beginning to advanced players, under the tutelage of Phil Green's Tennis Academy.

Phone 800-BEST-SPA (800-237-8772).

Sanibel Harbour Resort and Spa, Florida
$$$
Sp F R

Located on a 1,000-foot stretch of sandy beach, Sanibel Harbour is a resort for sun lovers, tennis lovers, and spa lovers. The tennis program, offered on eight lighted clay courts, features clinics for individuals and groups, match making, and round robins. Guests can even play in the 5,500-seat Centre Court Stadium, site of the 1989 and 1992 Davis Cup tournaments.

The Spa and Fitness Center offers the latest in health, nutrition, beauty, and fitness programs. Cybex training equipment is featured, as well as an aqua-fit pool and aerobics classes. A wide variety of massage and body therapies is available; skin and hair treatments are offered in the beauty salon. Sanibel Harbour also has a complete program for children. The resort chefs prepare a variety of cuisines, including healthy spa dishes.

Call 800-767-7777.

The Spa at Doral, Florida
$$$$
L F S W R Sp

Inspired by the great spas of Europe and designed to resemble a Tuscan villa, The Spa is located on the grounds of the famed Doral Golf Resort in Florida. The Spa offers an extensive array of therapies, including massages, wraps, anti-cellulite treatments, facials, skin-care treatments, and hydrotherapy. The Spa's fitness programs are wide-ranging enough to accommodate both the weekend jogger and the professional athlete. The Spa's Mental Edge fitness training program, in particular, challenges the serious exerciser physically and mentally.

Spa guests are welcome to enjoy all of the facilities of the Doral Golf Resort, including five championship courses and 16 tennis courts. Guests are accommodated in 48 lavish marble-decorated suites, many with two bathrooms.

Contact 800-331-7768.

Turnberry Isle Resort and Club, Florida
$$$$
R F Sp L

Turnberry Isle's 300 landscaped, tropical acres are home to a yacht club, two Robert Trent Jones 18-hole golf courses, a marina, a country club, 24 tennis courts, four swimming pools, restaurants ranging from elegant to poolside casual, and a health spa. The accommodations themselves are a major attraction: The large, luxurious rooms have ocean or golf course views.

Each guest receives a personalized diet/nutrition consultation by the staff physician, plus unlimited access to the Swedish sauna, Turkish steam baths, Nautilus machines, free weights and cardiovascular equipment, whirlpools, and racquetball courts. A wide selection of beauty treatments is available, with spa packages offering a generous sampling.

Phone 800-223-1588 for more information.

Central

The Elms Resort and Spa, Missouri
$$
R F Sp

With its majestic facade of Missouri limestone and its beautifully landscaped grounds overlooking the bluffs of the Fishing River, The Elms is one of America's great historic hotels—everyone from Presidents Truman and Roosevelt to Marilyn Monroe has stayed here. The Elms has recently been restored with every modern amenity, including a spa and fitness center.

Spa facilities include Swiss and Vichy showers, body treatment rooms for mud, sea-weed, and aloe wraps, studios for hydrotherapy and massage, whirlpools, and mineral baths. The fitness center features an indoor European swim track, a banked jogging track, a sauna, and steam rooms.

The Elms' 153 guest rooms and suites have all been meticulously restored and up-graded to preserve the hotel's grace while providing all the amenities of a high-tech world. For entertainment away from the hotel, downtown Kansas City, with its famous 18th and Vine Jazz District and riverboat gambling, is only minutes away.

Contact The Elms at 800-843-3567.

The Broadmoor, Colorado
$$$$
L Sp F R

The Broadmoor is the grande dame of Colorado Rockies resorts. Built on 3,000 acres in 1891 by a Silesian count, it began its colorful life as a hotel and gambling casino. Parts of the original hotel survive and are now incorporated into the architecture.

The Broadmoor spa has 16 massage rooms, six facial rooms, and wet treatment rooms for wraps, hydrotherapy, aromatherapy, and Vichy showers. Mountain water is used for cascading showers and relaxing baths and whirlpools. There are also traditional sauna, steam, deluge, and inhalation rooms; elegant locker rooms; and relaxation rooms with fireplaces.

The Broadmoor's fitness center has indoor and outdoor pools, an aerobics studio with a spring-loaded wood floor, and a gym with Cybex weight resistance and cardiovascular equipment. For outdoor activity, there's 54 holes of championship golf, 12 tennis courts, horseback riding, hiking, and cross-country skiing. The Broadmoor also has nine restaurants and a special children's program.

Phone 800-634-7711 for more information.

The Lodge and Spa at Cordillera, Colorado
$$$
L F A Sp R

Cordillera is a luxurious, secluded hideaway, set on 6,800 private acres of forest and meadows, that boasts stunning mountain views. There is more to do at Cordillera than at resorts many times its size, including guided hikes, cross-country skiing, mountain biking, snowshoeing, fly fishing, white-water kayaking, rafting, hot-air ballooning, golf, and tennis. For downhill skiing, the slopes of Vail and Beaver Creek are nearby.

Cordillera's modern spa offers more than 35 treatments, including massages, hydro-therapy baths, beauty therapies, and a variety of wraps. Fitness classes, weight training, and meditation are also featured. Healthy gourmet cuisine is served, and most of the resort's 56 guest rooms have fireplaces and terraces.

Call 800-87-RELAX (800-877-3529).

The Peaks Resort and Spa, Colorado
$$$
L A Sp S M R

For scenery, sports, and culture, there's nothing quite like The Peaks in the Rocky Mountains near Telluride. The resort looks out on mountains, valleys, and forests of aspen trees. In wintertime, the fine powdered snow makes The Peaks a skier's dream; in summertime, Telluride, a quaint Victorian town, hosts many cultural events, including the Telluride Film Festival.

Sports are king in this part of Colorado, especially Alpine, Nordic, and heli-skiing. Also popular are skating, sleigh riding, snowmobiling, mountain climbing, fly fishing, hang gliding, hiking, biking, horseback riding, and rafting. At the Peaks, you'll also find tennis, other racquet sports, and the golf course with the highest elevation in the

United States (9,450 feet). The Peaks' Kiva Spa has 44 treatment rooms for massages, body and beauty treatments, and a state-of-the-art fitness center.

Contact Phone 800-789-2200 for more information.

Loews Ventana Canyon Resort, Arizona
$$$$
L Sp F S R M

The Loews Ventana Canyon Resort blends so easily into the landscape of the Catalina Mountain foothills that it seems to always have been part of the environment. The resort's secluded paths and terraces are laced through virgin groves of mesquite, squawbush, and blue paloverde.

The newly opened spa offers a wide range of massage and beauty treatments featuring Florian spa products. The glass-enclosed workout center features Cybex cardio and resistance equipment and mountain views. A wide range of mind-body classes are offered, including yoga and meditation.

There are two Tom Fazio–designed 18-hole PGA championship golf courses only steps from the lobby. Hikes in the desert and excursions to the town of Tombstone, the Colossal Cave, the ponderosa forests of Mt. Lemmon, and the centuries-old San Xavier Mission on the Papago Indian Reservation are other popular activities. The resort has 400 luxury accommodations.

Contact 800-234-5117.

Marriott's Camelback Inn Resort, Golf Club, and Spa, Arizona
$$$
L Sp F R S M

The Spa at Marriott's Camelback Inn has everything you would expect to find in a first-class, European-style spa, plus all the amenities of a major resort. Featured is an outstanding range of aerobic and wellness-testing programs pioneered by Dr. Kenneth H. Cooper, creator of the aerobic movement and president of the Institute for Aerobic Research in Dallas. You can undergo a computerized body composition analysis with cardiovascular, abdominal, and flexibility testing, as well as nutrition analysis, wellness assessment, and lifestyle evaluation. Daily classes include high- and low-impact aerobics, Pilates method, water aerobics, power walks, boxing aerobics, body sculpting, yoga, and tai chi.

The spa has over two dozen treatment rooms, indoor and outdoor massage studios, a lap pool, Finnish saunas, Turkish steam baths, exercise machines, circuit weight training, free weights, and a full-service salon. Resort activities include golf, swimming, biking, horseback riding, tennis, and other racquet sports.

Call 800-228-9290.

The Phoenician and The Centre for Well-Being, Arizona
$$$$
L S M F Sp R

High in the Sonoran Desert, where the rugged Arizona landscape reaches toward a sun-drenched sky, you'll find the Phoenician resort and its spa, The Centre for Well-Being. The Centre features Southwestern body treatments adapted from Native American cultures, using desert plants and minerals such as aloe vera, jojoba, clay, and sage. The spa also features the Shirodhara Scalp Massage Treatment, an Ayurvedic therapy from India that dates back 5,000 years. Skin-care treatments, including facials and body masks, are also specialties. Classes are offered in aerobics, yoga, and meditation.

333

The resort features hiking, golf, tennis, horseback riding, biking, suites with Italian marble bathrooms, a $1.7-million art and antiques collection, and an exotic garden with 350 varieties of cacti and succulents. Each of the resort's several restaurants features specially prepared gourmet dishes that are low in fat, sodium, and cholesterol. The Phoenician is a resort for the whole family.

Reach them at 800-888-8234.

California

The Claremont Resort and Spa, California
$$$
F R Sp M

Located 20 minutes from San Francisco, the palatial Claremont with its 22 acres of manicured gardens has been a favorite vacation destination for 80 years. The world-class spa offers a fitness program, health and beauty treatments, and programs promoting wellness and lifestyle enhancement. Featured are personal mind-body sessions such as relaxation therapy, restorative yoga, and therapeutic stretching.

The Claremont has heated lap and recreational pools, tennis courts, saunas, steam rooms, Jacuzzis, weight training, and aerobic studios. Golf is available nearby. In the evening, many guests like to hop across the bridge to San Francisco for a night on the town.

Call 800-551-7266 for more information.

La Costa Resort and Spa, California
$$$
Sp F R L

Thename La Costa has become synonymous with luxury hideaway, especially as it applies to the California movie colony.

La Costa's masseurs specialize in traditional Swedish massage, reflexology, shiatsu, aromatherapy, reiki energy therapy, and European water treatments. Guests also can enjoy herbal wraps, relax in a whirlpool bath, have a loofah treatment to exfoliate the surface skin, or be wrapped in moor mud or seaweed algae.

For recreation, there are pools, saunas, tennis courts, and two championship golf courses. La Costa also features a special program for lifestyle enhancement, designed in affiliation with Scripps Memorial Executive Health Center. Guests can choose from a number of elegant restaurants featuring spa cuisine. Accommodations include single, double, and suite configurations and special spa rooms.

Contact La Costa at 800-854-5000.

La Quinta Resort and Spa, La Quinta, California
$$$$
L Sp R M

In the fall of 1998, this legendary California resort opened a magnificent new spa. The designers created a luxurious environment featuring celestial showers, hydro tubs, wrap and massage studios, facial rooms, a skin-care and beauty salon, a fitness studio, outdoor massage areas, and a relaxation garden. Guests can enjoy massages, body scrubs, facials, aromatherapy, underwater massage, and many more treatments, as well as yoga, tai chi, nutrition counseling, and personal training. La Quinta also has a world-class golf program, 30 tennis courts, 25 secluded swimming pools, and 38 hot spas.

La Quinta is located among orange and lemon groves in the desert, only a stone's throw from Palm Springs. It has been a favorite getaway of the rich and the famous since the days of Garbo and Gable. Dining choices at La Quinta range from Mexican to Mediterranean. Guests stay in distinctive Spanish-style casitas.

Call 800-598-3828 for more information.

Ojai Valley Inn and Spa, California
$$$
L M R Sp F

Long recognized as one of the country's top resorts and golf destinations, Ojai has just added a state-of-the-art spa. The spa village contains 28 treatment rooms, many with fireplaces, wet rooms with water-wall fountains, an art studio, meditation garden, creekside reading areas, a Chumash Indian Interpretative Trail, weight room, and workout studio. In addition to a wide array of aerobic and water exercises, classes are offered in everything from tai chi to organic gardening.

Beyond golf (on a course designed by renowned golf architect, George C. Thomas Jr.), activities include tennis, horseback riding, hiking, mountain biking, boating, artist studio tours, wine tours, and shopping. There also is an Outward Bound course and a children's camp. The inn, created in the style of California Spanish Revival architecture, is situated on 220 acres of shady trees and exquisite gardens.

Phone 800-422-6524.

Sonoma Mission Inn and Spa, California
$$$
F R Sp

For 70 years this gracious country inn has been a favorite for people who appreciate the finer things in life. Situated in the lush wine country of Northern California 40 miles from San Francisco, the inn is famous for its pink facade, classic Spanish architecture, curative mineral waters, and, in recent years, for its high-tech spa.

The spa has a complete array of bathhouse facilities, exercise studios, and treatment rooms. During the week, packages are offered that include a variety of spa services, fitness classes, and the option of spa meals or regular dining. On weekends, all services are available a la carte. Guided wine country hikes and bicycle tours are a special attraction, and golf and tennis are always available.

Contact them at 800-862-4945.

Two Bunch Palms, California
$$$
R Sp

Two Bunch Palms is the oasis resort where the infamous Al Capone resided decades ago. For protection, he built a small stone fortress with a lookout tower (now a two-bedroom bungalow), and for amusement, he added a casino (now the resort dining room). Although the gangsters are gone, Two Bunch Palms is still a favorite hideaway for many Hollywood stars. Tall tamarisks, stately palms, and lush bougainvillea screen guests from prying eyes and provide shelter for romantic picnics and leisurely strolls.

The emphasis is on sensuous experiences, beginning with a soak in the natural artesian-fed mineral waters that surface at 148°F (though cooled slightly for bathers). Afterward, guests head to the spa for a mud bath, body wrap, or massage. Guests are accommodated in lavishly appointed bungalows and condominiums.

Call 800-472-4334 for more information.

Hawaii

Hilton Waikoloa Village, Hawaii
$$$
R Sp F M

This spectacular 62-acre oceanfront resort on Hawaii's big island offers guests the perfect fantasy escape plus a first-class spa in the Hawaiian tradition. Guests can relax in a private balneotherapy or Jacuzzi, detoxify with a seaweed wrap, or choose from a variety of massages, including the rhythmical ancient Lomi Lomi massage. The massages are all administered in a private cabana overlooking the Pacific Ocean. The spa also has a complete fitness facility where classes in yoga, tai chi, and meditation are held.

Other facilities include three pools, two golf courses, eight tennis courts, water sports, a children's camp, and six restaurants. Accommodations are available in one of three luxurious low-rise towers accessible from the main building via the Museum Walkway, which features the resort's $5 million collection of Pacific and Asian art.

Phone 800-445-8667.

Grand Wailea Resort, Maui, Hawaii
$$$$
L Sp R S M F

Many travelers consider this $800-million resort to be the most fabulous vacation destination in the world. Spa Grande is the centerpiece. Decorated in gold and marble, it is the setting for an East-meets-West philosophy blending Hawaiian healing techniques with European, American, Oriental, and Indian Ayurvedic treatments.

A highlight of the spa program is the Terme Wailea, a hydrotherapy circuit that includes a loofah scrub, a plunge in a Roman tub, a cool plunge, steam, sauna, waterfall treatment, aromatherapy, and a sampling of the spa's specialty baths, including mud, papaya enzyme, limu, and mineral salt.

The resort boasts golf, tennis, world-class restaurants, a full array of water sports, a 3,000-foot river pool, the only squash and racquetball courts on Maui, and an art collection featuring Botero, Leger, Picasso, and Warhol. Every room in the hotel has a private terrace, sensational views, and marble bathrooms with separate glassed showers and large bathtubs. There is even a day camp for kids.

You can reach the resort at 800-875-1234.

Canada

The Hills Health and Guest Ranch, British Columbia, Canada
$$
R S W Sp A

If unwinding beneath a Cinemascope sky in a wilderness setting reminiscent of a John Ford western appeals to you, then pack up your gear and head for The Hills, located on 20,000 acres of unspoiled lakes, mountains, and forests in British Columbia. The Hills offers a selection of spa and fitness packages, including massage and beauty treatments. There's also a supervised weight-loss program, a daily schedule of exercise classes, and beauty treatments. The Hills is home to the Canadian Wellness Center, which promotes an integrated approach to health education, fitness activities, nutritional planning, lifestyle enhancements, and body treatments.

The Hills features horseback riding, sing-along hayrides, campfires, sleigh rides in winter, swimming, and over 20 miles of walking and hiking trails. In addition to comfortable accommodations in the two main lodges, deluxe country-style chalets are available.

For more information on The Hills call 250-791-5225 or contact Spa Finder at 800-255-7727.

Solace Spa at Banff Springs Hotel, Alberta, Canada
$$$$
R Sp A L F

From the moment you first spy its turrets and gables rising above the emerald forest, you'll be enchanted by the Banff Springs Hotel. Built in 1888 by the Canadian Pacific Railroad, it is a thriving remnant of a more elegant time when such travel was exclusively reserved for the rich and the worldly.

The hotel is located within the boundaries of a national park, near the raging Bow Falls and the unmatched beauty of glacial Lake Louise. Activities include skiing, fishing, swimming, tennis, golf, hiking, biking, and skating. It's not at all unusual to see enormous elks strutting down Banff's main street or to spot a fox, lynx, or bighorn sheep on the golf course.

At the Solace Spa, you may indulge yourself with body wraps and scrubs, mineral and herbal baths, facial treatments, and massages. With three fireplace lounges and cascading waterfall pools, the spa is also a wonderful place to just relax.

For more information contact Spa Finder at 800-255-7727.

The Caribbean and Mexico

Island Outpost, Strawberry Hill, Jamaica
$$$
R M Sp

Island Outpost Hotels has teamed with Aveda to open the first Aveda Concept Spa in the Caribbean at Strawberry Hill. A mountain retreat nestled into the side of the Blue Mountains, it offers sweeping vistas of the surrounding mountains, the verdant valleys, and the city of Kingston below. Guests stay in a dozen nineteenth-century, Jamaican-style wooden villas, each featuring louvered windows, mahogany furniture, and a wide, private veranda.

Most of the island-born spa staff has been trained at the Aveda spa in Minnesota. They offer a wide variety of spa services for the face and body, as well as extractions, skin-care consultations, back treatments, and therapies for the hair and scalp. Tours of the surrounding Blue Mountains can be arranged, including the Old Tavern Mountain Coffee Estate, the Fairy Tale Glade, the National Gallery, and Spanish Town, Jamaica's original capital.

For more information contact Spa Finder at 800-255-7727.

Round Hill Hotel and Villas, Jamaica
$$$$
R Sp L

From its inception in 1952, Round Hill has been one of the world's most celebrated retreats for international celebrities. The resort's intimate 36-room hotel is called Pineapple House. Guests also stay in the resort's 27 villas, each of which is owned by a shareholder, many of whom are quite famous. You might end up staying in Noel Coward's former cottage (no. 3) or being a neighbor to Ralph Lauren, who owns no. 26.

Spa services include many kinds of massage, reflexology, body wraps, and facials. Stretching, muscle toning, and step aerobics classes are offered. There is also a fully equipped fitness center.

Activities at Round Hill include nature hiking, snorkeling, swimming, scuba diving, tennis, and golf. You also can enjoy mountain valley rafting on the Great River, a Black River Safari through mangrove swamps, and tours of the surrounding plantation houses.

For more information contact Spa Finder at 800-255-7727.

Privilege Resort and Spa, St. Martin, French Antilles
$$$
R S Sp

This intimate Caribbean hideaway has 43 rooms and suites offering stunning views of Marcel Cove, one of the island's most private beaches. The Balneotherapy Health Spa has a variety of massages, lymphatic drainage, thalasso baths, hydrojet showers, slimming treatments, anti-stress therapies, seaweed body masks, hot mud treatments, steam baths, and bubble baths.

The Institute of Aesthetic Medicine, also on the resort's grounds, is dedicated to providing relief from the premature effects of aging and offering treatments for wrinkles, circulation problems, and cellulite.

The Privilege Resort Sports Center houses six tennis courts, four squash courts, three swimming pools, a bodybuilding center, and a gymnastics studio where aerobic, stretching, and dance classes are held. For the evenings, the island's hottest nightspots are not far away. The resort's two restaurants—Le Privilege, located atop a hill, and La Louisiane in the marina—offer French cuisine and local delicacies.

For more information contact Spa Finder at 800-255-7727.

Le Sport, St. Lucia
$$
R Sp F S M

Le Sport is an all-inclusive resort for couples and singles who want a Caribbean vacation with sports, night life, and a pampering spa. In addition to almost every water sport imaginable, the resort has tennis, golf, fencing, archery, biking, dance, and a fitness center with personal trainers. Le Sport is an excellent place to learn scuba diving. The all-inclusive vacations offer professional instruction in all sports.

High on a hill, the Oasis Spa is a fantasy of Moorish architecture. A staff nurse consults with all guests after their arrival, and a personalized spa schedule is devised. A well-rounded program of treatments is included in the price of your stay; however, additional services may be booked a la carte.

For more information contact Spa Finder at 800-255-7727.

La Source, Grenada
$$
R Sp F M

This all-inclusive resort is located on a long stretch of sandy coastline named "Pink Gin Beach." When guests arrive, they put their wallets away because everything is included in the price of their stay: accommodations, food, wine served with meals, drinks at two bars, the use of all sports equipment, instruction, evening entertainment, and a complete schedule of spa treatments.

The spa offers massage, yoga, meditation, skin-care treatments, aerobics and stretching classes, and cardiovascular and weight training with personal trainers. Water activities at La Source include snorkeling, windsurfing, water-skiing, Sunfish sailing, and swimming. For scuba divers, there are over 20 dive sites within easy reach. On land, there is a nine-hole golf course, tennis courts, fencing, archery, volleyball, and badminton.

For more information contact Spa Finder at 800-255-7727.

Harbour Village Beach Resort, Bonaire, Dutch Antilles
$$$
R F S Sp

This romantic resort is located on a private white sandy beach only a short stroll from the island's quaint capital, Kralendijk. The spa offers a wide range of services, including indoor and outdoor massage, health-management training, indoor and outdoor exercise classes, and beauty treatments.

You will also find four lighted tennis courts, as well as bicycles on which to explore this friendly island. Great Adventures Bonaire is an on-site dive operation providing certified divers access to the island's top-ranked dive sites aboard the resort's two customized boats. A complete water sports program also features snorkeling, windsurfing, and complimentary use of Lasers and Sunfish sailboats and kayaks. Guests are accommodated in 64 private rooms, suites, and apartments in two-story villas whose terraced balconies overlook the beach, the marina, or a Caribbean garden.

For more information contact Spa Finder at 800-255-7727.

Hosteria las Quintas, Cuernavaca, Mexico
$$
A R F Sp

Average temperatures of 72°F, breathtaking scenery, and fascinating historic sites have made this area a favorite of Mexico's elite. One of its lavish estates has been transformed into this 60-room resort situated on 7,000 square meters of lushly landscaped grounds.

Though not large, the spa offers an extensive range of treatments, including deep-cleansing facials, Swedish and shiatsu massage, detoxifying Dead Sea fangotherapy, algae wraps, and exfoliating body scrubs. Classes in yoga, meditation, fitness, and weight training are also offered.

Hosteria las Quintas conducts ecological and cultural excursions to the Valley of Cuernavaca; to Xochicalco, a local archaeological site where guests can explore a pyramid, ancient ball court, steam caves, and an astrological observation post; to the pyramid of Tepozteco; and to "The Thousand Waterfalls of Granada," reachable by car and horseback in the mountains. There are also shopping excursions to the famous silver town of Taxco.

For more information contact Spa Finder at 800-255-7727.

Ixtapan Hotel and Spa, Estado de Mexico, Mexico
$
R W F Sp A

This large resort is located on the site where the Aztec emperor Montezuma came to enjoy the therapeutic mineral springs. Today, visitors are still coming, attracted by the springs, the spa, the resort's extensive facilities, and the excellent value.

A week's stay at the Ixtapan Hotel and Spa includes a daily massage and facial, additional beauty treatments, meals in the spa dining room, and participation in the daily exercise programs. A variety of packages are available, including the Diet Package for guests who want to lose weight, improve fitness, and receive beauty treatments; the Relax Package, which features yoga classes, shiatsu massage, and acupuncture sessions; and the Sports Package, offering mountain bike rides and excursions balanced with sports-intensive massages. Tennis and golf facilities are on the property, and instruction from pros in both sports is included in the spa packages.

For more information contact Spa Finder at 800-255-7727.

Las Ventanas al Paraiso, Los Cabos, Mexico
$$$$
R L

Las Ventanas al Paraiso is located at the tip of the Baja Peninsula, where the Sea of Cortez meets the Pacific Ocean. The resort's architecture combines Mediterranean and Mexican styles. The standard rooms are extraordinarily large; suites are up to 900 square feet. A unique touch is a telescope in every room so that guests can watch for whales during the day and view the stars at night.

Spa services include the "Hot Stone Therapy Massage," and eight other varieties of massage, a host of body treatments, and every type of facial imaginable. A few steps from the hotel's entrance, guests will find the 18-hole Robert Trent Jones II championship course. Las Ventanas guests also have privileges at two nearby Jack Nicklaus–designed courses. Yachting excursions, deep-sea fishing, snorkeling, and scuba diving are also available.

For more information contact Spa Finder at 800-255-7727.

Paradise Village, Beach Resort and Spa, Nayarit, Mexico
$$
R Sp F

Located on a tiny peninsula, this distinctively Mayan resort offers guests spacious accommodations, a wide array of land and water sports, and the most complete resort spa in Mexico. Every kind of water sport is offered, from sailing and jetskiing to boating and deep-sea fishing. There are championship tennis courts on the premises and an 18-hole golf course is nearby. Puerta Vallarta, with its charming cobblestone streets and quaint shops, is a half-hour away.

The Paradise Village Spa features a new medical area with a computerized natural diagnostic and preventive treatment program. Other facilities include an exercise studio, a cardiovascular and weight-training room, treatment studios, whirlpools, saunas, steam rooms, a Vichy shower, a lap pool, a full-service salon, and a boutique.

Special therapies include the silk-body treatment, anti-stress therapy, mud massage, and herbal hydromassage. Spa packages feature a fitness evaluation, exercise classes, beauty and wellness treatments, and one-on-one training.

For more information contact Spa Finder at 800-255-7727.

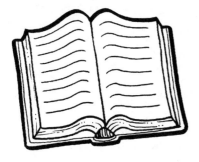

Glossary

aerobic   Activity that conditions your heart and lungs because you are taking in large amounts of oxygen to help your body cope with high levels of exertion.

affirmations   Positive statements that you repeat throughout the day and over many days until the content of the words becomes established habits and beliefs. The words send the message to your mind telling you what you want to accomplish.

aromatherapy   Using essential oils therapeutically by applying them to the skin or inhaling them through various methods. The term also describes scent-oriented therapies that use plant oils.

arrhythmia   A condition when the heart does not beat in a regular rhythm. It may skip a beat or two.

atom   The basic unit of all matter. Each atom is made up of three main particles: electrons, which have a negative electric charge; neutrons, which have no charge; and protons, which have a positive electric charge. The neutrons and protons are located in the nucleus, or center, of the atom, and the electrons orbit, or circle, the nucleus.

aura   The dictionary definition is a subtle quality or atmosphere that emanates from a person, place, or thing. My definition is a vibrating field of energy that engulfs the body. It is over, under, around, and through each of us.

B complex   Group of 10 vitamins that primarily works with enzymes to change the food you eat into nutrients your body can use.

beauty mask   Create a beauty mask by covering the face (not the eyes) with a product such as mud or facial cleanser that dries on the skin. Masks penetrate pores, absorb dirt, exfoliate dead skin cells, and tone skin tissue. When dry, the mask is washed off with warm water.

biofeedback   During a biofeedback session, a special machine gives the individual continuous information about her biological responses. She uses the information to learn to control her body's responses.

bodywork   Therapies such as massage, deep tissue manipulation, movement awareness, and energy balancing, which are used to improve the structure and functioning of the body.

bubbler   A small submersible pump, often used in home fountains or water gardens. It may be adjusted to create a quiet or a vigorous bubbling action in the water.

chakras (wheels)   Centers of energy from which rays of life-giving light and energy radiate. They are located between the base of the spinal column and the top of the head. Even Western medicine accepts them, but it calls them the nerve plexus. During meditation, the soul rises upward through the seven centers to connect with the Infinite.

chi   According to ancient Chinese medicine, chi is the universal energy that flows through the body's vital organs, bones, bloodstream, and other parts. The Japanese call it ki.

circumambulation   A pilgrim walks in a circle around the object of the pilgrimage. This circular pilgrimage leads nowhere, yet in the act of going, the pilgrim leaves behind the old life and is renewed.

compulsion   A basic driving force in one's personality that is hidden or unknown to the individual and causes him to be blind to the real motives for his actions. The Enneagram uses the idea of compulsion to help people with self-healing.

convent   The residential house of a religious community of women.

cosmetic scrubs   Creams or lotions containing small particles used to cleanse your skin.

day spa   A drop-in facility where you'll usually spend a few hours getting beauty and spa treatments.

detox or **detoxification plan**   Helps the body get rid of toxins that may accumulate from preservatives in food, caffeine, alcohol, environmental pollution, secondary smoke, pesticides, and other harmful chemicals.

directed retreat   A retreat that includes private individual interviews with a spiritual director.

dis-ease   Any condition that affects your body and causes pain, discomfort, or ill health.

distress   Excessive and extended stress that may cause bodily or psychological harm.

epiphany   A moment of sudden intuitive understanding; a flash of insight.

essential oils   Fragrant oils made from plant sources, including flowers, leaves, and bark. Only oils made by steam distillation are technically pure essential oils. Different essential oils are thought to have different, potent effects on body, mind, and spirit.

eustress   Good stress that may result from creative endeavors, heroic acts, or enjoyable activities, such as athletic competitions.

exercise   Activities that offer mental or physical release of tension and thereby promote relaxation, stress reduction, and a sense of peace.

exfoliant   A substance that sloughs off excess cells from the skin.

fast   A complete or partial abstinence from nourishment.

Feng Shui   Pronounced *fung shoy,* it's the Chinese art of placement that considers the movement of energy in a living space.

goal   A broad statement, similar to a mission statement, of what you intend to do, be, and achieve.

haiku   A Japanese verse form which, in English, consists of three unrhymed lines of five, seven, and five syllables, respectively (totaling 17 syllables), often on some subject in nature.

Hajj   Annual pilgrimage of Muslims to Mecca.

hedonists   These folks believed that the highest aim of society or the individual is to seek pleasure. Hedonism has come to be described as the self-indulgent pursuit of pleasure as a way of life.

HEPA air filter   A high-efficiency air filter that removes potentially harmful particles from the air.

herbal wraps   Wrapping sheets around the body that have been soaked in teas made from herbs steeped in water.

hermitage   A place where a person lives away from other people; secluded retreat.

holistic health   Emphasizes wellness, prevention, and patient education. It focuses on the whole individual and his environment and emotions, his capacity to heal himself, and his role as an active partner in his health.

homeopathy   Based on the idea that "like cures like." Consequently, a patient is given a very diluted solution of a substance that causes symptoms of his disease.

hydrotherapy   Water therapy that uses the healing power of water in concert with massage or movement or simply for soaking, steaming, spraying, or otherwise applying water to the body.

hypoglycemia   The condition caused by having too little sugar in your blood.

inspired   When referring to writings, this term means that God guided the writers so that their words were God's words. God speaks to us through these writings.

ions   Small, charged (either positive or negative) particles found in the air. Ions are produced by radioactivity, cosmic rays, the movement of hot, dry winds, and water-falls.

kachinas   Ancestral deities of the Pueblo Indians who spend half the year in the sacred mountains or a sacred lake and the other half in the villages of their human descendants. You may be familiar with the kachina dolls that represent the deities.

mantra   Hindu for a word or phrase that is said or chanted repeatedly. The sound vibrates in the body (each chakra has its own sound) and facilitates meditation.

meditation   An altered state of awareness during which the person is in a type of trance state, experiences relaxation, and is able to tune out all external activity in order to go within himself or herself.

monastery   The building or group of buildings that house monks, men who have withdrawn from the world for religious reasons.

mud bath   Immersing your unclothed body into mud or spreading on mud and letting it dry for benefits similar to a mask.

Myers-Briggs Type Indicator (MBTI)   This test is used to establish individual preferences in daily behavior. The MBTI is one of the most widely used psychological tests today.

nirvana   In Buddhism, the state of perfect blessedness reached when the individual soul becomes one with the supreme spirit.

nonaerobic   Activity that does not raise your heart rate, is more serene, and does not require great amounts of oxygen to fuel your body's active needs.

non-directed retreat   One where a spiritual advisor is not present or available.

novitiate   The building which houses novices, who are individuals beginning their study in a religious order and who have not taken final vows to become full members.

objectives   The details or the steps you need to take to make your goal become reality.

osteopathy   A system of medical treatments based on the belief that physical manipulation of bones and/or muscles can alleviate problems by realigning body parts into their proper positions.

personal trainer   An individual who works with you to create a personal fitness routine.

pilgrim   A believer in any culture who looks beyond the local temple, church, or shrine, feels the call of some distant holy place, and answers the call by journeying there.

pilgrimage   Some outer action with inner meaning; a journey taken to become closer to God or to touch the holy in life.

pitch   The highness or lowness of a tone.

prana   According to the Indian yogic tradition, a form of energy that animates all physical matter, including the human body.

programmed retreat   Has a leader who takes the group through a set program schedule for the duration of the retreat.

puja   Name given to certain Buddhist prayer rituals.

pumice   A light volcanic rock used in solid or powdered form for smoothing, scouring, and polishing skin.

quiet day   Follows a typical retreat day format but lasts only the one day, whereas a traditional retreat lasts at least three days.

reflexology   Massage done on one part of the body (typically the feet, hands, and ears) to affect the health and function of other areas.

relic   An object associated with a saint, such as a fragment of the saint's bones or part of a saint's article of clothing. Relics were used in prayer and for healing.

REM   The stage of sleep in which there is rapid eye movement. REM phases occur at regular intervals and are associated with dreaming.

retreat   A place that, whether it uses physical activity or not, aids guests in reaching higher personal goals or spiritual renewal. In addition, the facility offers none, or very few, of the services generally associated with spas.

Sabbath   The seventh day of the week in the Hebrew calendar, the name is derived from the root *sbt,* which means "to cease from or rest." This root word evokes the most characteristic trait of the Sabbath, which is the cessation of all activity that fills ordinary, everyday life.

sacramental   A holy object that is infused with divine power. In the field of comparative religions, the word sacramental is sometimes used as a general term for anything that represents a hidden reality that is sacred or mysterious.

self-healing   You accept responsibility for and make the lifestyle changes necessary for your own emotional, mental, physical, and spiritual health. Another aspect of self-healing for many is belief in and use of mind-body techniques such as biofeedback and meditation.

self-talk   What you say to yourself. How much positive or negative self-talk you do affects your moods, your outlook, and your health.

shamans   Priests or medicine men who contact and influence the good and bad spirits of their traditions.

shrine   A fixed location that has strong associations with significant religious persons or events. It might house a sacred object, such as a relic, or stand at a sacred location.

silent retreat   Everyone must observe absolute silence at all times, or speak only during specified times in permitted places.

spa   A place that offers a variety of beautifying body treatments and often other services and activities.

stress   The sum total of normal and abnormal pressures of living that test the individual's ability to cope and that change a person's mental, emotional, or physical state.

stress response   A reaction that creates a release of hormones that in turn initiates a series of changes in the functioning of the body.

synchronicity   A term coined by Carl Jung to describe moments of meaningful coincidence, a coming together of seemingly unconnected events.

tachycardia   A condition in which the heart beats faster than normal.

tai chi   A Chinese martial art form with a constant flow of energy, combining mental concentration, slow breathing, and graceful dance-like movements.

tirtha   The Hindu word for pilgrimage, which means a sacred crossing, and may apply to many different aspects of an individual's life. Tirtha is the intermediary step toward a more ideal state.

Type A personality   Type of person who experiences high levels of stress. This personality type is hard-driving, competitive, verbally aggressive, easily angered, and time-conscious.

Type B personality   Type of person who is easy-going, relaxed, restrained, and more or less the opposite in behavior of a Type A person.

unstructured retreat   You plan your entire time at a retreat as you wish. The retreat facility may or may not have a spiritual advisor available.

vacation spa   More like a vacation: You travel, stay perhaps a week, and enjoy more services.

wellness   The intentional and consistent effort to stay healthy and to achieve your highest potential for well-being.

wellness centers   Places where people come to learn about wellness and how to change their attitudes and their behavior so they can be as healthy as possible. Neighborhood wellness centers offer drop-in classes and programs; others welcome guests for days or even weeks at a time.

wellness retreats   A new mix of spa services and retreat services.

yoga   A practice developed in the East, using postures and controlled breathing to stretch and tone the body, improve circulation, calm the central nervous system, and experience a meditative and whole state of being.

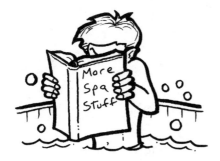

Further Reading

Directories and Listings of Spas and Retreats

For finding spiritual retreats, the best starting point is to contact a place of worship that will have or know where to obtain directories of retreat facilities of that denomination. Most retreat houses are open to people of any faith or none. If you have Internet access, use one of the search engines and log on to sites of specific religious affiliations. Also read about the spiritual retreats described in Chapter 22, "A Sampling of Retreats," and check some of the periodicals, directories, and books listed in the following sections.

Periodicals

These periodicals list spas and/or retreats in each issue, and most have special annual directory issues:

Getaways
(also *New England Getaways*)
Insider's guide to escapes, including weekend retreats and hideaways.
Phone: 401-421-2552
E-mail: getaways@getawaymag.com

Healing Retreats & Spas
Nurturing and healing alternatives worldwide.
Phone: 805-962-7101
Fax: 805-962-1337

Hideaway Report
Small, secluded resorts and executive retreats around the world.
Phone: 208-622-3183

Hot Springs, Mineral Waters
Listings of hot springs and mineral waters locations.
Phone: 303-575-5676

Hotel, Resort, Cruise Ship and Spa Report
A review of the latest in resorts, cruises, and spas.
Phone: 212-755-4363

New Age
New Age thinking from visionaries.
Phone: 617-962-0200
Email: editor@newage.com

Outside Travel Guide
Information for family vacations.
Phone: 505-989-7100
E-mail: outside@starwave.com

Spa Finder Directory
Lists more than 250 spas, fitness resorts, and New Age retreats worldwide.
E-mail: allspas@spafinders.com

Spa Finder Magazine
Spas and related health news.
E-mail: allspas@spafinders.com

Spa Magazine
For the health-conscious female traveler.
E-mail: subs@spamagazine.com

Spa Vacations
Travel guide to resorts, retreats, and sanctuaries for the spa traveler.
Phone: 801-628-8060

Women's Traveller
City and resort destinations from lesbian perspective.
Phone: 415-255-0404
E-mail: damron@damron.com

Yoga Journal
Spas and retreats focused on health-conscious living.
Phone: 800-600-9642
E-mail: yoga@pcspublink.com

Books

Baji-Holms, Karin. *101 Vacations to Change Your Life: A Guide to Wellness Centers, Spiritual Retreats, and Spas.* Secaucus, New Jersey: Carol Publishing Group, 1999.

Benson, John. *Transformative Adventures, Vacations, and Retreats: An International Directory of 300+ Host Organizations.* Portland, Oregon: New Millennium Publishing, 1994.

Benson, John. *Transformative Getaways: For Spiritual Growth, Self-Discovery, and Holistic Healing.* New York: Holt, 1996.

Bischoff, Matt C. *Touring California and Nevada Hot Springs.* Falcon Publishing Co., 1997.

Bowler, Gail Hellind. *Artists and Writers Colonies: Retreats, Residencies, and Respites for the Creative Mind.* Mercer Island, Washington: Blue Heron, 1995.

Burt, Bernard. *Fodor's Health Escapes: 244 Resorts and Retreats Where You Can Get Fit, Feel Good, Find Yourself, and Get Away from It All.* Fodor's Travel, 1997.

Catholic Shrines and Places of Pilgrimage in the U.S. U.S. Catholic Conference Staff, Jubilee Edition. Washington, D.C.: U.S. Catholic, 1998.

Christian-Meyers, Patricia. *Catholic America: Self-Renewal Centers and Retreats.* Junction City, Oregon: Beacon Point Press, 1993.

Hagen, Jeff. *Northern Retreats: A Guide to Unique Lodging in the Upper Midwest.* Northward Press, 1991 (out of print).

International Spa Guide. Flushing, NY: BDIT Inc. Travel, 1999.

Joy, Janet. *A Place Apart: Houses of Prayer and Retreat Centers in North America.* California: Source Books, 1995.

Kelly, Jack, and Marcia Kelly. *Sanctuaries: A Guide to Lodgings in Monasteries, Abbeys, and Retreats of the US: The Northeast.* New York: Bell Tower, 1991.

Kelly, Jack, and Marcia Kelly. *Sanctuaries: The Complete US Guide to Lodgings in Monasteries, Abbeys, and Retreats.* New York: Harmony Books, 1996.

Kelly, Marcia, and Jack Kelly. *Sanctuaries: West Coast and Southwest: A Guide to Lodgings in Monasteries, Abbeys, and Retreats of the US.* New York: Bell Tower, 1993.

Kelman. *Jewish Family Retreats.* New York: Jewish Theological Seminary of America, 1992.

Lederman, Ellen. *Vacations That Can Change Your Life: Adventures, Retreats, and Workshops for the Mind, Body, and Spirit.* Naperville, Illinois: Sourcebooks, 1998.

Levick, Mebla, and Stanley Young. *Paradise Found: The Beautiful Retreats and Sanctuaries of California and the Southwest.* San Francisco: Chronicle Books, 1995.

Martin, Craig. *Enchanted Waters: A Guide to New Mexico's Hot Springs.* Boulder, Colorago: Pruett, 1998.

Matson, Robert W. *Havens, Retreats, and Hideaways North of San Francisco.* Sea Wolf Publishing, June 1989.

Miller, Jenifer. *Healing Centers and Retreats: Health Getaways for Every Body and Budget.* Santa Fe: John Muir, 1998.

Morreale, Don, ed. *The Complete Guide to Buddhist America.* Boston: Shambhala Publications, 1998. (The 1998 revised edition supersedes the 1988 edition, *Buddhist America: Centers, Retreats, Practices,* which is out of print but may be found in some libraries.)

Navaretta, Cynthia, and Donna Marxer. *Artists Colonies, Retreats, and Study Centers.* New York: Midmarch Arts Press, 1998 (revised).

Official Catholic Directory 1997: Pilgrimage Destinations Guide (180th edition). Washington, D.C.: U.S. Catholic, 1997.

Rudee, Martine, and Jonathan Blease. *Traveler's Guide to Healing Centers and Retreats in North America.* Santa Fe: J. Muir. Distributed by Norton, 1989.

Stockley, Tom, and B.G. Olson. *Umbrella Guide to NW Natural Hotsprings.* Kenmore, Washington: Epicenter Press, 1992.

Zagat Survey Staff. *Zagat Survey Hotels, Resorts, and Spas.* New York: Zagat Survey, 1998.

There are a few other books that may be available in your library, but which are out of print, including Judith Brode Hirsch's *The Spa Book: A Guide to the Top 101 Health Resorts in America* (Perigee Book, 1988).

On the Web

Adventure Health Travel
List includes some spa and retreat facilities.
www.adventurehealthtravel.com/

Satya: Great Getaways in Upstate New York and New Jersey
Spas, retreats.
Web site: www.montelis.com/satya/backissues/feb97/getaways.html
E-mail: stealth@interport.net

Spa and Fitness Vacation Planners
Member of the International Spa and Fitness Association.
www.resort2fitness.com/

Spa Finders
More than 200 listings worldwide.
www.spafinders.com

***Spa* Magazine**
Destination, day, and resort spas worldwide; over 235 spas in United States listed.
www.spamagazine.com

www.itiaccess.com/~merkaba/retreat.html
For retreats for healing, spiritual training, and meditation.

www.modlife.com/
Has 1,200 destinations in 38 countries in database, including spas, resorts, and retreats.

www.retreats.org.uk.
The National Retreat Association for retreats in the United Kingdom.

www.syncreny.org/F59P25.html
For retreats in Canada.

www.syncreny.org/F59P27.html
For retreats around the world.

If you still want more, use one of the search engines like Yahoo! and Alta Vista with key words such as "spas," "retreats," and related topics like "alternative medicine," "fitness," and "religion/spirituality," or specific sites with religious affiliations such as Buddhist, Catholic, Jesuit, or Jewish.

Books About Self-Healing

Anderson, Sherry Ruth, and Hopkins, Patricia. *The Feminine Face of God: The Unfolding of the Sacred in Women.* New York: Bantam Books, 1991.

Angell, Jeannette L. *All Ground Is Holy: A Guide to the Christian Retreat.* Pennsylvania: Morehouse Publishing, 1993.

Appleton, Nancy Ph.D. *Lick the Sugar Habit.* Garden City Park, New York: Avery Publishing Group Inc., 1988.

Bausch, William J. *Pilgrim Church*. Connecticut: Twenty-Third Publications, 1995.

Bardey, Catherine, and Zeva Oelbaum. *Secrets of the Spas: Pamper and Vitalize Yourself at Home*. New York: Black Dog & Levanthal, 1999.

Beesing, Maria O.P., et al. *The Enneagram: A Journey of Self-Discovery*. New Jersey: Dimension Books, Inc., 1984.

Bender, Sue. *Everyday Sacred Journal*. San Francisco: Harper, 1997.

Black, Sara. *The Supple Body: The Way to Fitness, Strength, and Flexibility*. New York: Macmillan USA, 1995.

Borysenko, Joan, Ph.D. *Minding the Body, Mending the Mind*. Reading, Massachusetts: Addison-Wesley Publishing Company, 1987.

Budilovsky, Joan, and Eve Adamson. *The Complete Idiot's Guide to Massage*. New York: Alpha Books, 1998.

Budilovsky, Joan, and Eve Adamson. *The Complete Idiot's Guide to Meditation*. New York: Alpha Books, 1999.

Budilovsky, Joan, and Eve Adamson. *The Complete Idiot's Guide to Yoga*. New York: Alpha Books, 1998.

Capellini, Steve. *The Royal Treatment: How You Can Take Home the Pleasures of the Great Luxury Spas*. New York: Dell, 1997.

Chakravarty, Amiya, ed. *A Tagore Reader*. Boston: Beacon Press, 1961.

Charles-Edwards, T. *Saint Winefriede and Her Well: The Historical Background*. Holywell, Wales: W. Williams & Son (undated).

Chopra, Deepak, M.D. *Creating Health: Beyond Prevention, Toward Perfection*. Boston: Houghton Mifflin Company, 1987.

Chopra, Deepak, M.D. *Quantum Healing: Exploring the Frontiers of Mind/Body Medicine*. New York: Bantam Books, 1989.

Chuen, Master Lam Kam. *Feng Shui Handbook: How to Create a Healthier Living and Working Environment*. New York: Henry Holt & Company, 1996.

Clift, Jean Dalby, and Wallace B. Clift. *The Archetype of Pilgrimage: Outer Action with Inner Meaning*. New York: Paulist Press, 1996.

Collins, Louise. *Memoirs of a Medieval Woman: The Life and Times of Margery Kempe*. New York: Harper & Row, 1964.

Cooper, David A. *Renewing Your Soul: A Guided Retreat for the Sabbath and Other Days of Rest with David A. Cooper*. San Francisco: Harper, 1995.

Cooper, David A. *Silence, Simplicity, and Solitude: A Complete Guide to Spiritual Retreat*. Woodstock, Vermont: Jewish Lights, 1999.

Cornwell, John. *The Hiding Places of God*. New York: Warner Books, 1991.

Cottrell, Randall R. *Stress Management*. Guilford, Connecticut: Dushkin Publishing Group, Inc., 1992.

Cousins, Norman. *Anatomy of an Illness*. New York: Norton, 1979.

Cox, Jeff. *Landscaping with Nature*. Emmaus, Pennsylvania: Rodale Press, 1991.

Dadd, Debra Lynn. *Home Safe Home*. New York: Tarcher/Putnam, 1997.

Davidson, Jeff, M.B.A., C.M.C. *The Complete Idiot's Guide to Managing Your Time*. New York: Alpha Books, 1999.

Dearling, Robert, ed. *The Illustrated Encyclopedia of Musical Instruments*. New York: Schirmer Books, 1996.

Deiss, Lucien, CSSp., and Gloria Gabriel Weyman. *Dancing for God*. Ohio: World Library of Sacred Music, 1969.

Doner, Kalia, et. al. *The Wellness Center's Spa at Home*. New York: Berkley Publishing Group, 1997.

Editors of *Vegetarian Times*. *Vegetarian Times Cookbook*. New York: Collier Books, 1984.

Eliade, Mircea, ed. *The Encyclopedia of Religion*. New York: Macmillan Library Reference USA, 1995.

Eliot, Robert S., M.D., and Dennis L. Breo. *Is It Worth Dying For?* New York: Bantam Books, 1984.

Estés, Clarissa Pinkola. *Women Who Run with the Wolves*. New York: Ballantine Books, 1997.

Garber, Greta Breedlove. *The Herbal Home Spa: Naturally Refreshing Wraps, Rubs, Lotions, Masks, Oils, and Scrubs*. Vermont: Storey Books, 1998.

Gawain, Shakti. *The Path of Transformation: How Healing Ourselves Can Change the World*. Mill Valley, California: Nataraj Publishing, 1993.

Gibran, Kahlil. *The Prophet*. New York: Alfred A. Knopf, 1970.

Gill, Elaine, and David Everett. *Celtic Pilgrimages: Sites, Seasons, and Saints*. London: Blandford, 1997.

Gordon, Marcia, M.D., and Alice Fugate. *The Complete Idiot's Guide to Beautiful Skin*. New York: Alpha Books, 1998.

Gurvis, Sandra. *Way Stations to Heaven*. New York: Macmillan, 1996.

Harris, Maria. *Dance of the Spirit: The Seven Steps of Women's Spirituality*. New York: Bantam Books, 1989.

Hart, Thomas N. *Coming Down the Mountain: How to Turn Your Retreat into Everyday Living*. Mahwah, New Jersey: Paulist Press, 1988.

Hattatt, Lance. *The Water Garden*. Bristol, England: Parragon, 1996.

Hay, Louise L. *Heal Your Body A–Z: The Mental Causes for Physical Illness and the Way to Overcome Them*. Carlsbad, California: Hay House, 1988.

Henegar, Bill. *Pilgrimage of the Heart: Finding Your Way Back to God*. Joplin, Missouri: College Press Publishing, 1997.

Hesse, Hermann. *Siddartha*. Translated by Hilda Rosner. New York: New Directions, 1957.

Hirsch, Gretchen. *Womanhours*. New York: St. Martin's Press, 1983.

Hirsch, Anne, and Janice Biehn. *Home Spa*. Buffalo, New York: Firefly Books Ltd., 1997.

Hoffman, Lawrence A. *Israel: A Spiritual Travel Guide: A Companion for the Modern Jewish Pilgrim*. Woodstock, Vermont: Jewish Lights, 1998.

Housden, Roger. *Sacred America: Travels of an Englishman Through a Promising Land*. New York: Simon & Schuster, 1999.

Huddleston, Mary Anne. *Spring of Spirituality*. Liguori, Missouri: Triumph Books, 1995.

Junger, Sebastian. *The Perfect Storm*. New York: Harper Collins, 1997.

Justice, Blair, Ph.D. *Who Gets Sick: How Beliefs, Moods, and Thoughts Affect Your Health.* Los Angeles: Jeremy P. Tarcher, Inc., 1988.

Keating, Charles. *Who We Are Is How We Pray.* Connecticut: Twenty-Third Publications, 1991.

Knaster, Mirka. *Discovering the Body's Wisdom.* New York: Bantam Books, 1996.

Kroeger, Otto with Janet Thuesen. *Type Talk at Work: How the 16 Personality Types Determine Your Success on the Job.* New York: Delacorte Press, 1992.

Kushner, Harold S. *When Bad Things Happen to Good People.* New York, Schocken Books, 1981.

Lappé, Francis Moore. *Diet for a Small Planet.* New York: Ballantine Books, 1982.

Lee, Mary Price, and Richard S. Lee. *Coping Through Effective Time Management.* New York: Rosen Publishing Group, 1991.

Lindley, David, and T. Harvey Moore, eds. *Webster's New World Dictionary of Science.* New York: Macmillan USA, 1998.

Linn, Dennis, et. al. *Sleeping with Bread: Holding What Gives You Life.* New Jersey: Paulist Press, 1995.

Lorie, Peter, and Manuela Dunn Mascetti, eds. *The Quotable Spirit: A Treasury of Religious and Spiritual Quotations, from Ancient Times to the 20th Century.* New York: Macmillan USA, 1996.

Louden, Jennifer. *The Woman's Retreat Book: A Guide to Restoring, Rediscovering, and Reawakening Your True Self in a Moment, an Hour, a Day, or a Weekend.* San Francisco: Harper, 1997.

Magazinar, Allan, O.D. *The Complete Idiot's Guide to Living Longer and Healthier.* New York: Alpha Books, 1998.

McDonald, Kathleen, and Robina Courtin, eds. *How to Meditate: A Practical Guide,* revised edition. Massachusetts: Wisdom, 1994.

Moran, Elizabeth, and Val Biktashev. *The Complete Idiot's Guide to Feng Shui.* New York: Alpha Books, 1999.

Morse, Donald R., D.D.S., M.A., and M. Lawrence Furst, Ph.D, M.P.H. *Stress for Success: A Holistic Approach to Stress and Its Management.* New York: VanNostrand Reinhold Company, 1979.

Moyers, Bill. *Healing and the Mind.* New York: Doubleday, 1993. (Also available on audio and video cassette.)

Myss, Dr. Caroline. *Why People Don't Heal and How They Can?* New York: Harmony Books, 1997.

O'Hara, Tom S.J. *At Home with the Spirit: On Retreat in Daily Life.* Mahwah New Jersey: Paulist Press, 1994.

Otto, Rudolph, and John Harvey (translator). *The Idea of the Holy.* New York: Oxford University Press, 1958.

Payne, Joseph A. *Befriending: A Self-Guided Retreat for Busy People.* Mahwah New Jersey: Paulist Press, 1993.

Perring, Stefania, and Dominic Perring. *Then and Now.* New York: Macmillan Publishing Company, 1991.

353

Peters, F.E. *The Hajj: The Muslim Piilgrimage to Mecca and the Holy Places*. Kazi Publications, 1996.

Phillips, J.B. *Your God Is Too Small*. New York: Collier Books, 1961.

Pierpont, Margaret, and Diane Tegmeyer. *The Spa Life at Home*. Marietta, Georgia: Longstreet Press, 1997.

Pliskin, Marci C.S.W., A.C.S.W., and Shari Just, Ph.D. *The Complete Idiot's Guide to Interpreting Your Dreams*. New York: Alpha Books, 1999.

Rush, Anne Kent. *The Modern Book of Massage: Five-Minute Vacations and Sensuous Escapes*. New York: Dell Publishing, 1994.

Russell, Francis, et al. *The World of Dürer, 1471–1528*. New York: Time Inc., 1967.

Sachs, Judith. *Nature's Prozac: Natural Therapies and Techniques to Rid Yourself of Anxiety, Depression, Panic Attacks & Stress*. New Jersey: Prentice Hall, 1997.

Schulz, Mona Lisa. *Awakening Intuition: Using Your Mind-Body Network for Insight and Healing*. New York: Crown Publishing Group, 1998.

Sherwood, Keith. *Chakra Therapy: For Personal Growth & Healing*. St. Paul, Minnesota: Llewellyn Publications, 1988.

Spencer, Anita. *Seasons*. New Jersey: Paulist Press, 1982.

Sykes, Homer. *Celtic Britain*. London: Phoenix Illustrated, 1998.

Takoma, Geo, and Eve Adamson. *The Complete Idiot's Guide to Power Yoga*. New York: Alpha Books, 1999.

Taub, Edward A., M.D. *The Wellness Rx: Dr. Taub's 7 Day Program for Radiant Health & Energy*. New Jersey: Prentice Hall, 1994.

The Burton Goldberg Group. *Alternative Medicine: The Definitive Guide*. Puyallup, Washington: Future Medicine Publishing, Inc., 1993.

The Home Spa Aromatherapy Massage Set. United Kingdom: Quadrillion Publishing, 1997.

The Treasury of Christian Spiritual Classics. Nashville, Tennessee: Thomas Nelson Publishers, 1994.

Trott, Susan. *The Holy Man*. New York: Riverhead Books, 1995.

Valles, Carlos G. *Mastering Sadhana: On Retreat with Anthony DeMello*. New York: Doubleday, 1988.

Walpole, Brenda. *Macmillan Revised Encyclopedia of Science*. New York: Macmillan Reference USA, 1991.

Weed, Joseph J. *Wisdom of the Mystic Masters*. New York: Parker Publishing Company, Inc., 1968.

Weil, Andrew M.D. *8 Weeks to Optimum Health*. New York: Fawcett Books, 1998.

Weissman, Steve. *With Compassionate Understanding: A Meditation Retreat*. St. Paul, Minnesota: Paragon House, 1999.

Westwood, Jennifer. *Sacred Journeys: An Illustrated Guide to Pilgrimages Around the World*. New York: Henry Holt and Company, 1997.

Wiederkehr, Macrina. *The Song of the Seed: A Monastic Way of Tending the Soul*. San Francisco: Harper, 1997.

Wilson, Colin. *The Atlas of Holy Places & Sacred Sites.* New York: DK Publishing, Inc.,1996.

Witkin-Lanoil, Georgia, Ph.D. *The Female Stress Syndrome: How to Recognize and Live With It.* New York: Newmarket Press, 1984.

Witkin-Lanoil, Georgia, Ph.D. *The Male Stress Syndrome.* New York: Newmarket Press, 1986.

Yogananda, Paramahansa. *Man's Eternal Quest.* California: Self-Realization Fellowship, 1975.

Periodicals About Self-Healing

***Body, Mind, Spirit* Magazine**
Resource for men and women for practical, creative tools to improve the body, mind, and spirit.
Phone: 401-351-4320
Fax: 401-272-5767

Common Boundary
Explores the sources of meaning in human experience.
E-mail: connect@commonboundary.org

Conscious Living Magazine
Guide to enlightenment and seeking your higher self.
Phone: 203-454-0201
E-mail: conscliv@sprynet.com

For Men Only
Everything to ensure you outlast your Volvo.
Rodale Press
Phone: 212-967-8639

Friends of Omega
Omega Institute for Holistic Studies newsletter.
Phone: 914-266-4444

Men's Digest
Expert advice from fitness to life's hassles.
Rodale Press
610-967-5171

Men's Fitness
For men who aspire to lead an active lifestyle.
Weider Publications
818-884-6800

Men's Health Magazine
Fitness, nutrition, self-care, relationships, and work.
Rodale Press
215-967-5171

Men's Journal
Adventure, travel, fitness, and sports for men.
Wenner Media
212-484-1616

New Age
New Age thinking from visionaries.
Phone: 617-962-0200
E-mail: editor@newage.com

Spa Finder Magazine
Spas and related health news
E-mail: allspas@spafinders.com

Yoga Journal
For health-conscious living.
Phone: 800-600-9642
E-mail: yoga@pcspublink.com

Index

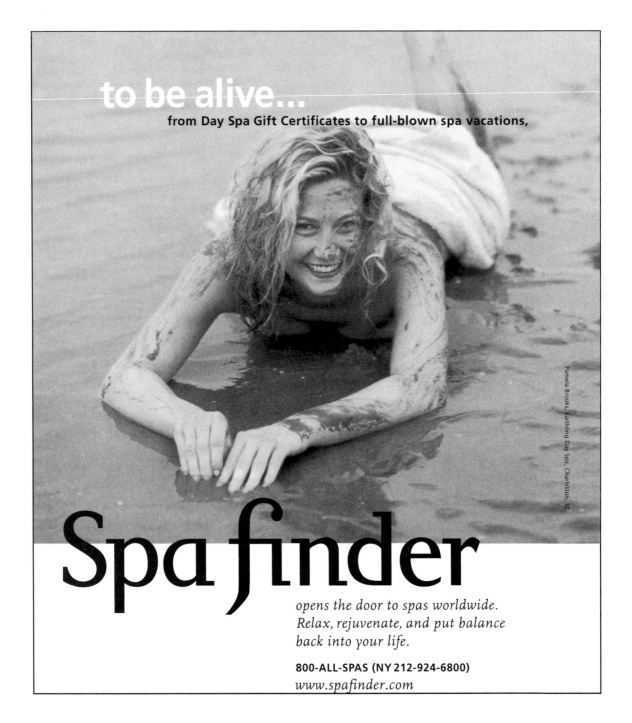

to be alive...
from Day Spa Gift Certificates to full-blown spa vacations,

Pamela Brooks, Earthling Day Spa, Charleston, SC

Spa finder

opens the door to spas worldwide.
Relax, rejuvenate, and put balance
back into your life.

800-ALL-SPAS (NY 212-924-6800)
www.spafinder.com